D1480140

Health Informatics

Lyle Berkowitz • Chris McCarthy
Editors

Innovation with Information Technologies in Healthcare

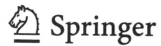 Springer

Editors
Lyle Berkowitz, M.D., FACP, FHIMSS
Feinberg School of Medicine
Northwestern University
Chicago, IL
USA

Chris McCarthy, MPH, MBA
Kaiser Permanente
Innovation Consultancy
Innovation Learning Network
Oakland, CA
USA

ISBN 978-1-4471-4326-0   ISBN 978-1-4471-4327-7 (eBook)
DOI 10.1007/978-1-4471-4327-7
Springer London Heidelberg New York Dordrecht

Library of Congress Control Number: 2012950460

Printed on acid-free paper

Springer is part of Springer Science+Business Media (www.springer.com)

Lyle's Dedication
This book is dedicated to the memory of friend, patient, creative genius and inspirational guru Peter Szollosi, whose motto resonates throughout this book: "Don't tell me what you can't do".

Chris' Dedication:
This book is dedicated to my father who taught me the power of process and to my mother who taught me the power of prayer. And to the memory of Galen Howell, whose struggles with healthcare are not forgotten.

Foreword

I was sitting in the Institute for Healthcare Improvement (IHI) Board meeting last September when I realized I needed this book. We held that meeting in the Simulation Lab at North Shore Long Island Jewish's Center for Learning and Innovation in Lake Success, NY. We were immersed in the space where North Shore-LIJ's President Mike Dowling and other leaders innovate, create, design, and train. The Board discussion centered on the science of improvement and the science of learning, and they asked me how IHI is preparing to teach to Generation Z. "Who?" I asked. Members of Generation Z – aka the Internet Generation – are about 8 years old today, and their relationship to the world is and will be fundamentally different from ours. Our Board's conversation that day highlighted and enforced the vital importance of innovation, integrating technologies, moving from reaction to prediction, and the need to lead from a new place in the years ahead. Some call the Gen Z folks "Generation M" (for Multitasking), and I left that Board meeting last year determined to envision how we will teach, learn from, and care with this new generation of multitaskers.

I began testing some of the ideas that came out of that wonderfully rich day on Long Island. I invited a group of innovative physicians, clinicians, and patients to IHI to "occupy" an innovation room we call the "sandbox." The challenge we took on was this: if we are spending $2.7 trillion on health care each year in the USA, and if over 75 % of that is spent on chronic disease management, and if all the metrics on chronic disease are going the wrong way... what should we do? My colleagues Dr. Kedar Mate and Kate O'Rourke led the conversation and discussion, which produced various ideas, data, and models drawn all over the walls and windows of the "sandbox." In 8 hours, this vibrant and diverse team, who had never met each other, co-designed a path forward that promises an integrated, continuous, and patient- and family-centered model for primary care.

I was so encouraged by that day and the way innovators from diverse backgrounds came together and inspired each other. But the challenges we face in health care are large, and there are so many questions. Questions about how best to innovate; questions about which innovations are working; and questions about how the explosion of technology can be used to transform health delivery. This book has the answers. Lyle Berkowitz and Chris McCarthy have laid out the changes for us in a compelling and instructive way. They define the need, give helpful and practical examples, and lead us into the future… a future that is happening today.

Maureen Bisognano

Preface: Why Did We Write This Book?

The idea hovered and shimmered delicately, like a soap bubble, and she dared not even look at it directly in case it burst. But she was familiar with the way of ideas, and she let it shimmer, looking away, thinking about something else.

Phillip Pullman, The Golden Compass

The reasonable man adapts himself to the world. The unreasonable one persists in trying to adapt the world to himself. Therefore, all progress depends on the unreasonable man.

George Bernard Shaw

Never doubt that a small group of thoughtful, committed people can change the world. Indeed, it is the only thing that ever has.

Margaret Mead

You have spent a lot of money on your electronic health record (EHR) systems and other healthcare information technology (HIT) projects... and you want to see results! You know that simply recreating paper-based processes on a computer will not significantly improve quality, efficiency or your financials. But what if you had access to a book that described how others in your position have used information technology systems in an innovative fashion to solve the types of problems you face every day? We wanted that book!

However, we could not find it. We did find some pretty fantastic books on implementing information technology in healthcare and others that detailed how innovation strategies could be used in healthcare. But we could not find a book that provided real life examples and explanations of how to combine these two powerful tools. Fortunately, when we asked around, what we did find were stories from our colleagues across the nation. We found stories of success, brilliant and innovative uses of healthcare IT to improve quality, efficiency and value. We found stories from multi-hospital organizations and small clinics. We found stories right out of the headlines and stories which have been succeeding outside the spotlight for many years. And we knew these stories should be shared to help guide the way for others.

We first thought about writing each chapter ourselves, but we quickly realized that it was the *Voice of the Innovator* which would be most revealing. We wanted the real people in the trenches who were involved with the innovations from the start to write their stories as only they could. And we asked them to provide the full arc of their story, to start with the origin of the innovation, to explain how it evolved from an idea to reality, and then to share both in the results as well as the lessons learned along the way.

We strongly believed that this robust rendering would be the most informative and powerful way to ensure that our readers could understand the innovations best, as well as visualize how they themselves could do something similar. So we invited a group of these innovators to tell us their amazing stories. We asked them to write their chapter with the passion which made their innovations great and they came through spectacularly.

Of course, we made sure that authors used a similar chapter structure for easier reading, but we relished in the fact that each chapter also has its own voice. Because of this, the book can be read cover to cover, or you can pick any chapter and read it on its own (although we suggest that all readers start off with Chaps. 1 and 2 to get a good background). Hopefully, you will find that the more you read, the more you will be inspired, educated and empowered to help move your own organization towards the intersection of innovation and healthcare IT which we call *The Healing Edge*!

Lyle Berkowitz, M.D., FACP, FHIMSS
Chris McCarthy, MPH, MBA

Acknowledgements

The writing of a book is an odyssey to see a vision fulfilled, and it only succeeds with the help, support, patience, friendship, trust, respect, loyalty and love from so many who circle around and within our lives.

I would like to first offer a big thank you to my incredible co-editor Chris McCarthy, who I knew would be the perfect partner in writing this book as he has helped guide me on my innovation journey for many years and inspires me on a regular basis. And a special thanks to my friend and colleague Marion Ball who surprised me one day by asking me to write a book about the intersection of healthcare IT and innovation... and convinced me I could do it!

Next, I could not do this without the support of those who work with me and support my craziness in trying to change the healthcare world. This is especially true for all my colleagues at NMPG as well as my right hands, Cathy and Amy. And a special thanks to the support provided by the Szollosi Healthcare Innovation Program and to Gerry, who believed in a little doctor with big ideas.

Immense gratitude to my family, Dana, Blake and Devyn, who have watched me disappear all too often to work on this labor of love. I hope my children grow up seeing that I truly do mean it when I say that it takes hard work to succeed, but if you are passionate about something, it does not feel like work at all. And special thanks to my Mom, who remains an eternal cheerleader for her rebel son; and my Dad, the ultimate physician role model.

Finally, a big thank you to the innovators in this book who have spent their own time helping others understand their "babies", those projects which they imagined, nurtured and grew because they realized there was a better way to do something.

They are the dreamers that do, the idealists that improve, the fantastic that fail, and the visionaries that are victorious. Thank you for inspiring us and making us want to keep reaching for The Healing Edge.

Lyle Berkowitz, M.D., FACP, FHIMSS

What a journey! When I signed on to do this with my friend and colleague, the amazing Lyle Berkowitz, the concept seemed simple and straightforward: let's find a bunch of the most promising HIT innovations and have the innovators themselves tell the story of their creations. The premise was very much like the organization I founded, the InnovationLearningNetwork.Org (ILN). Its purpose, like this book, is to bring together diverse healthcare innovators to share ideas. The difference is that the ILN is a near "free form" construct; books are not. And so, it was neither simple nor straightforward. And this book was taken to completion because of some amazing people. Here is our cast of characters:

Adrienne Smith: Project Manager, Cheerleader #1
Christi Zuber: Innovator, Confidant, Co-Author
Marilyn Chow: Chief of Inspiration
Michael Griffin: Publisher Project Manager, Chief "Feel Good" Guy
Penny Ford Carleton: Proof Reader, Cheerleader #2
Tim Kieschnick: Persona Guru
Will Dogan: Partner, Lost-Weekend Warrior, Cheerleader #3

To all the amazing chapter authors, who gave up nights and weekends to write their story for you. And in loving memory of Vivian Distler, our amazing Chap. 20 co-author, who helped show us the future.

Keep innovating. Keep sharing. And we'll all be the better for it.

Chris McCarthy, MPH, MBA

Contents

Contributors

Susan Anthony California HealthCare Foundation, Oakland, CA, USA

David Aron, M.D., MS Louis Stokes Cleveland, Department of Veterans Affairs Medical Center, Case Western Reserve University, Cleveland, OH, USA

Peter Basch, M.D., FACP MedStar Health, Ambulatory EHR and Health IT Policy, Columbia, MD, USA

Lyle Berkowitz, M.D., FACP, FHIMSS Department of Medicine, Northwestern University Feinberg School of Medicine, Chicago, IL, USA

Northwestern Memorial Hospital, Chicago, IL, USA

Szollosi Healthcare Innovation Program, Chicago, IL, USA

April R. Daugherty, B.S. Business, M.S. Technology Beacon Health System, South Bend, IN, USA

Erin DeMarce Leff, B.A., M.B.A. Specialty Services, Group Health Cooperative, Seattle, WA, USA

Vivian Distler, JD Health Horizons, Institute for the Future, Palo Alto, CA, USA

Lloyd D. Fisher, M.D. Department of Pediatrics, Fallon Clinic/Reliant Medical Group, Worcester, MA, USA

Steve Flammini, B.S., Computer Science Partners Healthcare, Inc, Wellesley, MA, USA

Mark S. Gagnon, PharmD Via Christi Health, Inc, Wichita, KS, USA

Thomas R. Graf, M.D. Community Practice Service Line, Geisinger Health System, Community Practice Service Ling, Danville, PA, USA

James Hereford, M.S. Mathematics Palo Alto Medical Foundation, Mountain View, CA, USA

Stacey Hirth, B.A. Department of Education, Louis Stokes Cleveland Department of Veterans Affairs Medical Center, Cleveland, OH, USA

James L. Holly, M.D. SETMA, LLP, Beaumont, TX, USA

Department of Family and Community Medicine, School of Medicine, UT Health Science Center, San Antonio, TX, USA

Steve Huffman, M.B.A. Beacon Health System, South Bend, IN, USA

Debra J. Hurd, RN, MS, NEA, BC Nursing Administration, Maplewood, MN, USA

Brian R. Jacobs, M.D., M.S. Pediatric Intensive Care Unit, Children's National Medical Center, Critical Care Medicine, Washington, DC, USA

Julie K. Johnson, MSPH, Ph.D. Faculty of Medicine, University of New South Wales, Sydney, NSW, Australia

Bradley Kreit, M.A., Anthropology Health Horizons, Institute for the Future, Palo Alto, CA, USA

Renée H. Lawrence, Ph.D. Medical Service Office, Louis Stokes Cleveland Department of Veterans Affairs Medical Center, Cleveland, OH, USA

Margaret Laws, MPP California HealthCare Foundation, Oakland, CA, USA

Chris McCarthy, M.B.A., MPH Innovation Learning Network/Innovation Consultancy, Kaiser Permanente, Oakland, CA, USA

Tamra E. Minnier, MSN, RN Donald D. Wolff, Jr. Center for Quality, Safety, and Innovation, University of Pittsburgh Medical Center, Pittsburgh, PA, USA

Janell Moerer Via Christi Health, Inc, Wichita, KS, USA

Marc Mora, M.D. Consultative Specialty Services, Group Health Medical Centers, Seattle, WA, USA

James W. Noga, B.S., M.S. Partners HealthCare, Inc, Boston, MA, USA

Gwendolyn B. O'Keefe, M.D. Group Health Permanente, Quality and Informatics, Seattle, WA, USA

David D. O'Neill, J.D., MPH California HealthCare Foundation, Oakland, CA, USA

Brian D. Patty, M.D., VP, CMIO Department of Health Informatics, HealthEast Care System, St. Paul, MN, USA

George Reynolds, M.D., MMM, FAAP, CPHIMS IT Department, Children's Hospital and Medical Center, Omaha, NE, USA

Tim Scearce, M.D. Department of Neurology, Group Health Permanente, Group Health Cooperative, Medical Informatics, Seattle, WA, USA

David T. Sharbaugh, B.A. SmartRoom, LLC, Pittsburgh, PA, USA

Ajay Sood, M.D. Department of Endocrinology, Medicine, Louis Stokes Veterans Medical Center, University Hospital Case Medical Center, Cleveland, OH, USA

David C. Stockwell, M.D., M.B.A. Pediatric Intensive Care Unit, Children's National Medical Center, Critical Care Medicine, Washington, DC, USA

Valerie M. Sue, Ph.D. National Market Research, Kaiser Permanente, Pleasanton, CA, USA

Alex Tam, BS Creative, frog, San Francisco, CA, USA

Katherine S. Thweatt, M.A., Ed.D. Research, Department of Communication Studies, Louis Stokes Cleveland VA Medical Center, West Virginia Wesleyan College, Cleveland, OH, USA

John W. Trudel, M.D. Department of Family Medicine, Fallon Clinic/Reliant Medical Group, Westboro, MA, USA

Karen Tsang National Market Research, Kaiser Permanente, Oakland, CA, USA

Jonathan S. Wald, M.D., MPH, FACMI Director, Patient-Centered Technologies Center for the Advancement of Health IT, RTI International, Waltham, MA, USA

Sharon A. Watts, DNP, MSN, BSN Medical Service Office, Louis Stokes Cleveland Department of Veterans Affairs Medical Center, Cleveland, OH, USA

Christi Dining Zuber, BSN, RN, MHA Innovation Consultancy, Kaiser Permanente, Oakland, CA, USA

Chapter 1
The Healing Edge

Lyle Berkowitz and Chris McCarthy

The Rocky Springs Healthcare system is a pretty typical American healthcare organization, owning two hospitals and a multispecialty physician group of 400 providers. Three years ago, they invested over $100 million dollars in an electronic health record (EHR) system and associated healthcare information technology (HIT) infrastructure upgrades – and their management team expected to see their baby soar! However, two years after implementation they were faced with abysmal results. They were taking care of fewer patients, making less money, and were not improving the quality of care they delivered. They were also mortified to find that physicians, staff and patient satisfaction levels were actually going down. This was not what all the marketing hype had promised!

They realized they needed to make some meaningful changes and learn to be "innovative" in using the IT products and the infrastructure they had in place. They just were not sure what that meant. Fortunately, the management team at Rocky Springs was open to new ideas and sharing stories, so they each went on a journey across the United States to find other places that were using IT tools in innovative ways. And they found them! They found hospitals and physician groups, big and small, who had used their EHR and HIT systems in an innovative AND reproducible fashion to better fulfill their vision of providing better care,

L. Berkowitz, M.D., FACP, FHIMSS (✉)
Department of Medicine,
Northwestern University Feinberg School of Medicine,
Chicago, IL, USA
e-mail: lyle@drlyle.com

C. McCarthy, MBA, MPH
Innovation Learning Network/Innovation Consultancy, Kaiser Permanente,
1800 Harrison Street, 17th Floor, Oakland, CA 94612, USA
e-mail: chris.mccarthy@kp.org

L. Berkowitz, C. McCarthy (eds.),
Innovation with Information Technologies in Healthcare, Health Informatics,
DOI 10.1007/978-1-4471-4327-7_1, © Springer-Verlag London 2013

decreasing medical errors, increasing patient access, improving satisfaction for all involved, and much more. But instead of just learning about the innovations themselves, they also asked to hear about the stories that led to their success. They wanted to understand the "why", the "what" and the "how" from all these great organizations.

They learned that a lot of innovative ideas came from the bottom up, beginning as simple ideas from providers and staff based on their passions for making the patient experience better. They also learned that these innovations succeeded best when the leadership team supported the concept of trying new things and continuing to persevere when the goal was the right thing to do. They found that many of these "innovations" were common sense ideas which leveraged the existing HIT infrastructure, and just needed some nourishment and support to grow. Now and then they also saw innovations that were remarkably new and exciting, but which required a significant amount of time and money to succeed.

So they went back to Rocky Springs and started sharing these stories and ideas. They let everyone in the organization know it was okay to try new things and to think differently, and they reassured them that failures are often the best way to learn how to do things right. They asked them to look to other healthcare and non-healthcare organizations for inspiration and ideas. And they reiterated a mantra they heard in many forms, that "the day before something is a great idea, it is a crazy idea".

They told physicians and other providers that if they thought their HIT systems should do something better, they should sit down with the IT staff to explain their needs and vision. And they equally encouraged their IT staff to partner more closely with providers, and to replace any "we can't do that" answers with a resounding "how can we do that" attitude.

A year later, Rocky Springs had become a different place. The EHR and other IT systems were no longer looked at as necessary evils thrust upon providers and staff, but were seen as critical tools in helping innovate care processes to improve the quality, efficiency and cost of care. Providers and staff were happier as they realized how easy it had become to deliver the right care at the right time by the right people. The IT staff was feeling truly appreciated and enjoyed being problem solvers instead of naysayers. Patients loved the superior experiences making their lives healthier and better in so many ways. And of course, the management team was pleased to see that by bringing together the right mixture of innovation and HIT, their organization was running smoother than ever and had become known as the place to get the best care and the best value around.

Does Rocky Springs Healthcare sound like your organization? Most likely parts of it do, although perhaps the happy ending is a little further away than you care to think about. Rocky Springs is fictional of course, but it comes from the stories we heard and lessons we learned along the way in assembling this book. However, before we share these stories and lessons, let's set the stage from which Rocky Springs and presumably you are starting this journey.

Why Should YOU Read This Book?

This book is a critical read for today's healthcare executives, managers, providers, consultants vendors and others who want to better understand how to design, implement and leverage their use of IT to improve quality and efficiency in the organizations they serve. Let's explore why this is so critical:

- **First, information technology is an increasingly important part of everyday life in healthcare, but there is a large gap between reality and potential**. We spend many, many millions on implementing EHRs and other HIT systems, but we have not always experienced the success we are expecting.
- **Second, healthcare innovation is HOT**. You probably wouldn't be reading this book if you didn't think so. It's hot because it is so badly needed. Innovation allows us to think differently, take risks, and drive for something far greater than what currently exists. Innovation is also becoming an increasingly well-established science, but healthcare innovation experts are rarely HIT experts and vice-versa.
- **Finally, the delivery and reimbursement of healthcare is in the midst of major changes**. People and organizations throughout the world are struggling to determine how to best balance the value equation of cost and quality of care. We all need more stories and better tools to help guide us in the evolution of our healthcare system.

Can YOU Really Do This?

We know our world is already a connected and high-tech place. We live in a smartphone and cloud-enabled environment where we can instantly check our credit scores, buy whatever we need with one click, get a bid from multiple mortgage companies overnight and book our travel across the world in minutes. And healthcare is high-tech in many ways as well. Mobile devices help us track our health and refill our medications, radiology machines allow us to see precise 3D images of organs, operating room robots help make surgery safer and quicker, nanotechnologies and genetic engineering help us develop more effective drugs, and big computing helps us analyze vast amounts of data in our systems.

However, the use of healthcare IT to support the actual process of healthcare is not usually of the same caliber as the use of IT for devices, medications, and analytics. For example, patients who come to a clinic because of a cough are leaving without ever having been told they are past due for a diabetes check or mammogram exam; nurses struggle to explain sophisticated laparoscopic surgery to patients who have minimal comprehension of English; and physicians prescribe advanced antiretroviral therapies and order imaging tests using a static EHR system which offers minimal value outside of legibility and rudimentary interaction checking.

Let's face it, most of our healthcare clinical processes are so last century. However, a revolution is brewing. More and more providers are slipping into the Twenty-First Century quietly and without fanfare. They are figuring out how to deliver care that is not only medically superior, but is operationally modern as well. And they are creating stories which are helping to awaken our spirits and move the rest of us forward. And this is good news for everyone!

These stories range from a rural healthcare system leveraging telemedicine strategies to an academic medical center using EHR decision support tools in a novel way. They span from a small clinic using a new type of home monitoring device to one of the largest healthcare organizations in the world trying new and exciting ways to manage and relate to their patients. What these organizations have in common is their relentless pursuit of making healthcare delivery better for patients and providers alike. They are defining a new type of health system, where technologies are seamless and delivering perfect care is easier and more cost-effective than the alternative.

Most of the innovations in this book are not revolutionary nor radical. In fact, they are expected and obvious in many ways. Consumers in other industries have demanded far more than they have of healthcare. Imagine if a bank told a customer that it would take a few weeks to see a bank balance. Imagine if an airline wouldn't let you book your own flights. Imagine if there was no way to compare car features or prices.

We in healthcare have just moved beyond the start line, and have a long way to go. Fortunately, healthcare organizations which are already innovating in this space are setting the pace and moving in the right direction, towards their own "*Healing Edge*". And hopefully this book will help you get there too!

How Did We Organize the Chapters?

This first chapter introduces readers to why we need to learn more about innovating with information technologies in healthcare, and the structure we have created to deliver this information. The second chapter provides an overview of innovation methods, many of which are discussed throughout the book. They serve as important primers to get you started. The remaining chapters, which can be read in any order, come from a wide variety of organizations that are doing something special with healthcare IT – something innovative which sets them apart from the pack. We found that these innovations coalesced into three major sections and so divided them appropriately.

The first section answers the question "*What Can I Do After I Implement an EHR?*" With so much focus on getting an EHR into place, some organizations have forgotten that the purpose isn't simply the implementation, but the ability to care for patients and make decisions faster, cheaper and better. Those on the *Healing Edge* are taking advantage of EHR functionality ranging from system-wide messaging to structured data collection to complex decision support tools. The results are improved care coordination, increased adherence to quality metrics and better detection of adverse events. These innovations come from places like Northwestern

Memorial Physicians Group, MedStar, Southeast Texas Medical Associates (SETMA), Fallon Clinic, Geisinger, and Children's National Medical Center.

The second section looks at several variations and novel approaches to *Virtual Interactions and Telemedicine*. Care delivery is a rapidly evolving concept. It used to be so simple, happening in the doctor's office on the doctor terms. Now delivery is happening in unique ways ensuring that the patient needs and desires are core to the equation. The results are better care delivered at the right time and the right place. These innovations come from places like Partners Healthcare, Group Health, the Veteran Affairs (VA) system, Indiana's Memorial Health System, the California HealthCare Foundation, and Via Christi.

And the final section in the book is a tour of new: *New ideas, New visions, and New Approaches*. And not just new – super cool! Smart rooms, mobile systems, real time business intelligence and dashboards, gaming technology and wisdom of the crowds are a few of the ideas that will take us to a better future. These innovations come from the University of Pittsburgh Medical Center, Partners Healthcare, HealthEast Care, Nebraska Children's Hospital, Kaiser Permanente, and more.

How Did We Structure This Book?

Even a book about innovation needs some structure. When we decided to have almost 20 organizations write about their healthcare IT innovations, we knew we needed to provide guidance to ensure both an educational and pleasurable experience for our readers. Each chapter of this book thus has the following elements:

- *An Opening Story*: We asked each author to start their chapter with a story which explains how their innovation is being used in their organization and how it affects both patients and providers. We provided the authors with the personas of a "model family" (See Appendix A) and asked them to create their story around the experiences of at least one member of that family.
- **Background:** A description of the healthcare organization where the HIT innovation was developed and is being used.
- **What is the Innovation**: An overview of the actual innovation itself.
- **Why did you Create this Innovation**: The backstory of the innovation. Was there a triggering or precipitating event? Was it someone's specific idea? Was there a specific systemic problem to be addressed?
- **How did you Succeed**: What techniques, methods or approaches were used in developing and spreading this innovation? What people, processes or technologies helped make the innovation successful?
- **Results**: Both formal success metrics and anecdotes to help explain the outcome of the innovation.
- **Lessons Learned**: A review of insights learned from any failures or problems, and how they helped guide the team to eventual success.
- **The Future**: What's next for the innovation? Are there plans to evolve the innovations, spread them or do something new?
- **Conclusion**: The author's final thoughts.

Through the Eyes of the Patient

Organizations on the *Healing Edge* know that their HIT innovations are much more than fancy technology or new processes – they are vehicles of care and cure focusing on our patients. To honor this philosophy, our book presents these innovations through the eyes of the patient. As described above, each chapter thus opens with how an organization's innovation will be felt by a group of very special patients, the Martinez Family.

So who is the Martinez Family? They are a very ordinary family. Typical Americans, who love typical things, are in typical shape, and have typical health conditions. However, they will experience quite a bit throughout the course of this book. They will be in and out of the hospital, see multiple providers, experience the latest technologies and they will get to experience some awesome HIT innovations which are available today in health systems around the country.

For those who are wondering, let's be clear, this is a fictional family (personas) and thus no personal health information (PHI) is involved. Personas are a powerful tool for innovators. They allow the innovator to have a fictional representation of real users to design towards, and best of all, they continually remind the innovator that they are designing for real people like you and me.

So let's meet them: The Martinez family starts with a core of four: Barbara the mom, Ray the dad, Cindy the eldest daughter, and Mike the youngest son. They also have some extended family that you will encounter along the way as well. They live in Anywhere, America. They are part Caucasian and part Latino. They are middle-class. They work hard, play as much as they can, but need to be careful with finances as most middle-class families do. They own two cars: a newish SUV and a beat up pickup truck. They live in a three bedroom, two-story home, and owe about $110,000 on their mortgage.

That is probably enough to give you a feel for the Martinez family. However, to better understand the use of personas, we encourage you to go deeper into who they are and what they are thinking via an interview and table of attributes which describe them in more depth in Appendix A. Feel free to use these personas when you think about the kickoff for your next innovation project.

Conclusion

Healthcare is a rapidly changing environment and nowhere is that more evident than in the use of healthcare information technology. Unfortunately, the use of HIT does not always result in better outcomes, increased efficiency or cost savings. In fact, the opposite is sometimes true.

Fortunately, innovation can bring out the best in any organization, especially in today's high tech world. That is why successful companies, ranging from real estate and investment banking to telecommunications and video gaming, invest heavily in the development of both information technologies and innovation to ensure they can consistently perform their missions better, faster and cheaper. We are excited for healthcare organizations to start doing the same.

And while innovative advances in science and healthcare products are being made every day, it is the final delivery of that care which is the real determinant as to whether an intervention is truly successful. In other words, while product innovation will always be important in healthcare, what is needed more than anything right now is process innovation to help ensure we are delivering the right care to the right people in the right time frame and right sequence. And there may not be a better tool to help achieve this vision than the information technologies which are changing every other part of our world on an escalating basis.

This book highlights that vision by sharing the stories of those who have combined innovative thinking with information technologies to improve their processes of care and solve a need at their organizations. It is meant to serve as both an educational platform for stimulating ideas in any organization, as well as inspirational read to help you realize that you too can innovate. Whether you are a CEO, a CIO, a department head, a clinic manager, a physician, a nurse, an empowered patient, an EHR vendor, an HIT consultant, or anyone else involved in the healthcare system, this book is meant to help you in your quest for *The Healing Edge*.

Chapter 2
Mad for Method

Chris McCarthy and Christi Dining Zuber

Innovation doesn't just happen by chance. It happens because smart, dedicated people work really hard. But arming innovators with an intelligent methodology to discover, test and spread innovations, certainly makes that job easier and more effective.

Every innovation featured in this book was the result of a concerted effort to solve a problem and every author in this book used various innovation methodologies to succeed. The most common was the PDSA (Plan-Do-Study-Act) experimental model. The PDSA model is a basic framework for solving problems., and it can be morphed depending on the nature of the challenge. It can morph into Lean[1] for efficiency challenges. It can morph into Six Sigma[2] for quality challenges. And it can morph into Human-Centered Design[3] to tackle experience challenges. There is powerful synergy when PDSA is combined with other innovation methods.

This chapter will focus on Kaiser Permanente Innovation Consultancy's brand of innovation method called Evidence Based Human Centered Design (EvHCD). The Innovation Consultancy (IC) is an internal design firm staffed by creative people who are part design, part strategy and part healthcare. They tackle complex, pervasive challenges when no known or acceptable solutions exist.

---

[1] See Wikipedia "Lean Manufacturing": http://en.wikipedia.org/wiki/Lean_manufacturing
[2] See Wikipedia "Six Sigma": http://en.wikipedia.org/wiki/Six_sigma
[3] See Wikipedia "Human-Centered Design": http://en.wikipedia.org/wiki/Human-centered_design

C. McCarthy, MBA, MPH (✉)
Innovation Learning Network/Innovation Consultancy, Kaiser Permanente,
1800 Harrison Street, 17th Floor, Oakland, CA 94612, USA
e-mail: chris.mccarthy@kp.org

C.D. Zuber, BSN, RN, MHA
Innovation Consultancy, Kaiser Permanente,
1800 Harrison Street, 17th Floor, Oakland, CA 94612, USA
e-mail: christi.zuber@kp.org

L. Berkowitz, C. McCarthy (eds.),
Innovation with Information Technologies in Healthcare, Health Informatics,
DOI 10.1007/978-1-4471-4327-7_2, © Springer-Verlag London 2013

EvHCD has six major buildings blocks or "anchors": Understand, Look for Patterns, Ideation, Prototyping, PDSA, and Piloting. The first four anchors were directly inspired by IC's work with IDEO (www.ideo.com), a world-renowned design and innovation firm, and PointForward (www.pointforward.com), gurus of innovation and masters of ethnography. The last two anchors come from the Institute for Healthcare Improvement (www.ihi.org), the nationally recognized healthcare improvement evangelists. This Kaiser Permanente blended method has been dubbed evidence-based human-centered design (EvHCD); meaning evidence is gathered to determine whether an idea should be adopted or abandoned.

It is important to note that each of these anchors is a complete method unto itself, and in fact can be a complete project. For example, a project might be in desperate need of Ideation in which case one could start at that anchor. But in combination, the power of their divergent and convergent natures have birthed many innovations for Kaiser Permanente, ranging from the *Journey Home Board* for new moms to the award winning shift change solution called *Nurse Knowledge Exchange Plus*.

Let's explore each of the six anchors (all techniques are more thoroughly described in Appendix B).

Understand: This anchor helps reveal the true needs within a system. Often this phase starts with desk research to rapidly explore what is known about the topic area. However, ethnography and other qualitative techniques are the signature tools to provide deeper understanding. Ethnography[4] is a technique whereby users are observed and interviewed in the context of where they work, play or live. Other techniques include "draw your experience", "fly-on-the-wall" observation, and "cultural probes kits".

Look for Patterns: This anchor creates meaning out of all the data collected in the Observation Phase. It is where patterns are identified and translated into models and frameworks to help project participants better understand the true needs and opportunities for innovation. Expert Clustering and Storytelling are just a few of the techniques used in this phase.

Ideation: Various idea-generating techniques, such as Brainstorming, Analogous Observation and Provocation, are used to produce a large amount of ideas-the good, the bad and the ugly. In this divergent phase, liberating rules are employed to keep project participants on the creative and generative path. The most sacred rule is "defer judgment".

Prototyping: Through Storyboarding, Handmade Construction and Improvisation, ideas are turned into low-fidelity prototypes. Through iteration, the most promising low-fidelity prototypes are then turned into high-fidelity prototypes. Perhaps the most creative anchor, if not the messiest, prototyping is the poster child for innovation.

PDSA: In the context of the Innovation Consultancy methods, PDSA is used to take prototypes into a live environment (such as a hospital or clinic) to rapidly adapt, adopt or abandon. It is viewed as the perfect refining tool, using culture, context and creativity to shape and shave prototypes into real-world, workable concepts.

---

[4]See Wikipedia "Ethnography": http://en.wikipedia.org/wiki/Ethnography

Pilot: The pilot phase is when the most promising PDSA concepts are implemented and measured over time to understand the value impact on the system. Those concepts that show negative or no effect on the system are dubbed "failures", while those with a positive impact are called "innovations".

Although the IC method may seem sequential, it is more like a game of Shoots and Ladders® where data, insights and ideas move back and forth through the anchor activities, accumulating more and more knowledge. For example, when PDSA's are conducted, observations help to provide insight on how the ideas are working, and ideation and prototyping can continually add new and better ideas into the PDSA tests until solutions are found. This ability to move between these fundamental anchor activities is a key skill needed for organizations to innovate.

Mashing Innovation Methods with Health Information Technology

Now let's toss in the power of Health Information Technology (HIT). The benefits of innovating with HIT are exponentially greater than innovating without it. Data is accumulated faster. Results are more precise. Effects are detected quicker. HIT brings the innovation and the testing of innovation into the new millennium. However most organizations are still in the early stages of innovating with HIT. Let's explore each of the Innovation Consultancy's anchors again, but this time in the context of HIT.

Understand: By far the most powerful use of HIT for this anchor is in the gathering of Electronic Health Record (EHR) data to kickoff exploration. Before EHRs, observations were based on the availability of skilled people to provide hours of observations paired with pulling charts to obtain and aggregate data. Now imagine how many charts can be "reviewed" instantaneously and how much data can be swiftly aggregated.

Look for Patterns: At its core, synthesis is about identifying trends and patterns. Thus the use of HIT to analyze and display the massive amounts of data from the observation phase more easily and quickly identify both association and causation. Data warehouses, statistical packages, business intelligence tools and data visualization software will all be important components in this phase. Furthermore, as HIT systems continue to increase in sophistication, decision support functionality could additionally benefit innovation activities.

Ideation: This is where HIT goes wild. In this anchor innovation teams are hungry for inspiration. There are several types of ideation that the Kaiser Permanente teams have seen as valuable, including form factor and functionality. *Form factor ideation* involves generating ideas about the technical form. For example, if nurses need access to information, an innovation team would think about what form factor best fits into their workflow – a hand held device, a tablet, a mobile cart, or a wall mounted device?

Functionality ideation is more about the user's experience. This often involves optimizing the navigation involved in retrieving and entering data to make the most intuitive sense. Technology demonstrations as thought-starters for design sessions have been an excellent way to both expose teams to new types of technology as well as to inspire new thinking in ideation. And of course, these technology brainstorms help teams imagine far-future and fantasy-type solutions.

Prototyping: If Ideation is where HIT goes wild, then it's in prototyping that it becomes imaginative. Design teams often use proxies and substitutes to begin the build process. Many organizations use "sandbox" HIT environments that run a version of their organization's HIT system so that they can test changes and ideas in the HIT environment without interrupting the live care setting. There are also extremely advanced systems that take prototyping ideas in an electronic form to a new level. Archimedes, a company affiliated with Kaiser Permanente, has developed a full-scale simulation model of human physiology, diseases, behaviors, interventions, and healthcare systems. By using advanced methods of mathematics, computing, and data systems, the Archimedes Model can even run clinically realistic virtual trials.

PDSA and Piloting: Similar to the Prototyping Anchor, HIT for PDSA/Pilot anchors comes in two forms. The first is running a PDSA or a pilot with the proposed HIT solution. This may range from the introduction of new decision support rules, to creation of a data dashboard, to introduction of telemedicine tools. The second is to use the EHR or other IT systems to measure the impact of a solution. This requires not only understanding the final impact, but also being able to measure and support the creative process along the way. In other words, leaders and designers can more easily make evidence-based decisions if it is easier to tap into the data contained within EHRs and other systems, easier to gain real-time data-driven feedback during field testing, and easier to measure the impact of an idea.

Case Study 1: Using the EHR to Understand Need and Validate Impact

Kaiser Permanente is a leader in electronic health record (EHR) systems, having implemented KP HealthConnect, their EHR system powered by Epic Systems (Madison, WI), across all its care-settings and geographies. While there are significant benefits to using this EHR, there are some darker half-truths to consider. First, there is the concern that EHRs "lock down" the ability to innovate on the fly, and lock in the current workflows, whether they are the most effective or not. There is also concern that creativity will be further blunted by putting in systems that are difficult for the end-user to manipulate. While partially true, we believe that the full truth is that most organizations are simply inexperienced at innovating with these new and complex tools. The following examples include an explanation and lessons learned about using HIT in an innovative manner to better quantify the effects of changes made in our system.

Prior to KP HealthConnect being implemented, metric collection was a laborious task. The Innovation Consultancy clocked hundreds of people hours gathering metrics through chart audits, surveys and other "feet on the ground" process observations. For example, in 2004 the IC had to measure the success of their innovative nurse shift change. With no automated data to be found, the team had to design a paper-based observation tool to be used by two observers three times a day for several weeks. The data from the paper forms were manually entered into Excel spreadsheets so that information could be graphed. Imagine all the additional prototypes that could have been built if data gathering and metrics analysis had been automated and not been so time consuming.

Fortunately, with the introduction of KP HealthConnect, data collection became streamlined. The trick was being able to ask the right question of the data. One of those right questions came along in 2010, when the Innovation Consultancy set out to create a safer, more responsive nurse-patient pain approach to pain management, called KP PainScape, on medical-surgical units in two KP hospitals. Because data was already being collected in the EHR, the team was able to co-design several metrics reports with the in-house analytics team. Hundreds of people-hours were reduced to just a few. The new reports helped the team to identify the real opportunities to impact pain management and they also provided sensitive and real-time feedback to show the impact of the tests of change during the project. In the end, the reports helped build the case for at least one innovative concept, the automated pain medication recheck timer to be included in the next upgrade of the EHR, as well as created an innovative set of actionable measurements for pain management.

Case Study 2: Low-Fidelity HIT Prototyping

Learning how to incorporate nimbleness in prototyping and testing within the EHR and other HIT has been a journey, from "oh my, that'll never work" to "hmmmm… what if we tried it this way?" Let's use the same two examples mentioned above, the nurse shift change project and the pain management project, to illustrate.

For the nurse shift change project of 2004, the inpatient EHR was not yet implemented but it was coming soon. A solution was needed that would be both a bridge to the EHR and, eventually, an integral part of the EHR. Using the IC's EvHCD approach, it was discovered that nurses deeply desired to have information at their fingertips during the shift change, and that patients wanted shift change to happen at the bedside. Combining these desires meant that a real-time EHR would have to be a part of the solution.

The team worked through several prototypes, but settled on a Microsoft Access database to replicate what would eventually be replaced by the EHR. The off-going shift of nurses would do some basic documentation in the database. This information would then be used to print a report at shift change for the on-coming and off-going nurses to have the close-to-real-time patient info at the bedside.

This project demonstrated that there are many ways to prototype for an EHR, including creating the initial prototype outside the EHR. Too often teams get stuck thinking they have to build their ideas in the EHR to test. But it turns out that approximating the tool in another system, such as the Access database and paper print-outs, can allow for increased efficiency, cheaper cost, faster development and more creativity than trying to do so in the EHR system itself.

With the pain management project of 2010, one of the ideas that emerged from this process was a way to help address the nurses' feeling of "task overload". Specifically, the IC developed the idea of an automated pain medication reassessment timer, which would be used to remind nurses to reassess their patients' pain within one hour of administration. To test what the reminders would feel like and understand their effect, the team first used egg timers (PDSA Cycle 1) and then Apple iTouches with a multiple alarm app (PDSA Cycle 2). These tests and results provided enough understanding and knowledge to build a business case, which incorporated the concept of automated pain timers in a future release of the EHR.

Since the EHR did not initially have time functionality, the team could have gotten stuck in a "we can't do that" phase. But instead, the team approximated this function with lower-fidelity prototypes to inform whether or not to move forward with higher-fidelity prototypes and solutions within the EHR.

Conclusion

Innovating involves taking risks. Fortunately, there are innovation methodologies to help mitigate them. And while the PDSA method is the foundation for trying and learning, it can be augmented with more divergent and creative methods to push thinking into new territory. Who would have thought that egg timers could be the precursor to innovative EHR functionality? Go wild with methods, and you'll be sure to discover other outrageous but valuable ideas.

Section I
You Have an EHR. Now What?!!?!

Paper is really good at being paper. Computers are really good at being computers, but they are lousy at being paper. What if we really recognized all we could with EHRs?

Electronic health record (EHR) systems have such grand potential. But that potential is often not met if they are designed or implemented simply as replacements for the paper chart. It should come as no surprise that most people, including physicians, just want a system that is familiar to them. So they often try to force an EHR to behave like paper, instead of thinking in an innovative fashion about how IT can be used to actually make a system better, not simply mimic an established process.

Fortunately, once an EHR is in place, something interesting begins to happen. There is always someone who begins to wonder "what if we could do this"? A patient has a bad outcome, a nurse notices an inconsistent pattern, a physician never wants a mistake to happen again and minds start to ponder, wonder, and imagine all sorts of interesting possibilities for using EHRs to improve the care process.

These type of innovations can range from simple concepts, such as the ability to have instant and ubiquitous messaging and chart review across multiple sites, to more complex concepts, such as the ability to create decision rules which can be personalized and woven into the workflow of care, or to the advanced work of analyzing big data and presenting it in ways never before possible.

We start off this section of the book with a story about the use of an EHR to help address the eternal quest of honoring people's needs when they need it most. Northwestern Memorial's Inflection Navigator system helps patients at their most vulnerable moments by using basic EHR functionalities to empower a physician and their staff to create an efficient, high quality, and cost-effective system of care coordination.

The Fallon Clinic, Medstar Health System, and Southeast Texas Medical Associates (SETMA) then each explain how they use the decision support capabilities in their EHR systems to make it easy to do the right thing at the right time by using EHRs to automate and delegate various care processes. The result is that these healthcare systems transform into magical places where prevention and disease management are fully integrated into the daily workflow of care. And while their stories have similarities, it is fascinating and important for future innovators to understand the *differences* as well, so the best of all worlds can be combined to create the perfect solution for other organizations.

We conclude with two very important "beyond EHR" ideas which bring in the theme of how real time data transparency can lead to both increasing "always events" and decreasing "never events". The Geisinger Health System explains how they have redesigned the process of care by using their EHR system to track and display the bundles of care elements required for various disease processes. And Children's National Medical Center details how they use an automatically generated EHR report to help them more easily and quickly identify and fix occurrences of preventable harm in their hospital.

The key concepts in this section are system optimization and good ol' imagination. It has become clear that as EHR functionality and data sets grow, we have entered the wild west of healthcare informatics. Healthcare "imagineers" are rethinking and inventing all sorts of wonders and the potential for creative minds to improve what we do every day is both critically important and bewilderingly large. We hope these stories help you stop and think about how you can reinvent care at your organization with a little imagination of your own.

Chapter 3
The Inflection Navigator

Lyle Berkowitz

"Hey Doc, I have to tell you. I'm amazed. When I sent you that email about the blood in my urine I never would have imagined that so much would happen so quickly." Ray Martinez knew he wasn't the healthiest guy in the world, but he thought he did pretty good with what he had. He hated all the wasted time in going to the doctor. When he was initially diagnosed with diabetes years ago, it seemed they never had what they needed at his appointments; a missing lab here, a lost referral there. It amounted to a lot of running around and a lot of stress.

This time was different. He noticed some blood in his urine one morning and was not sure what to do, so he emailed Dr. Johnson. He quickly received a reply from his doctor saying someone from his team would call him to help coordinate the workup of this new problem. Seamlessly, labs were ordered, appointments made, insurance contacted, and most amazingly no one was surprised when he showed up for any of the tests or appointments. He really hated when he was told to go do some medical thing, and then when he would attempt to do it, the medical people would be clueless on why he was there.

Two weeks later, Ray had his CT scan done, but had to cancel his urologist appointment because something came up. He figured he'd get to it later, but wondered if it was really important anymore since the blood in his urine had gone away. Fortunately, his question was answered when he got a call a week later from the doctor's care coordination team making sure he made a new appointment. And it was a good thing, because it turned out Ray had early stage bladder cancer, which his urologist was able to treat quickly and easily.

L. Berkowitz, M.D., FACP, FHIMSS
Department of Medicine,
Northwestern University Feinberg School of Medicine,
Chicago, IL, USA
e-mail: lyle@drlyle.com

L. Berkowitz, C. McCarthy (eds.),
Innovation with Information Technologies in Healthcare, Health Informatics,
DOI 10.1007/978-1-4471-4327-7_3, © Springer-Verlag London 2013

When Ray saw Dr. Johnson the following month, he told him the story and said, "this really makes me feel your team is watching out for me!" Dr. Johnson smiled. He'd been hearing this same surprise for a while. "It's called the Inflection Navigator system. Basically it means that we, as doctors, get to focus on you and your care, and we let our care coordinators worry about handling all the paperwork and helping you navigate the system – I know how complicated it can get. It's great that they make sure every step is completed and they always let me know if something is missing." Ray liked the sound of that and hoped his others doctors started using this same type of system too!

Background

Northwestern Memorial Physicians Group (NMPG) is a multi-site practice of over 100 primary care physicians who are on the medical staff at Northwestern Memorial Hospital (Chicago, IL) and faculty members of Northwestern University's Feinberg School of Medicine. NMPG brings the exceptional quality of Northwestern Memorial Hospital to convenient locations throughout the Chicagoland area. NMPG has been live on an electronic medical record (EMR) system from the Cerner Corporation (Kansas City, MO) since 2003.

The Szollosi Healthcare Innovation Program is a charitable endeavor housed within Northwestern Memorial Hospital's nonprofit foundation. Its mission is to leverage creative thinking and information technologies to produce a better experience for patients, physicians and others associated with their care.

The Innovation

The Inflection Navigator system is a low-tech and low-cost innovation which empowers a care coordination team to help ensure patients receive a consistent and efficient workup for important healthcare issues. These health care related "Inflection Points" can range from a new lab finding (e.g. Hematuria or blood in the urine) to a new diagnosis (e.g. Atrial Fibrillation, Cancer).

A physician initiates the Inflection Navigator process by choosing a "Pathway" message in their EMR system and sending it to their care coordination team. These care coordinators, or Inflection Navigators, then notify patients about what to expect in the coming weeks, provide them with educational materials, obtain referral authorizations and help them set up tests and specialty visits in the correct sequence and timeframe. Additionally, the Inflection Navigators will close the loop in a few weeks by making sure patients complete all the tasks in the physician assigned Pathway (see Fig. 3.1 for an example of the Hematuria Pathway).

PATHWAY - Hematuria

CRITERIA (please choose at least one)
[ ] Microscopic Hematuria at least twice in an otherwise healthy patient
[ ] Microscopic Hematuria at least once in high risk pt (e.g. smoker, age > 50)
[ ] Gross Hematuria once (without an obvious explanation)
[ ] Other:
LABS: Please order Urine Culture (and ideally Urine Cytology)
NOTE: Hematuria should be from full UA (not dipstick)

PATIENT CONTACT INFO
Phone Number:

OTHER CLINICAL HISTORY (optional)
Comments:

HEMATURIA PROTOCOL
[x] CT of the Abd/Pelvis w/wo contrast (in the next 5–10 days)
[x] NMFF Urology consult + Cysto (after CT done)

Fig. 3.1 The hematuria pathway template

The result is an easy method to improve the quality and efficiency of care, while also offering financial benefits to patients, providers and payors.

Reason for This Innovation

History of the Szollosi Healthcare Innovation Program (SHIP)

In 2008, the Szollosi Healthcare Innovation Program (SHIP) was created in honor of Peter Szollosi, a well known "creative talent" and innovator in the Chicagoland area. As Peter was dealing with his medical illnesses, he was shocked at the paucity of innovative thinking in healthcare and would challenge the establishment in a friendly way, with his well known mantra, "Don't tell me what you can't do"! After Peter passed away, his friends and family helped create SHIP to take up Peter's challenge with the goal of utilizing innovative thinking and information technologies to improve the healthcare experience for both patients and their caregivers.

The Healthcare "Inflection Point"

One of the first areas that the SHIP team decided to explore was how to provide a better experience for patients newly diagnosed with a serious medical issue. The team defined this point in time as a healthcare "Inflection Point", analogous to the mathematical definition of the point on a curve where the curvature changes dramatically (See Fig. 3.2). A healthcare "inflection point" is thus defined as a significant change in a patient's health status and needs, such as the new diagnosis of cancer or diabetes, or a new finding such as a thyroid nodule or hematuria.

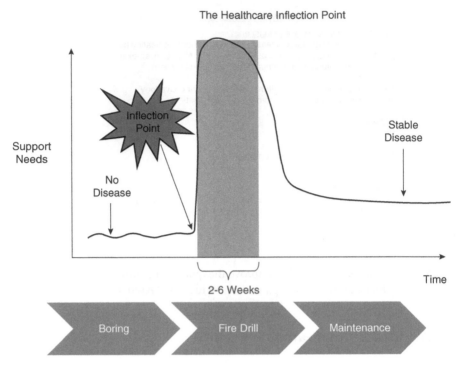

Fig. 3.2 The healthcare inflection point

Fire Drills and Black Holes

Most inflection points are unique and rare occurances for patients. The result is that all too often they result in "Fire Drills", when a lot of care has to happen quickly and without full knowledge of all data points. Additionally, a patient might experience "Black Holes", when care gets lost or slows down due to a variety of complexities.

During fire drills, a patient and physician spend a lot of time and energy tracking down what should be a consistent standard of care. The result can be delays in care, mistakes due to rushing things, and frustration on all sides.

But even more worrisome are black holes, where the patient never completes the entire care process. This might happen because patients or their physicians forgot to complete a step, or a physician is not aware of every step needed, or a patient does not complete all the steps for some other reason. The result can be devastating, as a patient may not be diagnosed with an important issue or does not get the care they need.

Peter Szollosi experienced these types of issues on a regular basis due to having multiple acute and chronic issues affecting him, and so working on inflection points was an especially good fit for this innovation program. Additionally, the traditional research world did not pay much attention to this area of inflection point management since it could be very complex and individualized, and thus not amenable to the standard style of research that could be applied to a new drug or surgical procedure. ***It was time for some innovation!***

Why This Innovation Succeeded

For the Inflection Navigator system to succeed, there were three main issues that needed to be solved: How to get physicians to want to use this system, how to build the infrastructure with essentially no budget and how to create the actual Pathways.

Physician Adoption

An important mantra concerning physician adoption is that "there is no quality without usage of a system" [1]. This section describes the physician friendly theories backing the Inflection Navigator system, as well as the educational and monitoring activities which helped ensure physician adoption of the system.

Getting Physicians to Like Checklists

In exploring this newfound area of care coordination addressing inflection point management, the SHIP team found that most primary care practices do not have a standardized process to deal with inflection points, thus creating potential delays or incomplete treatment. This is likely driven by the fact that physicians often eschew "cookbook medicine" tactics which try and automate their higher order thinking. So how could one get physicians to buy into the concept of standardizing some aspects of the care they delivered?

As fate would have it, as the SHIP team was pondering this issue, the New Yorker published Atul Gawande's "Checklist" article [2] which described the benefits of using a checklist to ensure a procedure was done in a consistent and complete manner. The team thought if someone can make a checklist for a procedure, why couldn't they do the same for a process?

The SHIP team was further influenced by two books on rethinking the standard care process, Christensen's The Innovator's Prescription [3] and Bohmer's Designing Care [4]. A key theme in both books was that while certain parts of healthcare require a physician's higher order thinking, there are other parts of the care process that are structured and consistent, and could be shifted to other members of the care team in an "assembly" line fashion.

Thus the idea was born to extend the checklist philosophy from procedure based care (e.g. surgical procedures) to the process based care which is done on a daily basis by primary care physicians. It additionally made sense that while physicians do not like the idea of standardizing their higher order thinking, they would be very happy to have someone standardize the structured or assembly line type of care and then delegating that to the correct person on their team. In other words, the hunt was on to figure out what parts of a care process could be "checklisted" and "task-shifted".

Initial Marketing: Make It Easy to Do the Right Thing

When the Inflection Navigator system was launched, providers received education via emails and group announcements which explained this new care process, as well as how using these bundled pathways would be much easier than placing each order separately. To help illustrate this point, physicians would be asked to imagine the story from a patient's perspective: "You are told you have a new and serious disorder. You don't need to be admitted to the hospital, but you will need to set up three tests, see two specialists and read about your new diagnosis on a specialized website – all in the next 10 days."

Physician communications would thus remind providers that most patients are usually overwhelmed when facing a healthcare Inflection Point, and would then propose an alternative scenario with the use of the Inflection Navigator system: "What if your physician told you someone from his team would contact you in the next 24 h to help you navigate the system – this person would have access to specific protocols for your situation and thus know who you have to see, what tests you need done, and what resources are available to you. Furthermore, your Inflection Navigator will make sure everything is done in a timely, efficient and complete manner – all at no cost to you." This type of communication turned out to be a powerful way to help providers quickly understand the power and importance of the Inflection Navigator system.

Ongoing Education and Feedback

To further encourage use, physicians would receive ongoing email updates about new pathways being implemented, as well as reminders about old ones. And every few months, they will receive a document they can print which lists all current Consults, Orders and Pathways they can access in the system, as well as future ones that are in the process of being created (see Fig. 3.3).

CONSULTS

    CONSULT – Behavioral Health/Therapy
    CONSULT – Dermatology (NMPG)
    CONSULT – Diabetes Education (NIW)
    CONSULT – Dietitian/Nutrition (NIW)
    CONSULT – General Surgery (NMPG)
    CONSULT – Health Learning Center
    CONSULT – NMFF Specialists
    CONSULT – Northwestern Integrative Medicine (NIW)
    CONSULT – OB/Gyne (NMPG: General)
    CONSULT – OB/Gyne (NMPG: Pelvic PT)
    CONSULT – OB/Gyne (NMPG: Ultrasound Appointment)
    CONSULT – Pelvic Health
    CONSULT – REHAB (RIC/Spine&Sports Rehab Center)
    CONSULT – Sleep Clinics
    CONSULT – Smoking Cessation (NIW)

Fig. 3.3 NMPG care coordination – consults, orders and pathways

ORDERS

    NMH ORDERS – Cardiology
    NMH ORDERS – Mammogram
    NMH ORDERS – Miscellaneous
    NMH ORDERS – Radiology

PATHWAYS

    PATHWAY – Atrial Fibrillation
    PATHWAY – Cancer (Lurie/NMFF)
    PATHWAY – Cancer/Heme (HemeOnc Associates
    PATHWAY – Chronic Disease, TuneUp
    PATHWAY – Chronic Kidney Disease (CKD)
    PATHWAY – Diabetes Tune Up
    PATHWAY – Hypertension
    PATHWAY – Lung Nodule
    PATHWAY – Obesity
    PATHWAY – Thyroid Nodule

COMING SOON

    PATHWAY – Asthma
    PATHWAY – Breast Lump
    PATHWAY – Cholesterol
    PATHWAY – DVT
    PATHWAY – Liver enzyme elevation
    PATHWAY – Low Back Pain
    PATHWAY – Rectal Bleeding

Fig. 3.3 (continued)

The Care Coordination team also reviews usage of the system and will contact individual physicians who are not consistently using the system so they can understand what is going on and make sure they understand how and why to use them. Low utilizers are often doctors who are so busy they never had time to learn the system, but they often become heavy users once they are aware of how it can make their lives more efficient.

Creating the Care Coordination Infrastructure

Unfortunately, even if a medical group agrees on the concept of an Inflection Navigator system, they might not have an infrastructure to allow for its easy activation due to both staff and technical issues. From a staffing perspective, there is concern that it is expensive and difficult to hire specialized care coordinators. From a technical perspective, the problem is that this type of team based care coordination functionality is not traditionally built into standard electronic medical record systems. For the Inflection Navigator project, the SHIP team converted the Referral Team staff into a robust care coordination team for no extra cost and discovered how most any EMR system could provide the basic messaging capability essential for this type of care coordination system.

Who Can Be an Inflection Navigator?

The NMPG Care Coordination program is staffed by a Director and five care coordinators. These individuals were previously known as the referral team, but were renamed the care coordination team as their responsibilities expanded. Members of the team all have at least high school or college degrees, good computers skills and strong social skills. While they are all medically savvy due to working in a medical group, only one had any formal medical training (as a Medical Assistant). In other words, even though the care coordinators were mainly non-clinicians, they could succeed in this type of role because the checklists only required them to follow directions, not make clinical judgments.

It also turned out that due to their experience as referral coordinators, they had the perfect set of skills needed for the care coordination activities required by the Inflection Navigator system. First, they knew how to obtain referral authorizations. Second, they were adept at using the EMR for both messaging and data retrieval. Third, they were very comfortable and facile in communicating with both patients and physicians. Finally, they understood and appreciated the concept of following a structured checklist. These skills made the transition from a basic referral team to a full-fledged care coordination team a seamless transition.

Building the Care Coordination Team Without a Budget

As stated, a new team did not need to be created since the referral team transitioned into the care coordination team without a change in size or salaries. They were able to perform their expanded duties without growing due to the following reasons:

- *Similar duties.* Much of their work remained referral authorizations and patient communication, which they were doing already.
- *Minimal extra work.* The extra work required around patient education and follow-up is relatively small.
- *Time Saving.* The team wound up spending a lot less time dealing with retroactive authorizations (which are needed if an authorization was not performed before a test or consult) since they were getting notified about all tests and referrals BEFORE they happened. And because it was always faster and easier to get authorization before a test or consult was performed, the care coordinators were able to spend more time helping patients navigate the system more easily, and less time dealing with insurance companies and upset patients.

Other cost savings related to the Inflection Navigator system included:

- *Decreased Overhead.* Because the care coordination process had become fully computerized, the majority of the care coordination team started to work from home, thus saving overhead costs.
- *Decreased Turnover.* It appears both the ability to work from home and the shift from negative to positive interactions (i.e. not having to deal with the retroactive

authorizations) has also helped staff morale, as no care coordinator has quit since the system has been in place.

Of course, as the number of care coordination pathways increase and the number of physicians using it expands, it is expected that additional staff will need to be hired. However, there are a variety of positive financial trade-offs which should make adding staff cost-neutral for the group and its related hospital:

- Anything which reduces time pressures on physicians by shifting work to lower cost staff creates a cost-effective "staffing arbitrage" with a good return on investment since physician are the highest paid employees in the group [5].
- Ensuring all the right tests and management are done lowers malpractice risk.
- Delivering a consistent high quality experience improves reputation in any market.
- Delivering consistent high quality experiences may improve reimbursement with certain insurance plans.
- Getting all the right tests in the right sequence with the right authorizations can have a positive economic effect for the hospital due to increased volume and more consistent authorizations.

Enabling Care Coordination Functionality in Any EMR

Fortunately, NMPG had started laying the groundwork for the Inflection Navigator infrastructure a few years earlier without fully realizing it. In 2006, NMPG addressed a long-term problem of ordering tests (e.g. Radiology and Cardiology testing) and setting up specialty consults by allowing physicians to send EMR-based messages to the referral team about these items [6]. This team would then obtain referral authorization for these requests and send them to the appropriate hospital schedulers to set them up for the patient.

By 2008, the infrastructure for ordering tests and requesting consults via EMR messaging was fully in place at NMPG and being used routinely by the majority of Internal Medicine physicians (as well as some of the other primary care providers, such as Ob/Gyn, Pediatrics and Dermatology). So when the SHIP team needed to create a system to accommodate the Pathway messages, they recognized that they could combine multiple tests and consults together into a single EMR message and add additional components for the care coordination team to carry out. The result was that the physicians could initiate a Pathway message in their EMR, choose which parts of a checklist applied to their patient, and then send it to the care coordination team to fulfill.

Do You Need More Than Your EMR?

Since the Inflection Navigation process required keeping track of multiple tasks, the SHIP team initially worked with the Northwestern University Biomedical Informatics Center to build a low cost, open source, web-based tool [7] to help the care coordination team track everything outside of the EMR. This web-based tool was used for the first year of deployment, and the team discovered the importance of being able to track results on specific patients over a specified period of time, as well the importance of having very well defined steps that anyone on the care coordination team could read and follow.

However, the SHIP team also recognized that this process was inefficient because it required the care coordinators to use two separate systems to track patients. Thus the decision was made to replicate the care coordination functionality within the EMR system as follows:

• Step by step instructions for the care coordination team: instead of being contained in a separate system, these were written out in detail at the bottom of the Pathway messages so that the care coordinator would know what to do when they received the message (see Fig. 3.4).

Physicians- Do not write anything below this line.
****
For NMH Radiology
* PATIENT DOB:
* TEST NEEDED: CT Abdomen/Pelvis WWO contrast; TIMING: 5–10 days
* RADIOLOGY SCHEDULING TO CALL PATIENT [x] YES [ ] No
NMPG Referral Department (Phone: 312–926–xxxx; Fax: 312–926–xxxx)
Insurance Authorization Number:
Additional Comments:
NMH Radiology Department (Phone: 312–926–xxxx; Fax: 312–926–xxxx)
Scheduled Date/Time:

****
For NMFF Consult Team Only
* Send an EPIC message to Urology: "P URO" – "Uro Nurse Pool"
* Once the Urology appointment has been set, please reply to both:
--- The Ordering Physician
--- NMPGPOOL, IMREFERRALS
* If no Urology appointment has been made after several attempts, please notify
  the Ordering Physician

****
For NMPG Referral Team Only
* Do chart review and make sure patient has UA, Urine Culture and Urine Cytology
  resulted (or ordered). If not, notify PCP that these are requested before the Urology visit.
* Get approval for CT Abd/Pelvis WWO contrast (Dx Hematuria, ICD 599.7)
* Fill in "Date of Birth" under NMH Rads
* Fax this Order to NMH Radiology: 312-926-2007
* Forward this PCO message to "NMFFPOOL, CONSULT"
* Let the patient know that the Radiology and Urology departments will
  call them to set up their appointments (but Urology will only call after the CT has been
  set up).
* Once you get appointment info from the NMFF Consult Team, get approval
  for Urology visit AND Cystoscopy (Dx Hematuria, ICD 599.7)
* In 4 weeks, review the chart and notify Ordering MD if the following have not been completed
--- CT Abd/Pelvis WWO contrast
--- Urology visit

Fig. 3.4 The Care Coordination Team view of the Hematuria Pathway

****

ADDITIONAL INFORMATION FOR ORDERING PHYSICIAN
* This protocol is for a finding of Hematuria
* Hematuria is defined by the AUA as two UAs with at least 3 RBC/HPF or one episode of gross hematuria. It also may be appropriate to use this protocol in a patient with one abnormal UA if the patient is a smoker, age > 50, or if you are clinically suspicious for any other reason.
* Please make sure the patient has a recent UA and Culture in the system, and try to do Urine Cytology before their GU visit.
* The urologist will review the CT ahead of time and has the option to cancel the Cysto, or change to a Surgical room cysto depending on those findings.
* The NMPG Care Coordination Team will review the chart and send you a message in a few weeks to let you know if the patient completed all the steps in the protocol.

Fig. 3.4 (continued)

- Reminder system for Chart Review: Initially, the care coordination team would forward the message to a separate Inbox they created in the EMR. In the title of that message they would put the date when the chart review was needed. They would then check that Inbox daily and do the chart reviews on those patients who were due. Fortunately, recent updates to the EMR system now allows the staff to more easily create reminders which show up in their inboxes on a designated date.
- Patient Education: The care coordination team stores any patient education handouts on a shared hard drive they can all access. They can then either mail these handouts or send them to the patient via NMPG's secure messaging system.

Developing Pathways

Picking the Initial Set of Pathways

The first three inflection points chosen for Pathway development were hematuria, atrial fibrillation and cancer. These were chosen in part because each one had afflicted SHIP's namesake, but mainly because they each represented a separate and important type of inflection point. As with the start of any innovation process, the next step was acquiring data. The SHIP team spent several months observing and talking with primary care physicians, specialists and patients to understand how to best manage these various healthcare inflection points in a patient's life. The result was the following:

- *The Hematuria Pathway* represented a new lab finding (blood in the urine) which requires an imaging study and a Urology visit. While this type of pathway is not an acute emergency, it does require a specific workup to rule out cancer. A primary care physician might see this a few times a year.
- *The Atrial Fibrillation Pathway* represented a new diagnosis (often discovered surreptitiously in the office) which requires various cardiac tests and then a consult with a cardiologist. This type of pathway requires a risk stratification by the physician and in some cases requires a very quick timeframe for evaluation. A primary care physician might identify this once or twice a year.

- *The Cancer Pathway* represented a much more vague situation in which a patient is either thought to have cancer (e.g. an abnormal CT scan), or has been definitely diagnosed with cancer. Initially, the SHIP team thought they would define all the common types of cancer and create checklists for each one. However, it became clear that this was over-managing the process and moving into the territory of higher level thinking where checklists were not appreciated. Instead, it was discovered that there were actually some very important items which all cancer patients needed regardless of the specifics of their diagnoses, but which they often did not get in a timely manner. The Cancer Pathway thus included a specialist appointment, as well as a referral to specific cancer support center on campus, information on how to gather all the information needed for a second opinion, and support for the notification of the patient's other physicians about their new situation. While all physicians agreed these were important issues, there had never previously been a process to ensure all patients received all this information in a consistent and timely manner.

The Pathway Components

A Pathway message includes the following three main components:
- *Background*: An introductory section explains when the Pathway should be used. It may also suggest lab tests to get before seeing a specialists, and it will often explain the exact criteria which should be met in order to launch the a specific pathway. For example, the hematuria pathway clarifies what type of hematuria scenarios require the Pathway workup (See Fig. 3.1), as well as suggests some labs tests to obtain. The atrial fibrillation pathway explains which patients should be sent directly to the emergency department instead of doing an outpatient workup. It also helps physicians risk stratify the patient for stroke (via use of the CHADS-2 score). The timing of the testing and consults are then based on this score, which puts a patient into a high-risk category (workup within 3 days) or a low-risk category (workup within 3 weeks).
- *Checklist*: The next section provides a standardized checklist of all suggested tests and specialist referrals for that inflection point, as well as the timeline in which they should be accomplished. For example, the hematuria pathway includes orders for a CT scan followed by a urology consult with cystoscopy; while the atrial fibrillation pathway includes orders for an echocardiogram and a 24 hour heart rhythm test using a Holter monitor, followed by referral to a cardiologist. Physicians can accept the entire bundle or order only those tests and referrals they deem necessary (i.e. by un-checking those they do not want performed). The physician can also change the timing of the workup if they feel it is clinically appropriate.
- *Care Coordinator Instructions*: The final section is for the care coordination team only. It provides detailed step-by-step instructions on how to fulfill each of the steps on the checklist they have been sent (see Fig. 3.4).

The Pathway Process

- *Initiation*: A physician initiates the Pathway in the EMR by creating a message on a patient, and then choosing the specific pathway they want from the list of available message types. The pathways naming convention is simply the word pathway (in capitals) followed by the name of the inflection point being addressed. Examples include "PATHWAY – Hematuria" and "PATHWAY- Lung Nodule".
- *Payer Authorizations*: The Inflection Navigator receives the pathway message in the EMR system and then obtains needed authorizations from the insurance company for any testing or consults ordered. It is important that the care coordinator be able to review the chart and print out the physician's recent note or other relevant data to send to the payor if needed.
- *Transmitting Orders and Consults*: The care coordinator electronically sends the order and authorization to the hospital scheduling department, who then calls the patient to schedule their appointment. The care coordinator also forwards the EMR message about any consults to the specialist's office, who reviews the record to see when testing will be completed and contacts the patient to schedule the appointment at the appropriate time.
- *Confirmation that care steps have been completed*: After a certain period of time, usually 4 weeks, the care coordinator reviews the patient's chart to confirm completion of all pathway elements, contacts the patient if needed, and notifies the primary care physician of any gaps in care. This review is done more quickly for an acute scenario like cancer or atrial fibrillation, but it can be longer for a chronic situation like a follow up for hypertension.

Results

The Inflection Navigator system improves the physician and patient experience by increasing process efficiencies and ensuring a consistent use of care standards. It has also resulted in a variety of financial benefits for patients, providers and payors of care.

Improving Efficiency, Quality and Access to Care

It makes logical sense that the care coordination process should improve the efficiency and quality of care by applying consistent standards to the type and timing of steps which need to be done for an inflection point. To help prove this point, an IRB approved research study [8] examined how the Hematuria Pathway impacted 100 patients with hematuria who were enrolled by NMPG physicians between May 2009 and May 2010. They were compared to a control group of 100 hematuria patients who were referred to the same urology group by a similarly sized internal medicine group during the same time period. The Hematuria Pathway provides an excellent example of how care coordination can improve efficiency by ensuring patients get their imaging studies before they see the urologist (See Fig. 3.5). The results for these "navigated patients" include several measures of improved efficiency:

- *Time to Imaging*: The time between the initial finding and completion of their CT scan averaged 22 days, less than half the 45.2-day average for similar patients not referred through the program.
- *Imaging completed BEFORE the urology visit*: Three-quarters (75.5 %) of navigated patients had their CT scan completed prior to the first urology visit, compared to just 28.8 % of other patients.
- *Time to Cystoscopy*: The time between the initial finding and completion of cystoscopy averaged 38 days for navigated patients, much quicker than the 70.6-day average for those not navigated. Cystoscopy is considered the final part of the hematuria evaluation.
- *Completion in one visit*: More than half of the navigated patients (56.6 %) had their evaluation completed in one visit, compared to only 21.9 % of the non-navigated patients. This is not only more efficient for patient but also demonstrates how certain care coordination activities can free-up capacity for specialists by ensuring appropriate testing is done before their visits. In other words, by streamlining the care process, the urology group had more appointment slots open, thus enhancing access to their care and theoretically allowing the group to increase revenues by attracting new patients and/or performing additional procedures in those time slots.

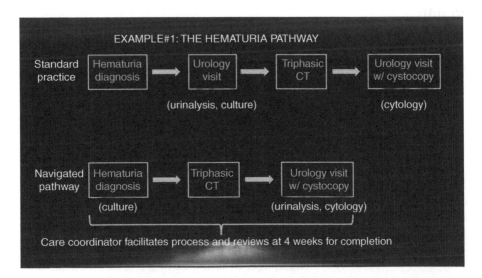

Fig. 3.5 The hematuria pathway

While an improvement in efficiency metrics should result in a better patient experience, it can also be an important quality metric. For example, around 10% of hematuria cases will result in a diagnosis of a life threatening condition [9], and thus a faster diagnosis could improve outcomes.

Financial Benefits

Care coordination has many potential financial benefits. This section describes both the measured and theoretical financial benefits attained in a primarily volume-based, fee for service reimbursement system. It is likely that the financial benefit in a value-based reimbursement system (e.g. capitation, accountable care organizations) would be even higher due to the decrease in extra visits and the earlier diagnosis of problems.

Decreasing Retroactive Authorization

Before the referral messaging system for hospital tests (e.g. Radiology, Cardiology) began in 2006, NMPG's referral team had to deal with approximately 25 retroactive referral authorization requests every month for patients who did hospital testing without getting them pre-approved. Within 4 years of implementing NMPG's care coordination system, the amount of retroactive authorizations needed dropped to under one per month (Fig. 3.6). This is significant for two main reasons:

- *They take a long time to do.* While a pre-approval authorization may just take 1 min, a retroactive referral may take many hours of the team's time, and might also require physician time, a very expensive activity. So cutting out 25 of these a month can create significant time savings for the care coordination team to work on other activities. This is one of the main reasons that the team was able to expand their duties with the same number of personnel.

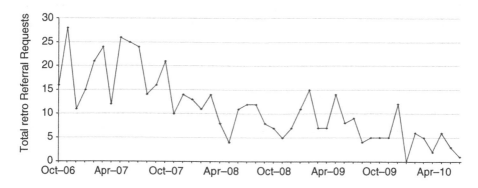

Fig. 3.6 Total radiology initiated retro-authorization requests – Oct-2006 to Jul-2010

- *Non-approved referrals cost money.* If a retroactive referral request is denied, then the team has to deal with an upset patient, and often the hospital will have to write off the charges. So if the hospital had to write off 25 tests a month that could account for a loss of $500,000–$1 million in revenue per year.

Decreasing Malpractice Risk

Malpractice risk can be decreased in at least two ways by using the Inflection Navigator system.

- *Decrease bad outcomes.* The system helps ensure that all patients get a consistent, consensus based level of care, meaning they do the right tests, see the right specialists, and do everything in the right time frame. Therefore, problems are found sooner, treatment is initiated more quickly, and patients feel better about the thoroughness of their care. Additionally, because the care coordination team strives to make sure that everything is completed, there is less of a chance of patient missing a test or appointment and thus not getting a timely diagnosis. This is a major quality issue as studies have shown that about 30% of patients fail to even set up the specialist appointment recommended by their primary care doctors [10]!
- *Documentation is better.* If a patient does not follow through with their recommended evaluation and management, the Inflection Navigation system ensures that the patient is notified multiple times and everything is well documented. For example, if a patient was referred to the Hematuria Pathway, but did not complete their evaluation, they would be called by the care coordination team, the radiology service, the specialists and later by their personal physicians. All of these communications would be documented, so if they still refused to finish their evaluation and later developed cancer, there would be ample documentation that they were told about the seriousness of their situation and offered timely access for their evaluation.

Mathematical Model of the Financial Effects of Care Coordination

As part of the Inflection Navigator project, the SHIP Team created a mathematical model to look at the potential financial impact of this type of care coordination from three perspectives:

- *The patient*, who is responsible for co-pay fees, as well as travel expenses and lost time from work. They will want to have as few visits as possible
- *The payor*, who also wants as few visits as possible to finish the evaluation.
- *The specialist provider*, who may get paid more for an office visit where they can perform a procedure vs. an office visit where they have to tell the patient to get another test and come back after that has been completed.

This mathematical model was created with the assumption that a patient needed to get a certain test before the specialist could render a final opinion. Therefore, seeing the specialist before getting a test was considered an "unnecessary visit".

Additionally, the model assumed that there might be a price differential between an unnecessary visit vs. a visit where the specialists could complete their evaluation because all the data was available. This price differential might be because they could appropriately use a higher complexity code and/or because they would perform a procedure at this more complex visit. For example, with hematuria, the research study confirmed that a non-navigated patient will be more likely to see a urologist first, then be told to get a CT scan and finally come back for a second visit with the urologist to get a cystoscopy. However, a navigated patient would be more likely to first get their CT scan and then see the urologist for their one and only visit, where the cystoscopy would be performed.

The result of this care coordination should thus be a clear cost savings for patients and payors since one visit was appropriately eliminated. Assuming there is a price difference between two types of visits, then there is also an economic advantage to the specialist, since it will decrease low-income visits, thus increasing the appointment slots available for higher income visits. This does assume there is high demand for the specialty services ensuring all their appointment slots are taken.

This model was applied to the Hematuria Pathway using test and visit costs which were identified as part of the research study discussed previously. The results (see Fig. 3.7) demonstrate that increasing the number of patients who are navigated produces three important financial outcomes:

The Mathematical Model
And how it can be applied generically to help predict the effect of other care coordination activities

Percent Navigated	Total # Patients Completed	Total # patient Slots	Payor Cost (per PT)	MD Revenue per pt	Total MD Revenue	Patient own cost (average)
(include % change from baseline)						
0%	100 (0%)	200 (0%)	$1000 (0%)	$600 (0%)	$60,000 (0%)	$180
25%	125 (+25%)	200	$975	$575	$70,000	$160
50%	150 (+50%)	200	$950	$550	$80,000	$140
75%	175 (+75%)	200	$925	$525	$90,000	$120
100%	200 (+100%)	200 (0%)	$900 (-10%)	$500 (-16%)	$100,000 (+66%)	$100, (-40%)

Example with the following assumptions

• Total number of visits reduced from 2 to 1 (the "Initial visit" is eliminated)

• Initial visit costs $100, Confirmatory Visit costs $500, Test costs $400

• MD has endless demand for this particular situation

Fig. 3.7 The mathematical model

- *Patients save money*. Because they have less office visits, the patients have less out of pocket expenses and less time away from work.
- *Payors save money*. They similarly benefit because they pay less per patient.
- *Specialty physicians might increase revenue*. For example, use of the Hematuria Pathways will result in a decrease of low cost visits for urologists. Therefore, they could use those appointment slots for more highly productive visits involving complex cases and/or procedures, which are reimbursed at higher rate.

This mathematical model can be applied to similar clinical scenarios and thus can be a useful tool for medical groups trying to prioritize the next Pathway to focus upon at their organization.

Lessons Learned

Getting Started with This Innovation

- **Expect it to take time**: Planning and piloting this type of process enhancement takes time, as there is a need to figure out current processes, develop protocols, and obtain physician support. Furthermore, getting consistent physician use can take several months or longer.
- **Incorporate relevant decision-makers**: Working with people who have relevant decision-making authority (e.g., the director of hospital scheduling) helps to ensure that new processes are appropriately developed and embraced by the various stakeholders. Similarly, there must be a specialist "physician champion" for each pathway developed to assist with the content and workflow needed to make sure it succeeds.
- **Quick wins by solving a pain**: A long-standing complaint from doctors was getting paged by the radiology technicians when a patient showed up without a written order. By creating the initial messaging system for test orders, the doctors recognized that they could substantially reduce the chance of this happening since the order would be available in an electronic format. And once they began using this consistently, adding further types of messages was a relatively straightforward evolution with built in physician understanding.
- **Make it easy to use**: Adding the order bundles into the typical EMR workflow made it easy for physicians to access and use at the right point in the care process. It was easier to use compared to paper because (1) It already had the patient information attached to it; (2) It had everything pre-checked, and (3) It explained the appropriate clinical situations for its use. Additionally, it was easier compared to paper or single electronic orders since it bundled multiple tests and consults together, and included extra educational components.
- **Systematize and shift tasks**: To make it as valuable and cost-effective as possible, it is important to shift as much work away from physicians and towards the care coordination team. As with any checklist, one wants to systemize all the steps involved with the healthcare inflection point, and then delegate as many as possi-

ble by making them clear and unambiguous steps that need to happen with all patients. This helps ensure that all steps will be followed in a consistent manner.

- **Make use optional but transparent**: Physicians never like to be told they have to use a system, so usage should be optional – but clearly should be made easier than the status quote. Additionally, it is important to start capturing usage and feeding it back to physicians so they can see how they compare to their peers.
- **Shared EMR access**: It is critical that the care coordination team have easy access to the EMR system, so they can easily and quickly handle referral management and chart reviews.

Sustaining This Innovation

- **Educate and educate some more**: To promote high utilization of the system, it is important to regularly remind physicians about the system, especially if there are new pathways implemented.
- **Set expectations**. Admit to physicians at the start that no system is perfect and that they still might get an occasional call from the radiology center or from a patient who didn't get called as expected.
- **Learn from failures.** It is important to make it easy for physicians to report any problems they notice, so they can be appropriately evaluated. A common complaint we heard early on was when they physicain would get paged about finding an order. By tracking these down armed with specific patient instances, we learned that not all the scheduling staff knew where to look for the orders - and so more education on their end was needed.
- **Positive feedback and physician champions**. Providing positive feedback to physicians about their usage is always a good thing to remember to build into your processes. It is additionally helpful to identify a physician champion at every office site who can make sure to promote this system to his colleagues and help if there is a low utilizer.
- **Explore reasons for non-use:** It is important to understand usage patterns for both specific pathways as well as specific physicians. Low usage of a pathway may mean it requires more education to physicians and/or needs to be redesigned. Low usage by a specific physician usually is simply due to them not knowing about a specific pathway because they were too busy to read the group emails that were sent. Thus contacting low usage physicians individually can result in a quick win.

Future Plans

Now that the Inflection Navigator system has helped establish the people, process and technical infrastructure for care coordination, future plans will be to go "deeper and wider".

Going Deeper: Adding More Pathways

NMPG is adding additional pathways on a regular basis. The initial ideas for pathways often come from an anecdotal experience with a patient, or from a physician who is passionate about a specific issue. The SHIP Team reviews requests to determine which pathways would be most appropriate, based on the number of people affected, as well as both the complexity and significance of the situation. Fig. 3.4 includes a list of pathways currently being developed for release in the near future.

Going Wider: Expanding to Other Practices

A pilot project has been initiated which extends the Inflection Navigator care coordination system as a service to other medical groups affiliated with the hospital. This will allow other physicians the ability to initiate a variety of consults, orders and pathways via their own EMR systems. The NMPG Care Coordination Team will then have access a special Inbox in these EMRs so they can manage the messages. This system will utilize the same content and workflows to assist with everything from referral authorization and scheduling to education and follow-up care. In other words, other medical groups will be able to leverage the economies of scale already created by NMPG. The result will be the ability to improve the quality and efficiency for all patients on campus while expanding the infrastructure that can work in current reimbursement models, but can thrive even further in potential future reimbursement models, such as accountable care organizations (ACOs).

Conclusion

Like many innovations, the Inflection Navigator came from humble origins, when a doctor and a patient simply asked, "how can we improve the experience for patients and providers when they need it most?" What began as a way to transmit a single radiology order evolved into a robust care coordination infrastructure which improves efficiency, quality and financial reimbursement across a wide spectrum of care activities, and sets the stage for many more things to come.

References

1. Berkowitz LL. Physician adoption strategies. In: Carter JH, editor. Electronic health records. 2nd ed. Philadelphia: American College of Physicians; 2008. p. 249–74.
2. Gawand A. The checklist. The New Yorker. 2007. Online at http://www.newyorker.com/reporting/2007/12/10/071210fa_fact_gawande. Accessed on 08 Oct 2012.

3. Christensen C, Grossman J, Hwang J. The innovator's prescription. New York: McGraw-Hill; 2008.
4. Bohmer R. Designing care. Boston: Harvard Business Review Press; 2009.
5. Dorr DA, Wilcox A, Burns L, Brunker CP, Narus SP, Clayton PD. Implementing a multidisease chronic care model in primary care using people and technology. Dis Manag. 2006;9(1):1–15.
6. AHRQ Health Care Innovations Exchange. Innovation profile: the inflection navigator. In: AHRQ Health Care Innovations Exchange. Rockville. Available: http://www.innovations.ahrq.gov. Accessed on 08 Oct 2012.
7. caBIG® and patients: navigating cancer complexities together. Cancer biomedical informatics grid newsletter. 2009. Online at http://cabig.cancer.gov/resources/newsletter/issueXXV/action.asp. Accessed on 08 Oct 2012.
8. Casey J, Cashy J, Tourne-Schwab A, Wickramasinghe N, Schaeffer A, Gonzalez C, and Berkowitz LL. New care coordination system improves the quality, efficiency and cost of care for patients with hematuria. In: American Urological Association annual conference proceedings, Washington, DC; 14 May 2011.
9. Khadra MH, Pickard RS, Charlton M, Powell PH, Neal DE. A prospective analysis of 1,930 patients with hematuria to evaluate current diagnostic practice. J Urol. 2000;163(2):524–7.
10. Weiner M, Perkins AJ, Callahan CM. Errors in completion of referrals among older urban adults in ambulatory care. J Eval Clin Pract. 2010;16(1):76–81.

Chapter 4
Making "Right" Easier

Peter Basch

It's 8 am on Friday morning, and Ray Martinez is ready to leave the doctor's office, even though his 8:15 appointment for a blood pressure check hasn't even started. He knows his wife Barbara will give him hell if he doesn't keep this appointment, and bring home something from the doctor that shows what the plan is for keeping his blood pressure under control. So he decides to stay. Five minutes later, he is called back by Nurse Betty, "Now let's take those vitals and see how your blood pressure is doing." She enters his vital signs into the computer. Ray is a bit surprised when she clicks a button on the display and asks, "Mr. Martinez, have you stopped smoking cigarettes yet?"

A few minutes later, Dr. Wright walks into the room and shakes his hand. "Mr. Martinez, I see you are here for a blood pressure check today. How are you feeling today, any problems?" Ray says he is feeling fine, and was sorry that he was wasting the doctor's time, but kept the appointment to please his wife.

"I'm glad you are feeling fine, but I am also glad that your wife convinced you to keep this appointment." After clicking a button on the computer screen, Dr. Wright adds, "In addition to checking your blood pressure, which by the way is still up – I can see we have a few other issues to deal with today. I see that you are still smoking, and before you leave here today I want to do whatever I can to help you make and keep a plan to quit. Also, because of your smoking history and your diabetes, you are also due for a pneumonia shot. Smokers are at higher risk for a certain kind of pneumonia, and according to your record you have never had this vaccine before. And speaking of your diabetes, you are overdue for a blood test and eye check. Also, because your father had colon cancer at age 56, we should start colon cancer screening on you now, rather than waiting till you are 50. I'll get you a referral for your first colonoscopy. Sorry. Please unbutton your shirt, take off your shoes and socks, and hop up on the table."

P. Basch, M.D., FACP
MedStar Health, Ambulatory EHR and Health IT Policy,
5565 Sterrett Place, 3rd Floor, Columbia, MD 21044, USA
e-mail: peter.basch@medstar.net

L. Berkowitz, C. McCarthy (eds.),
Innovation with Information Technologies in Healthcare, Health Informatics,
DOI 10.1007/978-1-4471-4327-7_4, © Springer-Verlag London 2013

Ray had been seeing Dr. Wright sporadically over the past 15 years. During these appointments, he came in with a reason for the visit (which was always attended to), and Dr. Wright frantically looked through his folder or more recently through several computer screens for something, and occasionally Dr. Wright asked him about some other issues. But today was different. Both Dr. Wright and his nurse both seemed to be able to zero in on everything that was due.

At the end of his appointment, Ray saw Dr. Wright click another button, and then said to him, "Mr. Martinez, please wait here for a moment, and Betty will be right in to give you that pneumonia shot. After you get it, please get dressed and come to the checkout desk; your lab slip and colonoscopy referral are there. I also have a visit summary there for you and your wife. It contains your lab orders for today; your referrals for the colonoscopy and diabetic eye exam, your medication list, today's blood pressure and weight, and the smoking patch we discussed during the visit. Please share this with your wife, because I know she will call me later if you don't let her see it. We'll see you in a few months."

"Ok doc, thanks I guess. A guy can't get away with anything anymore!"

Background

MedStar Health, the largest not-for-profit health system in the mid-Atlantic region, is comprised of nine teaching and non-teaching hospitals, outpatient medical practices, visiting nurse and home care, a research institute, and other health-related entities. Last year it saw more than 162,000 inpatient admissions and almost 1.5 million outpatient visits. Founded 13 years ago, MedStar is a relatively new health system, and like most new health systems has had to deal with connecting disparate IT systems as well as different versions of the same system. MedStar was the birthplace of the world-class health information system Azyxxi, which was purchased by Microsoft in 2006 and rebranded as Amalga. MedStar also recently started the MedStar Innovation Institute (along with a collaboration with the Cleveland Clinic) to stimulate and drive innovation that advances health.

The Innovation

The innovation is an overlay to the outpatient electronic health record (EHR), which allows for whomever is seeing the patient to easily identify and act upon relevant protocols that are due while still respecting visit workflows. In essence, it makes it easier for providers to always offer the right care to the right patient at the right time. The innovation is called "View all Protocols," and it presents to all credentialed and appropriate users of the EHR, all relevant care opportunities that the patient is due for, including presenting sufficient information by which to understand the protocol and why it is due; appropriate orders that may be executed to fulfill the protocol; and the ability to document why a protocol may not be otherwise addressed (such as a

Fig. 4.1 Protocols due for this patient

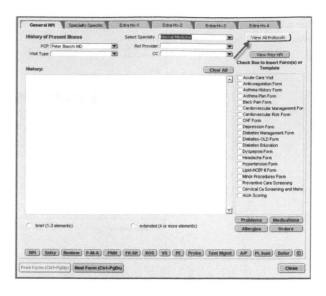

patient declining a test or procedure, or documenting that something was done else-where by another provider). This innovation allows for an unlimited number of protocols to be presented and acted upon as clinically appropriate, by clicking a yel-low button labeled "View all Protocols," as this button is present throughout the visit form (and protocols can thus be viewed by the provider and patient at multiple times during a visit). Protocols are determined by advisory groups within the health sys-tem, and as per those decisions, they are presented ONLY to the specialties and/or individuals for which the health system has decided that the protocol should be addressed. For example, cancer screening protocols are presented to Internal Medicine and Family Medicine, and only to providers.

This innovation is intentionally presented at multiple points during a patient visit, as it is seen as fulfilling multiple functions. Having an ability to see protocols due at the beginning of a visit allows for a provider to see what is due, and introduce these care opportunities to the patient then, creating a shared agenda for the visit. Seeing these same protocols due during the course of the visit allows for these care opportunities to be appropriately acted upon. And seeing the protocols due (if any remain due) at the end of a visit serves as a reminder if anything is left or forgotten at the end of a visit, or needs still to be scheduled for a future visit.

Here is what the provider (and the patient) sees when the EHR is opened to that patient's record (Fig. 4.1). The highlighted button "View all Protocols" is present on most of the EHR forms. When the button is glowing "yellow" it means that a proto-col relevant to the role and/or specialty of the logged on user is probably due. If there are no protocols due at that time for that patient or for the type of provider that the patient is seeing, the button is blue, providing a readily visible status indication (without having to be clicked).

Here is an example of what might be seen on a typical patient visit, where the chief complaint for the visit is "sinus infection." Again, the "View all Protocols" button is yellow, so while the history is being obtained and the button is clicked,

Fig. 4.2 Protocols due for a patient with a sinus infection

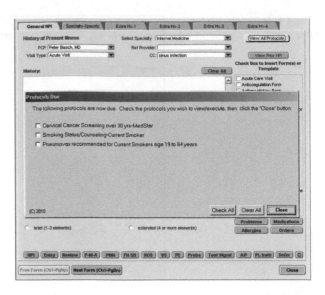

Fig. 4.3 Smoking status prompt

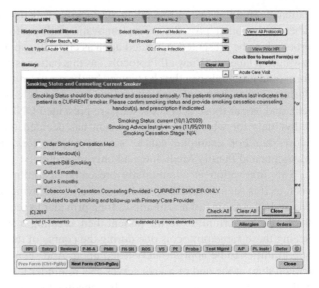

the doctor and patient see the following (Fig. 4.2). This global prompt could then be closed (it has raised awareness of the three protocols due) or one or more of the protocols could then be checked to open the next detailed, actionable screens. In this example, it would not be appropriate to interrupt the flow of the history of present illness to bring up the apparent lack of timely Pap smear. However, as smoking status and pneumococcal vaccination status are relevant at this point in the visit, a provider should click them both, and then click "close." While the patient is still providing history, the provider would see this (Fig. 4.3). In this instance, the provider can see that as of 10/13/2009 the patient was a smoker, and

Fig. 4.4 Pneumococcal vaccination prompt for current smokers

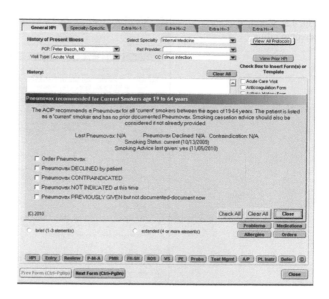

the provider can now appropriately ask if the patient is still smoking, and then click the appropriate boxes regarding smoking status. If the patient is still smoking, the provider can also provide smoking cessation counseling and generate a handout or prescription, if appropriate. Those actions will be documented whenever check-boxes are clicked.

As soon as the "close" button is clicked, this next screen comes up (Fig. 4.4). The provider might then tell the patient: "…whatever is going on with you now, as a current smoker you are highly susceptible to a particular type of bacterial infection that causes pneumonia, and I recommend you get vaccinated today. This vaccination should provide good protection for you against this particular infection, and won't have to be repeated until you turn 65." Depending on the patient's response, the provider would check the appropriate box, and either generate an order, refusal, contraindication, or documentation that it had been done elsewhere.

The provider would then review the patient's vital signs, do an appropriate physical exam and determine a course of treatment. Prior to the patient's leaving the office, the provider would see that the "View all Protocols" button is still glowing yellow, and could decide to choose the "Cervical Cancer" protocol that was not addressed earlier. After clicking on the checkbox for this issue, the provider would then see the following (Fig. 4.5). Since in this example the patient is here for an acute sinus infection, it would be very unlikely to actually perform the Pap smear that day. However, the provider could at least ask if she had it done elsewhere, determine if it is not due yet, or schedule her for an additional visit.

Thus, by creating or endorsing a set of clinical protocols and best practices, and then determining who should see them (specialty and role) and all allowable actions for each protocol, MedStar Health now has a system in place that permits the doctor and patient to be aware of what is potentially due, take appropriate action, and create relevant documentation – all with minimal effort.

Fig. 4.5 Cervical cancer screening due

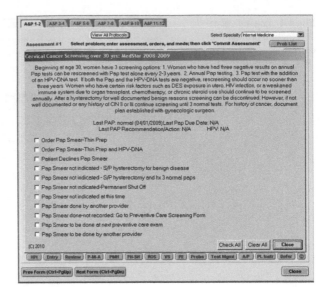

Reason for This Innovation

This innovation was driven by two very different but equally compelling needs: (1) improving compliance with existing protocols, thereby improving quality metrics, and (2) making it possible to get most of the benefit of multiple multi-page smart forms, without having to launch, read, interpret, and then act upon each form. Thus, in the example above, the provider could have found out the same information for this patient with a sinus infection by: opening the social history form and figuring out that the smoking status was old; opening the immunization form and seeing that this patient who smokes has never had a pneumonia shot; and opening the cervical cancer form and determining that the patient was due for a pap smear. That approach requires that the provider be able to focus not just on why the patient is there, but what the patient could be due for, and then manually opening up 10 pages or more of prior history and then documenting and ordering as appropriate. And after all that effort the patient ended up being due for nothing, it would seem like a lot of work for nothing. This approach dramatically reduces the burden by presenting upfront what is due. If nothing is due, the "View all Protocols" button does not glow yellow, and the provider can skip opening of preventive and chronic care forms.

MedStar Health created its Ambulatory Quality Best Practice Group in 2001 to vet and endorse protocols and best practices – primarily for primary adult medicine and pediatrics; and to conduct periodic chart reviews related to compliance with these protocols and best practices. As one might imagine, prior to the implementation of the EHR, chart review was such a laborious process that data collection and interpretation could take months.

With the implementation of the EHR (GE Centricity), MedStar Health began to use the GE data analysis and reporting tool – MQIC (Medical Quality Improvement Consortium). MQIC provided the ability to extract these reports on most of the clinical queries in hours instead of months. This dramatic lessening of the time it took to know how providers were doing on many clinical situations led to a paradigm shift of the work of this group. Instead of simply implementing the EHR and hoping that retrospective reporting coupled with the ability to more readily find information would result in care improvement over time, the group took a step forward, and began to work with a decision support expert to build into the EHR features that would make it more likely that best practices would be followed and the capability to easily track adherence.

Why This Innovation Succeeded

As is well known, adding additional functionality into an EHR does not guarantee that it will be used. To the contrary, unless workflow is concurrently addressed, any solution that adds significantly more time and effort (except where other business drivers dictate otherwise) is doomed to fail. At MedStar Health, the first iteration of attempting to use the EHR to improve compliance with preventive and chronic care objectives required that a different form be used for each condition (e.g. for preventive care, for each chronic disease state, for specific acute problems). In some instances this led to significantly improved compliance with protocols and best practices. However, to make this approach work consistently required that the provider know which forms to open, and then of course to open and use them. For example, if a patient came in for a diabetes follow-up, and the patient also had hypertension and heart disease, and several acute complaints, to optimize the benefit of the EHR would take so many pages of densely populated forms that seeing these patients in the typical time allotted for a follow-up visit was no longer possible. And of course if one forgot to open a form, one would likely not be aware of a care opportunity. MedStar Health had a dilemma; either implement longer and more complex forms – and hope that providers remembered to always use what was necessary (and were efficient enough to do this in a timely fashion); or come up with a different approach.

In 2007, MedStar Health entered into a contract with Clinical Content Consultants (CCC) of Concord, New Hampshire. The contract was both for traditional form design for multiple specialties, and more importantly to come up with an approach that would allow for improved compliance with known and yet to be determined best practices and protocols WITHOUT requiring additional forms. There was also a need for a process that would:

1. Put enough information on a single screen to allow for an informed decision coupled with the ability to act on that decision (e.g. documenting a refusal or contraindication, ordering a test or service);
2. Deliver that information and action ability to only certain people (based on role and specialty);
3. Track when these prompts were viewed and/or acted upon;
4. Allow easy modification or customization of these screens plus the ability to control who can customize them; and
5. Provide this information and action ability in unobtrusive or obtrusive ways (if hard stops are needed) at multiple times during a visit.

What CCC built for MedStar Health (and other groups and health systems with similar requirements) was a sophisticated protocol engine and delivery process. The process allowed MedStar Health to take a nearly unlimited number of protocols and best practices, and present them based on its business rules and clinical imperatives. For example, the Ambulatory Quality Best Practice Group discussed if preventive care services due should be prompted either during a preventive care visit, or any time a patient presented to a primary care provider for any reason. It opted for the latter, but built in flexibility such that providers and patients could decide to order or perform preventive screening services during a regular office visit. They could also note that they were due and schedule them for another time. It was also important to have this functionality present throughout the visit. While a patient was presenting her history of present illness, the provider could briefly click the protocols button and see what was due – and then close the protocols so that the patient was not interrupted.

This process has led to a fundamental change in most office visits. No longer were providers guided by the chief complaint of the patient and whatever the provider also remembered was due. The provider (and patient) could now develop a shared agenda for a visit, based on the chief complaint and the care opportunities the system identified.

Sometimes it would not be appropriate to interrupt a patient's history with the insertion of this new shared agenda; thus the benefit of being able to see and act upon this same information at the beginning of a visit, at multiple points during a visit, and before the patient was ready to leave. Similar to the new dynamic of the shared agenda at the beginning of the visit was a new dynamic at the end of the visit. Previously, an attentive and alert provider might ask a patient prior to leaving the exam room, "Do you have any other questions?" Now in addition to asking that, the alert provider will also check to make sure that he/she doesn't have any other issues to address before the patient leaves.

The Process for Keeping This Innovation Current

While the technology component of the protocol engine and delivery mechanism was viewed as crucial to the success of this work. Technology only provides the last components of the solution. What must occur first are the following:

1. A trusted and authoritative source must vet and endorse protocols and best practices;
2. A mechanism must be developed to ensure that protocols and best practices are reviewed and updated on a regular basis (or when new guidance is issued); and
3. A subgroup of the 'trusted and authoritative source' mentioned above, must work with the software developer to re-write (which sometimes means re-interpret) the protocols and best practices such that they can be operationalized as "good enough" within the existing practice environment and technology architecture.

MedStar Health was fortunate to already have had a group in place (the Ambulatory Quality Best Practice Group) that readily met conditions #1 and #2. They then used a subset of that same group to meet condition 3.

Fig. 4.6 HIV screening due

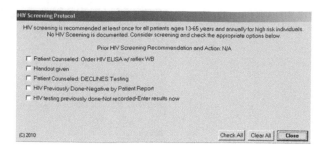

Here is one example of what is necessary to take a clinical protocol and operationalize it into an EHR system. The CDC has recommended that physicians ask all patients between the ages of 13–65 (who do not have HIV/AIDs) if they have ever been screened for HIV infection, and if not, offer screening. It further recommended that this be done annually for patients at high risk, and periodically for patients at normal risk. The Ambulatory Quality Best Practice Group asked its members what they considered to be a group of patients at high risk. One answer was "a history of sexually transmitted diseases." The process of creating the logic statements that precedes the coding process resulted in the following questions back to the committee members:

> Does this mean a current infection, or an infection at any time? For example, should a 70 year old healthy woman in a monogamous relationship be assigned to a high risk status for HIV testing because she had a Chlamydia infection once at age 17?

The group readily concluded that that approach would not work.

The Ambulatory Quality Best Practice Group then asked several HIV specialists how they would stratify a population into average and high risk. Their suggestion was to ask patients (at least once each year) if they had had sex for money. The Group felt that while this was a question that naturally fit into the workflow of the HIV clinic, it would likely not be consistently used outside of that situation, and thus would not result in meaningful risk stratification. The decision was then made to start with something much less ambitious, which was not to attempt to program "high risk" into the protocol. Rather, it was decided to create a simpler prompt that would appear for all patients in the appropriate age group (who did not already have HIV/AIDS or a prior test result in the EHR), regarding HIV status.

The prompt currently appears like this (Fig. 4.6). At this point the prompt is turned off permanently by having a HIV blood test result in the system, or a patient attestation of a negative result. If a patient declines testing, the prompt is turned off for a year. With this example, as with other prompts, MedStar Health may elect to modify the decision logic in the future.

Using the Protocol Alerts/Best Practices for Patient Safety

Shortly after releasing these first protocols to MedStar's primary care doctors, there was an urgent appeal from several endocrinologists to address the situation in which some providers (primarily new residents) were mistakenly ordering U500 insulin (5 × more potent than what they should be ordering), instead of U100 insulin.

Fig. 4.7 U500 insulin alert

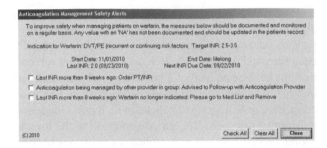

Fig. 4.8 Anticoagulation
management safety alerts

Using a process similar to that described above, MedStar Health had developed the following prompt, which appears once an order for U500 insulin is entered (Fig. 4.7).

Another example of a prompt developed to improve medication safety was one developed for warfarin use. After an initial analysis showed that warfarin was managed well by MedStar's anticoagulation clinics and inconsistently outside of these clinics, MedStar revised an anticoagulation form that would help to optimize its safe use. While use of this form did indeed make it easier to optimize warfarin safety, one had to (of course) open and use the form for it to add value.

MedStar Health also developed a CDS alert strategy that would prompt any clinician if a patient was on warfarin and certain parameters were otherwise not addressed, or not addressed in a timely fashion. Specifically, the prompt would appear if a patient was on warfarin, and if: there was no indication, no stop date, no target INR range, no INR within 8 weeks, or if warfarin was still on the active medication list AFTER the stop date had occurred.

Here is an example of what the prompt looks like (Fig. 4.8).

How This Innovation Was Spread

MedStar Health used a combination of messaging within the EHR, email, and bulletins to office managers to discuss this new approach with their providers. Additionally, they used their EHR implementation team to revisit practices to inform providers of this enhancement, and show them how to use it. Even then, they were not sure how widely it was being used until they conducted an analysis of quality improvement on four metrics described below for a subgroup of their primary care providers.

Fig. 4.9 Correlation between
use of protocols and quality
scores

Quality Score	4	3	2	1	0
Heavy – Consistent Use of Protocols	71%	29%	0%	0%	0%
Moderate Use of Protocols	57%	14%	29%	0%	0%
Occasional Use of Protocols	14%	14%	29%	43%	0%
Zero – Rare Use of Protocols	6%	9%	15%	15%	55%

Results

In August of 2010, approximately 4 months after releasing the prompts into the EHR, analysis was performed on quality improvement for 53 of MedStar's primary care providers. Performance on the following four metrics was analyzed: breast cancer screening, colorectal cancer screening, smoking status and counseling for current smokers, and pneumococcal vaccination for patients 65+. While some improvement was found in all four metrics, the results were not what were expected considering the ease of metric improvement that the prompt strategy enabled. As mentioned above, these prompts were built such that it was easy to track when they were used (or ignored). MedStar then looked at how consistently these prompts were being used, and found that they were only being used consistently by about one-third of these 53 providers. MedStar then looked at the quality data in comparison to use of the protocols application and found a striking correlation between consistent use of the protocols and scoring highly on these four metrics. To interpret the table below, a quality score of one point was assigned for each of the four metrics where the provider scored above the mean, and a score of zero for a result below the mean (Fig. 4.9). Note that while this study did not establish causality, it does show a high correlation between consistent use of the protocols and high quality scores. This finding has led the MedStar EHR team to adopt a much more aggressive educational campaign surrounding use of this protocol strategy. This approach calls for in-person visits to providers with lower quality scores and low use of the protocols tool, and showing them how to use the "View all Protocols" feature, and how using it consistently could rapidly and dramatically improve their scores on selected quality measures.

This innovation was also used with a point-of-care diabetes dashboard to attempt rapid-cycle improvement in diabetes quality measures with this same group of primary care providers. While the MedStar Health Ambulatory Quality Best Practice Group endorses best practice guidelines for outpatient diabetes care, it believed that to draw attention and clarity to quality improvement, it would use a nationally accepted subset of best practices – the NCQA Diabetes Recognition Program (DRP). The current metrics of the DRP are as follows:

- HgbA1C Control >9.0 % (Goal 15 % or Less)
- HgbA1C Control <8.0 % (Goal is 60 % or More)

Fig. 4.10 Diabetes
management alert

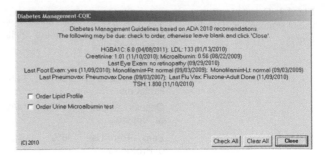

- HgbA1C Control <7.0 % (Goal 40 % or More)
- Blood Pressure Control >140/90 mmHg (Goal 35 % or Less)
- Blood Pressure Control <130/80 mmHg (Goal 25 % or More)
- Eye Examination (Goal 60 % or More)
- Smoking Status and Cessation Advice or Treatment (Goal 80 % or More)
- LDL Control ≥130 mg/dl (Goal 37 % or Less)
- LDL Control <100 mg/dl (Goal 36 % or More)
- Nephropathy Assessment (Goal 80 % or More)
- Foot Examination (Goal 80 % or More)

Essentially, it would use the EHR to gather DRP metric performance, and then submit this data electronically to the NCQA to seek DRP status for each of these primary care doctors.

As shown below, the "View all Protocols" approach also provides metric status and one-click ordering for diabetes tests and services. However, this view of diabetes information does not provide a clear view of DRP metric status for the provider, and does not provide a meaningful view of that same information for patients (Fig. 4.10). MedStar additionally elected to have a diabetes dashboard constructed to fill in those metric display needs. The diabetes dashboard automatically opens in every diabetic patient's visit note (regardless of reason for visit) for MedStar's primary care doctors.

Here is an example of the point-of-care diabetes dashboard currently in use at MedStar Health. Note that in addition to the NCQA DRP measures, the dashboard also contains other measures of diabetes quality (Fig. 4.11). Note also that clicking on a "?" provides a view of the last four numeric values, as well as the numeric mean (Fig. 4.12).

In 2008, while this entire group of primary care doctors had been fully implemented with the EHR, none of them had earned NCQA DRP status. Within 1 year of implementing the "View all Protocols" approach to care opportunities along with the Diabetes Dashboard for a meaningful view of diabetes quality metrics, 79 % of these doctors now meet or exceed the requirements for DRP status.

Identifying and Using Positive Deviance

The rapid cycle improvement in diabetes metrics such that MedStar Health went from 0 % of its largest primary care group reaching NCQA DRP status to 79 %,

Fig. 4.11 Diabetes dashboard

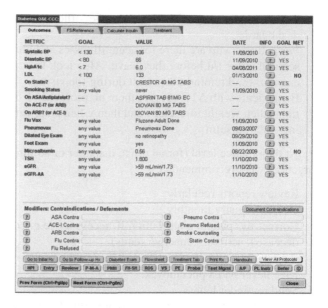

Fig. 4.12 A1C values over time

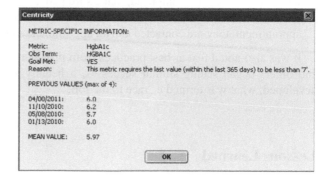

was not just a story of software development and implementation; it was also a story of provider and practice workflow improvement. However, while quality improvement programs typically seek early identification of and intervention with providers who are performing below designated thresholds and then initiate targeted educational processes to bring them up to the evolving standard care of care, MedStar Health took a different approach. It sought early identification of top performers (identification of positive deviance), and via interview, determined what practice workflow changes were being used to allow for such rapid improvement in diabetes metrics. It then took those interviews and created brief summaries and widely dispersed them across the primary care group. These local best practices included the following for point-of-care workflow:

- Every patient every visit – Click on "View all Protocols" button and the Diabetes dashboard.
- Review items that are labeled as NO in the dashboard, and aggressively treat BP, LDL, and A1C when out of compliance.

- Try not to let any diabetic leave the office without at least looking at the dashboard.
- For patients who are there for acute illnesses and are overdue for labs, get them scheduled for f/u before they leave. Also look to see what's due soon (like eye exams) – and remind the patient during the visit.
- For patients with A1C >9, give them no more than 6 months of adjusting medications, diet, weight loss, etc. – and then when it appears that they are not responding – start insulin

At the practice level (for an office manager or administrator), the following best practices were recommended:

- Review reports regularly
- Review registry monthly
- Correct the patient's attribution if necessary (e.g. correct responsible provider, deceased, active vs. inactive status)
- Review "services due" report to see if patients are overdue for A1Cs, LDLs, or have never had a pneumovax.
- Send reminder letters
- Refill Medication for only enough until due for next visit (usually 3–4 months) – when ANY refills are completed, make sure patient has a follow-up appointment in reasonable amount of time BEFORE refilling. If they do not have a follow-up appointment, they are contacted and an appointment is scheduled.

It was also noted that as best practices from providers and practices were spread and others began seeing similar successes, a healthy spirit of competition often developed, what was termed a "race to the top."

Lessons Learned

Developing an approach that makes it easier for providers to deliver the right care at the right time does work. It requires one to determine and prioritize protocols that matter for the practice or enterprise. It further requires their commitment to operationalize a protocol into logic statements that make sense for the providers, and that can be written into software code. It also requires a protocol editor and delivery mechanism that provides for flexibility and tracking. And lastly, provider education and feedback is crucial – as this implementation once again disproved the adage "build it and they will come." Providers will not use something just because it is easy. They need to know it's there, how to use it, as well as the implications of using it consistently.

Frequent feedback and correction to both providers and to the software developers also helped to drive success. Frequent and regular feedback seemed to be the most helpful, particularly when a workflow was dramatically different than before (i.e., replacing the traditional chief complaint with a negotiated shared agenda).

Feedback was also necessary to improve the prompts. Having a mechanism for providers to give feedback and then see that feedback inserted into the next version of the software was also viewed positively and added to providers' acceptance of the CDS prompt strategy.

Positioning the prompts as the source of definitive truth about a patient was never seen as a viable approach. In fact, even the perception by providers as "telling them what to do" led to negative comments and lowered use. However, framing the prompts in terms such as: "Pneumovax May be Due," and providing information within the prompt as to authorship and statements (where appropriate) as to prompts not being designed to override sound clinical judgment, added to positive perceptions and improved usage.

Delivering prompts selectively (by role and/or by specialty) makes clinical sense; although it is acknowledged that it is but one approach to improving adherence to recommended practices across a multispecialty system. Clinicians and leadership at MedStar Health viewed this approach favorably, as it respected accepted practice standards (e.g., dermatologists should not see prompts for colon cancer screening).

All lessons learned were not positive. Several specialties rejected prompts that were offered to them, either because they didn't seem to fit their workflow, or the advice or selection of choices was not granular enough to suit their needs.

Future Plans

MedStar Health is now leveraging the opportunity of Stage 1 of Meaningful Use to develop and promulgate one or more CDS prompts per specialty, and one or more prompts across all specialties. While the technologic approach and infrastructure is the same, the process of design and delivery are very different. And while Stage 1 of Meaningful Use only requires providers to attest that there is a CDS rule in place, it is fully expected that stages 2 and 3 will appropriately ask how these rules are used, and do they result in improved care. This will require even greater attention to CDS build, and build follow-up. Are prompts being used consistently? If not, why not? Too much alerting? Alerting when the ability to take appropriate action is impossible? Is there too little or too much information placed within a prompt?

Conclusion

MedStar Health is confident that carefully designed and delivered actionable prompts and alerts lead to significant improvement in quality metrics. It has shown what was already suspected – unobtrusive prompts without hard stops require that the provider know what the process is to use them, and then consistently use them in their everyday delivery of care. If the prompts are not consistently used – one should not expect to see significant improvement in quality metrics. As more practices and specialties begin to use this approach to address their own quality and/or safety priorities, MedStar trusts that this approach will be generalizable across these other environments.

Building a workflow-informed health IT system resonates with doctors and patients. Patients report feeling that they are well cared for and that they trust that their doctor is paying attention to their care needs. Physicians and other providers report that they also believe that they have more information available and the opportunity to readily respond to all relevant care.

How much time it takes to do the "right thing" for all of one's patients is still an open question in primary care medicine. In 2003, Yarnell et al. attempted to determine exactly how much time it would take for primary care doctors to carry out all recommended preventive care services on all patients [1]. Based on an average panel size of 2,500, it was determined that it would take 7.4 h per day.

In 2005, Ostby et al. did a similar analysis for the provision of necessary chronic care services [2]. Their conclusions: primary care doctors spent an average of 4.6 h per day on acute problems and their follow-up; and the provision of all necessary chronic care opportunities for the ten top chronic conditions would add an additional 3.5–10 h per day (this figure does NOT include the time it takes to determine what those services are, and assumes that another staff member would have to do so via chart preparation). The combined conclusions of both of these reports – doing the right thing for all patients requires primary care doctors to increase their average workday from 10 to 17 h – suggests something that is just not possible. However, our work suggests that similar benefits may be achieved with far less time extended. Based on interviews with consistent users of the "View all Protocols" feature, there was general agreement that it took an extra few minutes per patient to address all care opportunities, with the average workday extended about 45–60 min, not 7 h. This does not take into account further efficiencies that could be achieved via optimization of patient engagement, self-management, and non-visit based care.

The implications for health IT and EHR research are obvious. Looking at the work done here, one could conclude that using the EHR adds time to every visit and thus decreases provider efficiency. However, if one looks at the time providers could have spent to achieve an outcome of the right care to all patients seen on a consistent basis, and what the cost of that would be using paper records vs. the cost and upkeep of the IT systems along with the few extra minutes of provider time each visit, one would conclude exactly the opposite. Using an advanced EHR to produce consistently high quality is much less expensive and much more efficient than trying to achieve the same results with paper records. The implications for payment reform are obvious.

Most healthcare providers want to provide the very best care to their patients at all times. However, the fact that these efforts are not consistently and measurably visible is not because of ignorance or a lack of caring. They are due to factors of time, administrative and documentation distractions and burden; working within a misaligned payment system, and not having timely access to pertinent and actionable information. While our work cannot fix all that is broken within our healthcare system, it has at least made it easier to do the right thing.

Acknowledgements I would like to thank the MedStar Health Ambulatory Quality Best Practice Group and the leadership of MedStar Health for its support and encouragement of this work; with a special thanks to the EVP for Medical Affairs and CMO, William L. Thomas, MD. and the MedStar Health EMR team for its technical support and patience with version changes. Particular thanks are due to Edward Miller, MD, the President and Medical Director of MedStar Physician Partners and the Co-Chair of the Ambulatory Quality Best Practice Group; and to my "co-conspirator" in any and all projects involving quality improvement using the EHR, Diane Hollingsworth, RNC, MAOM, CPHQ, Director of Quality Management and Education for MedStar Physician Partners. I would also like to thank John Janas, MD, the cofounder and president of Clinical Content Consultants, who regularly created a v1.0 of the prompts to my specs, and then graciously allowed me to suggest enhancements, that usually returned the prompts back to what he originally wanted to build.

References

1. Yarnel K, et al. Primary care: is there enough time for prevention? Am J Public Health. 2003;93:635–41.
2. Ostby T, et al. Is there time for management of patients with chronic diseases in primary care? Ann Fam Med. 2005;3:209–14. doi:10.1370/afm.310.

Chapter 5
Prevention Every Time

James L. Holly

"Nurses can do that now?" a skeptical, but pleased Juanita Hernandez asked. Juanita is a retired seamstress. Back in the day, nothing seemed to happen unless directly ordered by the doctor. She thought back to when her sister, Marta, was a nurse. Marta always felt she could do more, help more, and relieve some of the burden for the patients and doctor, but that was not to be. Marta especially loved prevention. She always said that with every immunization, with every foot exam, with every diet consult that she was making the world a better place, at least for one person. "So how do you know what I need? I haven't even seen Dr. Bob yet."

Nurse Linda smiled, "We've been working hard to figure out an easier way for our patients to keep up with their prevention needs. A lot like getting your car serviced, we know what you need and when you need it. Of course, having the electronic medical record allows me to rapidly know all this." Incredible that it's taken all these years to be able to provide these proactive services, and we're ahead of the curve, Linda thinks shaking her head slightly. "Juanita, I see that you need your pneumonia vaccine and mobility assessment. How about we take care of them right now?"

Background

Southeast Texas Medical Associates (SETMA) was formed in August, 1995 by four physicians who had been in practice in Beaumont, Texas for more than 20 years. It is now a multi-specialty group of 24 physicians and 13 nurse practitioners spanning

J.L. Holly, M.D.
SETMA, LLP, Beaumont, TX, USA

Department of Family and Community Medicine,
School of Medicine, UT Health Science Center, San Antonio, TX, USA
e-mail: jholly@setma.com

L. Berkowitz, C. McCarthy (eds.),
Innovation with Information Technologies in Healthcare, Health Informatics,
DOI 10.1007/978-1-4471-4327-7_5, © Springer-Verlag London 2013

four offices and seeing 87,000 outpatient visits a year. In 1999 SETMA started using the electronic medical record (EMR) system from NextGen. Since that time, SETMA has become a leader in the innovative use of information technology and EMRs for the improvement of healthcare outcomes. SETMA has received numerous awards including the HIMSS Davis Award and the HIMSS Stories of Success designation. As a multi-specialty group SETMA is recognized as an NCQA Patient-Centered Medical Home and is accredited as an AAAHC Medical Home. In 2010, SETMA became the first multi-specialty group to be designated an affiliate of the Joslin Diabetes Center Affiliated with Harvard Medical School. SETMA's model of care has been reviewed by numerous national organizations and SETMA has been designated by the Office of National Coordinator of Health Information Technology as 1 of 30 exemplary practices in the USA for clinic decision support. The Agency for Healthcare Research and Quality lists the SETMA-LESS Initiative on their Innovation Exchange. SETMA is the first healthcare organization to be a semi-finalist for the Gartner Award for the use of business intelligence analytics in healthcare.

The Innovation

SETMA has created a series of innovative tools using their EMR system to maximize the preventive and disease management care they deliver in the most time-efficient and cost-effective manner possible. The three main innovative tools SETMA created were:

- **A Pre-Visit Preventive Screening Tool**, which allows providers to quickly assess the preventive and screening health care needs of an individual patient (See Fig. 5.1). This is the starting place for every patient encounter at SETMA. This tool allows the nurse to independently assess the preventive health and screening health needs of each patient evaluated. Once the nurse completes the intake of a patient, the provider briefly reviews this tool to make sure that all screening and chronic health preventive tests are performed or ordered. Because this is done at every visit for every patient no matter why they are being seen, SETMA's performance on all of these metrics is outstanding and consequently the patient's healthcare quality is enhanced.
- **An Instant Quality Measures Tool**, which provides a snapshot of an individual patient's disease management metrics at the time of their visit. SETMA tracks 200 metrics in a variety of tools from these three organizations:

  - The National Quality Forum (NQF): General Health Measures, Care for Older Adults, Comprehensive CHF Care, Diabetes, Female Measures, Medication Measures and Pediatric Measures. See Fig. 5.2 for an example.
  - The Physician Consortium for Performance Improvement (PCPI): Diabetes, Care Transitions, Hypertension, Chronic Kidney Disease, and Lower Urinary Track Symptoms. See Fig. 5.3 for an example.

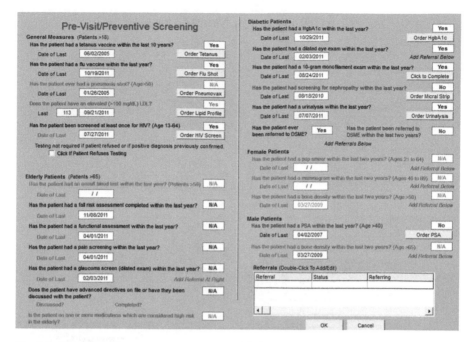

Fig. 5.1 The pre visit/preventive screening tool

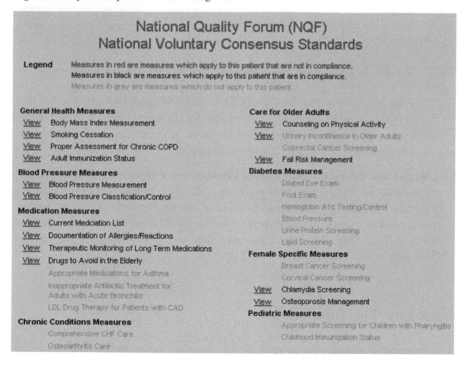

Fig. 5.2 National quality forum national voluntary consensus standards

PCPI Diabetes Management

Has the patient had a Hemoglobin A1c within the last year?	Yes	Order HgbA1c
Date of Last 10/29/2011		
Has the patient had a Lipid Profile witin the last year?	Yes	Order Lipid Profile
Date of Last 09/21/2011		
Has the patient had a urinalysis within the last year?	Yes	Order Urinalysis
Date of Last 07/07/2011		
Has the patient had a dilated eye exam within the last year?	Yes	*Add Referral Below*
Date of Last 02/03/2011		
Has the patient had a flu shot within the last year?	Yes	Order Flu Shot
Date of Last 10/19/2011		
Has the patient had a 10-gram monofilament exam within the last year?	Yes	Click to Complete
Date of Last 08/24/2011		
Is the patient on Aspirin?	No	*Add Medication Below*
Is the patient allergic to aspirin? ⦿ Yes ◯ No		
Is the patient's blood pressure controlled (<130/80 mmHg)?	Yes	
Today's Blood Pressure 60 / 60		
Does the patient have at least one visit schedule for the next six months?		Follow-Up Visit
Has the Diabetes Treatment Plan been completed with the last year?	Yes	Click to Complete
Date Last Completed 11/08/2011		

Fig. 5.3 Example of a PCPI instant quality measures tool for diabetes

- The National Committee for Quality Assurance (NCQA): Diabetes Recognition Program, as well as HEDIS measures for Effectiveness of Acute Care, Effectiveness of Chronic Care, Comprehensive Diabetes Care, and Effectiveness of Preventive Care. See Fig. 5.4 for an example.

- **A Real-Time Provider Performance Feedback tool**, which allows both providers and executives to know how well any individual provider is doing on their preventive and disease management metrics across populations. These performance feedback tools are aggregated on the Medical Home Coordination Review in Fig. 5.5 and they also display on each disease management tool, such as the Diabetes Disease Management tool (Fig. 5.6).

Reason for This Innovation

In 1999 SETMA started using an electronic medical record (EMR) system. In the first year of use, one of the physicians noted, "This is too hard and too expensive, if all

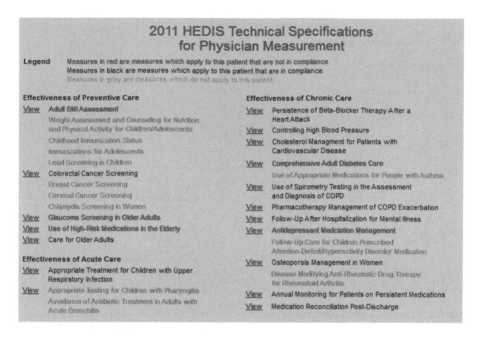

Fig. 5.4 Example of an NCQA instant quality measures tool

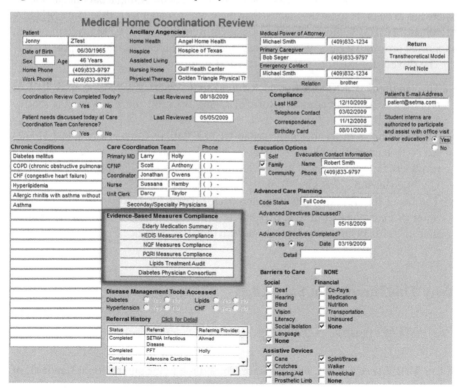

Fig. 5.5 Medical home coordination review template

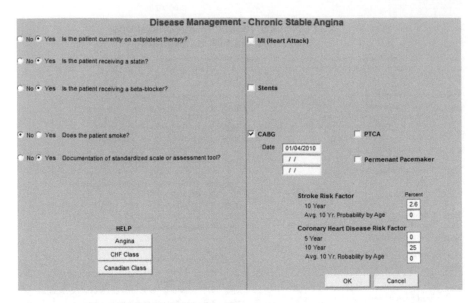

Fig. 5.6 Example of a real-time provider performance feedback tool for chronic stable angina

we're going to get out of it is an electronic means of documenting a patient encounter. There has to be more to EMR systems than there was to paper records". Thus, SETMA morphed their EMR into an "electronic patient management" (EPM) system, which supported preventive care, disease management and clinical decision support.

The drivers for this move towards an EPM were:

- The landmark RAND study which found that Americans receive only half of recommended medical care. (Ref. [1]). This inspired the Pre-Visit Preventive Screening Tool.
- The fact that in order to qualify as an NCQA Patient-Centered Medical Home, ten NQF-endorsed quality measures must be fulfilled and must be reported to the providers in the group and to an external organization. This inspired the Instant Quality Measures Tracking Tool.
- The belief that real-time auditing and performance feedback to providers at the point-of-care changes provider behavior and overcomes "treatment or clinical inertia." This inspired the Real-Time Provider Performance Feedback Tool.

Why This Innovation Succeeded

Pre-visit Preventive Screening Tool

Every Visit, Every Time. Using evidenced-based medicine and national standards of care, the pre-visit quality measures screening and preventive care tool was designed

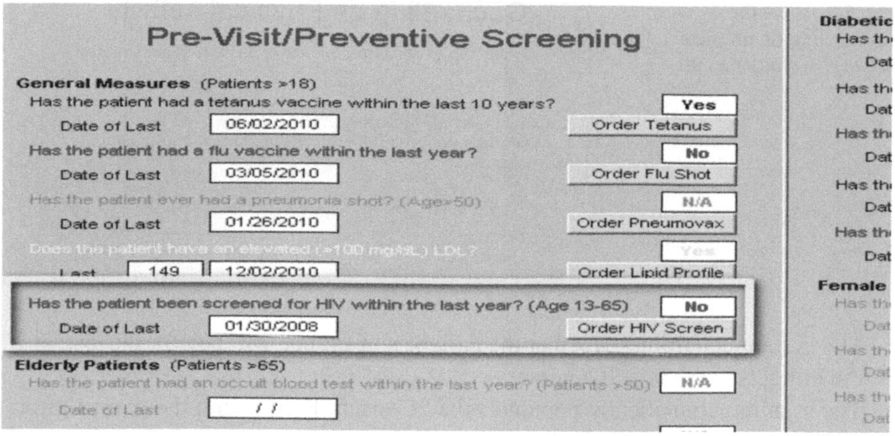

Fig. 5.7 Close-up of the pre-visit/preventive screening screen

to be used at every single visit. A key attribute of the design was the concept of "intentionality", which means that the provider and support staff "intentionally" address preventive and screening health needs at every visit. Consequently, the nurse and healthcare provider begin every patient visit at SETMA with the Pre-visit Preventive Screening template. While SEMTA's nurses are excellent in performing this screening, it is still the healthcare provider's responsibility to review this template and to make certain that all appropriate screening and preventive health standards have been met

Nurse Empowerment. Through training, the nurses are empowered to give any immunizations, order any tests or procedures and create any referrals which are needed in order for each patient to have their measures completed at each visit. Needs are quickly identified through color coding. It is not uncommon for a new patient to present with no prior screening or preventive care and for that patient to leave the first visit to SETMA with all their care having been completed or started.

Easy to Use. The tools were designed to be very easy for both reviewing and ordering. As seen in Fig. 5.1, all measures in black mean a measure is up to date, while all measures in red indicate the patient may be due. Grey measures do not apply to the current patient. If a measure is not up to date, it can be ordered or completed with a single click of a button.

To demonstrate how this works, it is helpful to review the example for HIV screening, which is advised for all patients between the ages of 13 and 64 (see Fig. 5.7).

In this case, the red "No" button highlights a problem - the patient has not had an HIV test documented at SETMA since 2008. A provider thus needs to either manually update the date of the last test if done outside the SETMA system, or click on the "Order HIV Screen" button and the following steps will then automatically happen:

• The HIV test is ordered and appropriate data is sent to the chart, billing and lab systems.

Fig. 5.8 View for
"counseling on physical
activity" for older adults

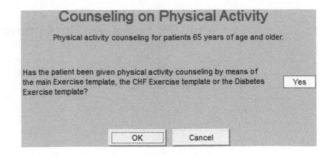

- The system determines whether the patient's insurance will pay for the test, or if the bill gets paid via a State grant.
- The system automatically populates the "Consent Form" with the patient information and then prints it for the patient to sign.

Shared Database. Because the same database is used for care of patients across the clinic, hospital, nursing home, emergency department, home health and provider's home, the documentation is immediately available at all points of contact. Thus, using this tool, a systemic solution can be easily infused throughout all SETMA clinics and placed into the providers' workflow with minimal effort.

Instant Quality Measures Tracking Tool

Automated Tracking. While preventive care and screening care is done intentionally as a part of excellent care, all quality-measure tracking is done automatically behind the scenes as part of the care that is being delivered. The philosophy is that the goal of care is health for all patients, not simply the fulfillment of quality measures. In other words, the quality measures are only a guidepost toward the final goal. So when the provider completes their evaluation of the patient, any of the "Quality Measures Tracking Tool" can be easily accessed so the physician can act upon them if they wish.

Easy to Use. Similar to the preventive care tool, the tracking tools are color coded for easy review (See Fig. 5.2). The color black indicates a metric is up to date, red indicates it is incomplete, and grey means "does not apply". If the provider wishes to see details, they click on the "View" button to see the details of the quality metric and what data is needed to fulfill it. For example, a provider can expand the view for "Counseling on Physical Activity" for Older Adults (See Fig. 5.8).

Easy to Access. Many of the tools described can be accessed by providers when they use the Medical Home Coordination Review Tool (see Fig. 5.5). For instance, by clicking on the *HEDIS Measures Compliance* button the provider can, at the point of care, evaluate whether all applicable HEDIS quality metrics have been fulfilled. HEDIS assesses three categories of quality metrics: effectiveness of preventive care; effectiveness of acute care; and effectiveness of chronic care. SETMA often sees new patients who have no HEDIS measures fulfilled and after their initial visit, all of the measures are completed. And, rather than receiving a report from an insurance company's HEDIS audit 12–18 months after the care is given, the provider is alerted to any deficiencies immediately.

Performance Reviews. These quality metrics give SETMA providers an opportunity to compare themselves with national standards of care and allows SETMA to audit provider performance. Performance review is done monthly in half-day training and peer-review sessions with all SETMA providers present. Because SETMA publicly reports provider performance by provider name on our website, all providers are highly motivated to improve their performance. If a provider's performance is substandard, SETMA provides training and instruction, which has proven quite successful.

Real-Time Provider Performance Feedback Tool

Use of BI Technology. This tool adapted business intelligence (BI) software to provide real-time auditing and performance feedback to providers, staff and executives. Using digital dashboard technology, the tool allows SETMA the ability to analyze provider and practice performance to find patterns which can result in improved outcomes for an entire population of patients. Data can be analyzed by patient population, provider panel, practice panel, financial class, payors and even by season. Patients can be compared as to socio-economic characteristics, ethnicity, frequency of evaluation by visit and by laboratory analysis, numbers of medications, payer class, cultural, financial and other barriers to care, gender, and other variables. It is even possible to look at differences between the care of patients who are treated to goal and those who are not.

Training. Each provider is trained how to use this tool to evaluate and compare his or her own performance at the point of care. Additionally, these tools are discussed with the support staff as they share responsibility for successfully meeting all standards of care.

Stimulating Quality Improvements. SETMA uses the data from the feedback tool to better understand how it can modify care in order to get all patients to goal. For example, in an analysis of the period January 1, 2009 to December 31, 2009, trending data showed that beginning in late October many patients with diabetes began to have worsening of their glucose control. Additional analysis showed that not only did the holiday season (Halloween Thanksgiving and Christmas) correlate with an upward trend of HbA1c but the patients who were losing control had fewer visits and less testing during that period.

Once SETMA understood this data, a quality improvement plan was implemented in which all patients with diabetes were contacted by mail and telephone in the Fall of 2011. A "contract" was established with each patient for dietary control, activity, clinic visit and testing. The results were positive as patients maintained their glucose control in October, November and December 2010 (Fig. 5.9). This improved process will be repeated annually.

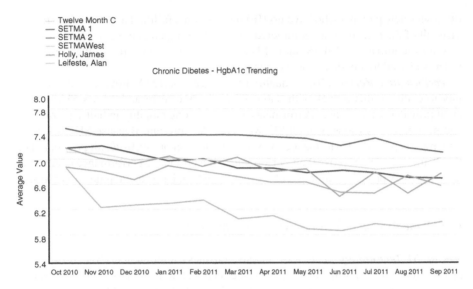

Fig. 5.9 HgbA1C trending for diabetics over time

In another example, the BI system identified some interesting data about patients with poorly controlled diabetes, which is indicated by a HbA1C value over 8 %. In an audit of HbA1C values, it was found that these poorly controlled patients were getting tested as often as the well-controlled patients and seeing their physicians almost as often. Thus, it was determined that simply increasing their testing or visit frequency would likely not have a big impact. So instead of focusing time and attention on those factors, SETMA was able to adjust their treatment regimen as well as focus on exercise and dietary-discretion support. In addition, attention was focused on getting patients into diabetes education classes and getting patients to keep a better log of their blood sugar readings.

The Power of Data Transparency. Periodically, executive staff will distribute special audits to the providers to be reviewed during peer review sessions and during quality improvement sessions. The organizational philosophy is that transparency of data is meant to empower, not embarrass. Transparency and public reporting by provider name have been paramount to the success of these innovations. The value of transparency in provider performance is that "once you open the door to provider-performance transparency, the only place to hide is excellence." When providers know that their performance is going to be quantified and then displayed, they pay more attention to the details which result in improved outcomes. When they know that public reporting is not going to be used punitively but educationally, they accept it and benefit from it. This is particularly true when systems approaches to healthcare delivery make it easy for them to know what the standards of care are and make it easy to comply with those standards. Without public reporting, the incentive for change diminishes.

Results

The result of these innovations has been to improve the quality of care delivered at SETMA, as measured by increased immunization rates, improved patient and provider satisfaction, increase in Quality Measure Score, and variety of other outcomes. Some specific examples of benefits include the following:

Improved Immunizations. Via prompting by the pre-visit prevention tool, SETMA has significantly improved vaccine compliance. Flu immunization rates increased from below 50 % up to 89 %. Pneumcococcal immunization rates which were below 20 % are now above 90 %. And Tetanus/Diptheria/Acellular Pertussis (TDAP) immunizations increased from below 30–95 % of all eligible patients. But more important is that these increased immunizations rates appear to have decreased the rates of disease. For example, while the incidence of Pertussis ("whooping cough") in Texas increased from 4.1 per 100,000 in 2005 to 13.4 per 100,000 in 2009, the county in which SETMA works had an increase of only 0.4 per 100,000 – very possibly due related to this high rate of TDAP immunization.

Improved Lab and Preventive Care Screening. After the first year of deploying the Previsit/preventive screening tool, the following metrics improved:

- HgbA1c testing compliance for diabetic patients increased from 88.5 to 91.9 %.
- LDL screening for diabetic patients increased from 84.3 to 90.0 %.
- For elderly patients, the screening for fall risk increased from 63.5 to 98.9 %.
- Screening for urinary incontinent in elderly patients increased from 32.8 to 94.7 %.

Improved Diabetes Outcomes. Four initiatives have resulted in improved outcomes for the SETMA's diabetic patients: (1) The deployment of the diabetes disease management tool in 2000, (2) The deployment of an American Diabetes Association recognized diabetes self-management education program in 2004, (3) The recruitment of an Endocrinologist in 2006 and (4) The public reporting by provider name of diabetes quality metrics 2008.

These four initiates have resulted in SETMA's mean HbA1C's decreasing from 7.5 % in 2000 to 6.5 % in 2011 and the standard deviation in the same period going from 2.0 to 1.2. Going forward, SETMA's strategy is to leverage these four initiatives to maintain the mean HbA1C results and to continue to improve the HbA1C standard deviation.

Superior Medical Home Results. In January, 2011, CMS contracted with RTI International to examine 312 Patient-Centered Medical Home practices and to contrast their Fee-for-Service results with 312 Benchmark practices with non-coordinated care. SETMA's results showed a total, annual cost per beneficiary which was 37.5 % less than the benchmarks (SETMA $8,134 versus Benchmark $12,919). The same study showed that SETMA had a rate of hospitalization of 24.5 per 100 beneficiaries while the benchmark was 47.4. The study also measured Potentially Avoidable Inpatient Hospital Payments, and found that the SETMA metric of $962 was significantly lower than the Benchmark metric of $2,259. (*Medical Home Feedback*

Report, October, 2011, SETMA II, 3,570 College, Beaumont, Texas, Prepared by RTI International 701 13th Street, NW, Suite 750 Washington, DC 20005–3967 CMS Contract No. 500-2005-00029I RTI Project Number 0209853.016).

Return on Investment. SETMA's innovations have resulted in a return on investment in both administrative and clinic ways. For an example of administrative savings, when SETMA began using an EMR in 1999, it was spending $16,000 a month on transcription services. SETMA management estimated that due to its size and multiple clinics, that amount would now be well over $40,000 a month. In other words, over the past 3 years, it would have spent $6,240,000 on transcription services, not accounting for space requirements for transcriptionists and record storage, paper costs, record retrieval and transportation, etc. Additionally, preparing reports such as PQRI measurements or the NCQA Diabetes Recognition would take weeks of work with paper records, rather than the few seconds it takes with electronic auditing.

From a clinical perspective, SETMA recognizes that the inefficiency of paper records would have made it impossible for SETMA providers to know how they were doing with their care management. But with automation of the medical record, SETMA has found that it can improve efficiency by making it easier for physicians and staff to do the right thing, such as alerting them to deficiencies in care at a point and place where the deficiency can be corrected. Additionally, SETMA has participated in the ePrescribing and in Physician Quality Reporting System, receiving the maximum reimbursement per provider for each program. On top of that, Blue Cross and Blue Shield currently rewards SETMA providers with an extra $500 per year per provider for the improved care of their patients with diabetes.

The result of these all these savings and extra reimbursement is that SETMA has been able to control expenses of health care as an aggregate and to decrease the cost of the delivery of care, thus increasing revenue while decreasing the unit cost of care. With the profits being largely returned to patient care, SETMA has remained debt free even while spending over $6,000,000 on HIT (for licenses, development, servers, computers, networking, etc.), contributing $1,500,000 to the SETMA Foundation for the care of patients who cannot afford it and spending $500,000 to adapt Business Intelligence software to healthcare.

Lessons Learned

The following principles have guided SETMA's EMR development and HIT Innovations:

- Pursue Electronic Patient Management rather than Electronic Medical Records – the electronic documentation of a patient encounter is not sufficiently valuable to justify the time, money and effort investment in EMR systems. Leveraging the computation, aggregation and integration of data power of electronics makes it worth the effort and cost.

- Bring to bear upon every encounter "what is known" rather than simply "what an individual provider knows." Display the appropriate data, use clinical decision support tools, implement process improvement and audit compliance to improve provider behavior in ways that can never be accomplished by education alone.
- Make it easier to do it right than not to do it at all – the power of this system creates efficiency and excellence in the practice of medicine. In fact, with well designed and deployed HIT, the more efficient the system, the more excellent the care.
- Transparency for Providers and Patients: Automatic summarizing of the patient's care as measured against evidenced-based criteria, including a summary of the provider's performance on quality metrics in the patient's plan of care and treatment plan creates a transparency for both the provider and patient. Encouraging the patient through the plan of care and treatment plan to ask for the care which the summary indicates that they need but have not received, allows the patient-centric care to be driven by the patient's request for evidence-based care.
- Continually challenge providers to improve their performance – Continuous quality improvement is a dynamic process as well as a goal and outcome. Innovative use of HIT allows providers to reach for excellence and to demonstrate where and when they achieve it.
- Promote continuity of care with patient education, information and plans of care – Continuity of care is most often identified with seeing the same provider most of the time.
- Enlist patients as partners and collaborators in their own health improvement – SETMA long ago abandoned the role of constable attempting to impose care upon an unwilling and unwitting patient. Instead, SETMA becomes a patient's collaborator, colleague and consultant, facilitating the patient's pursuit of the health they personally determined to have.
- Evaluate the care of patients and populations of patients longitudinally – without the ability to track, audit and analyze the care of populations of patients over time, quality improvement initiatives will be unfocused and often unsuccessful. The design of an EMR to facilitate these functions virtually guarantees the design, deployment and successful fulfillment of CQI.
- Audit provider performance based on the multiple quality performance sets – provider performance measurement is never punitive but always motivational. If you don't know where you are and how you are doing, it is impossible to know where you want to be and it is impossible to design ways in which to get there.
- Create disease-management tools integrated in an intuitive and interchangeable fashion, giving patients the benefit of expert knowledge while they benefit from a global approach to their health – pathways and guidelines are great tools for multi-specialty practice where there are varying degrees of expertise. EMRs with clinical decision and clinical process support embedded into disease management tools is a great lever of skill sets.

Future Plans

Innovation will be driven by problems that need solving. SETMA will continue to design solutions to new problems as they present themselves. Knowing that the demands upon healthcare providers will only increase and knowing that the time available to providers will not, SETMA will continue to innovatively use informatics to allow providers to perform more with less, and to do so in a professional and personally satisfying way.

Conclusion

Using a systems approach to create a logical and sequential process, SETMA has shown it is possible and rewarding for a provider to improve care for their patients in a real world manner. This process of tracking, auditing, analyzing, reporting and designing has set SETMA on a course for successful and excellent healthcare delivery that will provide cost-effective, excellent care with high patient satisfaction for years to come.

Reference

1. McGlynn EA, Asch SM, Adams J, et al. The quality of health care delivered to adults in the united states. N Engl J Med. 2003;348(26):2635–45.

Chapter 6
Logic Rules!

John W. Trudel and Lloyd D. Fisher

Ray Martinez is a busy man. His plumbing business is booming; so much so that he doesn't have much time to think about his diabetes. It really has always been a pain to get his checkups, so he is resigned to the fact that it is what it is. But he also doesn't mind complaining once in a while, "I hate getting my checkups. My doctor never seems to have the info he wants, he is always so rushed, and I end up having to go back or we try to catch each other on the phone."

However, when he calls up his clinic this time, he hears something he likes! "Mr. Martinez, I completely understand your frustration about our past workflows", says Michelle, the call center agent who answered his call. "It used to be such a pain...for you, me and for Dr. Smith. But we recently introduced some new functionality in our electronic medical record that helps solve your problem. Basically, with a simple click, I can get all the right labs ordered prior to your physical. That way, when you see the doctor, he WILL have the information that both of you need for the visit". Ray smiled knowing his experience would finally be more efficient, and Michelle thought to herself "I love having our Easy Button"!

And so on the day of Ray's visit, Dr. Smith was able to review his lab results before entering the exam room. "Hmmm... his HbA1C test is going up – meaning his diabetes is getting worse," he whispers to himself, "It's good to know that at this

J.W. Trudel, M.D. (✉)
Department of Family Medicine, Fallon Clinic/Reliant Medical Group,
106 East Main St, Westboro, MA 01581, USA
e-mail: john.trudel@reliantmedicalgroup.org

L.D. Fisher, M.D.
Department of Pediatrics, Fallon Clinic/Reliant Medical Group,
191 May Street, Worcester, MA 01519, USA
e-mail: lloyd.fisher@reliantmedicalgroup.org

L. Berkowitz, C. McCarthy (eds.),
Innovation with Information Technologies in Healthcare, Health Informatics,
DOI 10.1007/978-1-4471-4327-7_6, © Springer-Verlag London 2013

visit we'll have some objective, current data to guide our face to face discussions. Having our Call Center order the labs ahead of time is definitely saving us both time and helping with the quality of care".

At the visit, Dr. Smith seems more relaxed to Ray. He spent more time than usual with him. When Ray asks the doctor about this he replies, "In addition to having your labs done ahead of time, my workday has gotten easier since we also started using some new documentation tools. My staff brings up my documentation templates ahead of time and fills out what they are able to do. The result is that nothing is missed, and I can spend more time caring for my patients and less time punching buttons!"

Background

The Fallon Clinic is a 375 provider not-for-profit multispecialty group practice located in Central Massachusetts with a primary focus of providing high quality care along with appropriate cost containment and utilization management. The Clinic consists of 23 sites in Worcester and the surrounding communities, and it is the largest physician managed practice in the region. It began in 1929 when four physicians from the Mayo Clinic moved to Worcester and founded the first group practice in the area. In order to differentiate itself from a health insurance company in the community with a similar name, Fallon is now in the process of changing its name to Reliant Medical Group.

In 2006, the Fallon Clinic began a 2-year-long process of implementing the Epic Electronic Health Record into all clinical, practice management, and financial operations. While not always smooth, the roll-out has been very successful and physician satisfaction with the system remains high. Recognizing the success of this EHR implementation, the Healthcare Information Management Systems Society (HIMSS) awarded the Fallon Clinic the prestigious Davies award in 2011. The Fallon Clinic is also proficient at Lean and Six Sigma processes to further improve the quality and care management of the group's patients and the community at large.

The Innovations

This chapter will review two related innovations that have significantly improved the patient, provider and staff experiences at Fallon clinic by utilizing the conditional logic functionality built into the Electronic Health Record (EHR) system. One innovation helps staff pre-order lab tests before a patient's Annual Exam visit, and the other makes it easier for medical assistants to choose the correct documentation templates at a patient's office visit.

Reason for the Innovations

Lab Ordering Efficiency and Accuracy

Laboratory testing is traditionally ordered during a patient's routine annual exam at their physician's office. However, this workflow results in the need for time-intensive follow up, either by an additional office visit, phone call, mail or electronic messaging. Therefore, there is potential for increased efficiency if these labs could be ordered ahead of the visit, which can be done in one of several ways: physician directed, staff directed, or single standard. Unfortunately, each of these workflows has shortcomings in terms of efficiency and/or accuracy, and none of them truly leverage the power of an EHR system. Having the physician review the chart ahead of time requires significant non-reimbursable time and effort, and key information is often missed. Having a staff member ordering tests takes less physician time but extensive staff time, and there are risks of significant errors even when detailed paper-based algorithms are used. Finally, simply ordering the same thing for every patient is more efficient, but often results in unneeded lab work, false positives, excessive follow up testing and added cost.

At Fallon Clinic, the pre-visit lab order approach taken was the "staff directed" workflow, a complicated process whereby the call center staff reviewed the EHR for age, sex, medications, past labs and past history and then, using a set of personalized physician guidelines and a scratch paper process, ordered the appropriate labs when the patient called to set up their appointment (Fig. 6.1).

In April of 2010, a Fallon Clinic EHR team presented this workflow at the Epic Physician User's Group meeting as it did leverage the EHR to provide some efficiencies compared to the standard model of requiring all labs to be ordered at the visit only. It seemed as though the presentation had gone well until some negative comments were overheard. They included comments such as, "I expected much more out of them" and "That was not very efficient".

This feedback was taken as a challenge by the physicians and IT staff to utilize the power of the EHR to find a better, more efficient method. They recognized that the information needed to decide what pre-physical labs to order in most cases is already present in the system. And they knew that computers are particularly good at reviewing large amounts of data and is more accurate than humans at finding obscure information. So they thought, *"Why couldn't this information be compiled and used to automatically determine what lab work is due ahead of time?*

Documentation Efficiency and Accuracy

In 2009, the Fallon Clinic began implementing the Lean Management System to improve the efficiency and quality of health care delivery and rebranded it as the

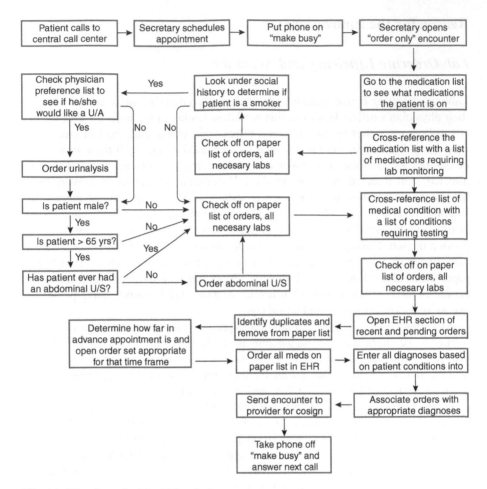

Fig. 6.1 Flowchart of original lab ordering process

Patient Care Improvement System (PCIS). The clinic had employed experts in the concepts of Six Sigma and Lean to improve all operations of the business in order to reduce waste, lower costs, and improve the patient experience. A Family Medicine site was used as the pilot site and significant resources were allocated to that site over a yearlong project to create a model for the rest of Fallon Clinic to follow.

An area the Lean team had hoped to improve was documentation efficiency and accuracy. The crux of their new process was to require medical assistants (MAs) to start a progress note template based on the chief complaint and fill in specified sections. Rather than the provider selecting a note from a list, the MA would select the note and complete the initial sections, thereby shifting some of the documentation work from the providers to the MAs.

This system worked well in pediatrics where most encounters were either acute, single complaint visits or well child checks. In adult medicine, the new process remained problematic for complex elderly patients with many different complaints. In addition, there were some physicians who wanted their own individualized templates, and others who did not want MA documentation or templates at all. The new method thus required the MAs to memorize close to 150 template names or have on hand a paper list for individual choices. This selection process required great accuracy or the MA would not choose the best option for the situation causing the provider to delete the note and begin again; a frustrating process for both MAs and providers.

Ultimately, it became obvious the "improvement" had inherent flaws that needed to be addressed before the process was disseminated throughout the company. The implementation of MA-initiated notes was quickly suspended and the EHR team was called in for assistance.

How These Innovations Succeeded

Improving the Lab Ordering Process

The physician and IT began experimenting with various tools available in their EHR and coming up with the logic required to create a rapid, comprehensive, accurate and efficient pre-physical lab ordering system. The key EHR functionality turned out to be a decision support tool called a best practice advisory (BPA) which could trigger individualized order sets. Specifically, the BPA tool is able to review a patient's data in the EHR database for the presence of items such as lab results, medications, diagnoses and the age or sex of the patient. Using these criteria, the system can automatically create an individualized order set which can be chosen by a user.

For the pre-visit lab system, the following four steps were required. First, a set of age, sex, and disease-related tests were decided upon by the physicians at a specific office. Second, the individual tests needed to be broken down further by the conditions with which they could be associated since all tests had to have an appropriate diagnosis and each disease needed to be stratified by importance. Third, extensive logic had to be created such that only one diagnosis showed for each test, each test was ordered only once, the diagnosis used was the most appropriate, the test was needed for that patient for that disease, the test wasn't already ordered and Medicare restrictions were respected. Finally, this all had to be packaged into an easy to use, reliable and efficient format such that secretaries could order these labs at the time of appointment booking without impeding their already busy workflows (Fig. 6.2). The solution devised was the "Pre-physical Lab Order Set" (Fig. 6.3).

Prototyping. Initially, a single test scenario was considered as a model to evaluate the viability of the process. The lipid test was chosen as it had several potential but well-defined and limited scenarios that would require testing. In addition,

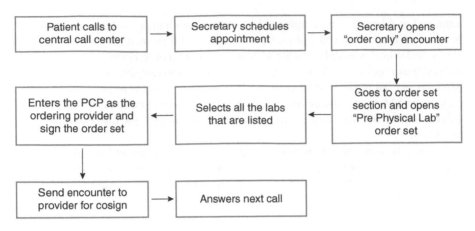

Fig. 6.2 Flowchart of new lab ordering process

guidelines were already well established at Fallon Clinic for when and why it should be ordered.

Although technically it was possible to customize by individual physician, it was decided that would be unwieldy and require excessive effort and maintenance. Fortunately, Fallon is organized into relatively small departments of 4–10 physicians and that was chosen as a reasonable level of customization.

Once this basic framework was decided upon (test, timing by age and condition, potential associated diagnoses), a test order set was created and the results evaluated. Test patients with different characteristics were chosen and the order set was validated and found to be acceptable and accurate on the small scale.

With this information in hand, the capabilities of the system were reviewed and any additional qualities that could be leveraged for ordering were considered. Indicators, such as the following, were all used to create filters that changed what orders would be presented to the secretary:

- Medication classes (antihyperlipidemics) or specific medications (Digoxin or Tegretol and all generic equivalents) on the active medication list
- The last available lab results (for example, if last LDL above 130, recheck lipids even if not due based on screening criteria),
- Demographics, including age, sex and the body mass index (BMI), which was based on the last available height and weight,
- Diagnoses on the problem list (e.g. hypertension, diabetes, vitamin D deficiency, hyperlipidemia, anemia),
- Existing unfulfilled orders

It was found that a given patient might have any 1 of 30 different orders written in various combinations.

The Pilot. Once the test scenario was found to be viable and the concept sound, a pilot site was identified for a trial run. The physician champion and builder of the order set chose his own office as the ideal site for several reasons. He would be there to monitor the process and correct any problems that arose, his colleagues were very

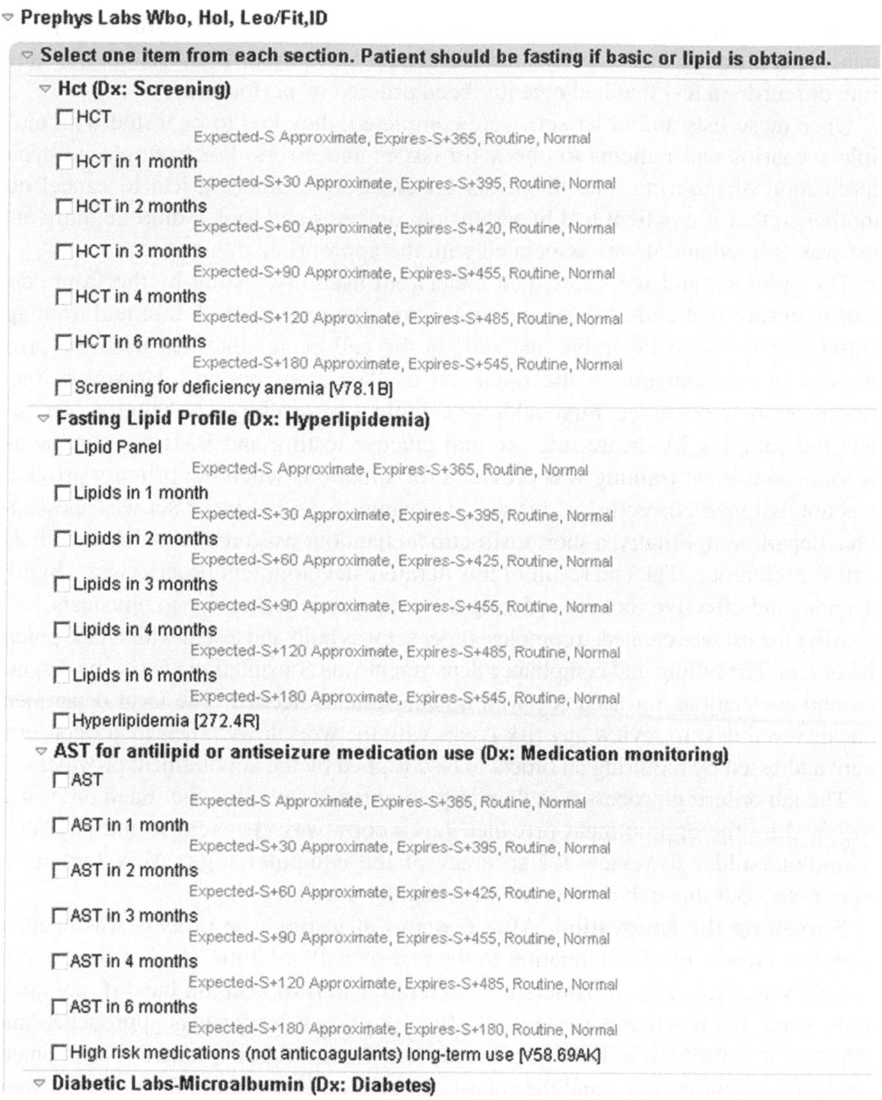

▽ **Prephys Labs Wbo, Hol, Leo/Fit,ID**

  ▽ Select one item from each section. Patient should be fasting if basic or lipid is obtained.

  ▽ **Hct (Dx: Screening)**
    ☐ HCT
              Expected-S Approximate, Expires-S+365, Routine, Normal
    ☐ HCT in 1 month
              Expected-S+30 Approximate, Expires-S+395, Routine, Normal
    ☐ HCT in 2 months
              Expected-S+60 Approximate, Expires-S+420, Routine, Normal
    ☐ HCT in 3 months
              Expected-S+90 Approximate, Expires-S+455, Routine, Normal
    ☐ HCT in 4 months
              Expected-S+120 Approximate, Expires-S+485, Routine, Normal
    ☐ HCT in 6 months
              Expected-S+180 Approximate, Expires-S+545, Routine, Normal
    ☐ Screening for deficiency anemia [V78.1B]

  ▽ **Fasting Lipid Profile (Dx: Hyperlipidemia)**
    ☐ Lipid Panel
              Expected-S Approximate, Expires-S+365, Routine, Normal
    ☐ Lipids in 1 month
              Expected-S+30 Approximate, Expires-S+395, Routine, Normal
    ☐ Lipids in 2 months
              Expected-S+60 Approximate, Expires-S+425, Routine, Normal
    ☐ Lipids in 3 months
              Expected-S+90 Approximate, Expires-S+455, Routine, Normal
    ☐ Lipids in 4 months
              Expected-S+120 Approximate, Expires-S+485, Routine, Normal
    ☐ Lipids in 6 months
              Expected-S+180 Approximate, Expires-S+545, Routine, Normal
    ☐ Hyperlipidemia [272.4R]

  ▽ **AST for antilipid or antiseizure medication use (Dx: Medication monitoring)**
    ☐ AST
              Expected-S Approximate, Expires-S+365, Routine, Normal
    ☐ AST in 1 month
              Expected-S+30 Approximate, Expires-S+395, Routine, Normal
    ☐ AST in 2 months
              Expected-S+60 Approximate, Expires-S+425, Routine, Normal
    ☐ AST in 3 months
              Expected-S+90 Approximate, Expires-S+455, Routine, Normal
    ☐ AST in 4 months
              Expected-S+120 Approximate, Expires-S+485, Routine, Normal
    ☐ AST in 6 months
              Expected-S+180 Approximate, Expires-S+180, Routine, Normal
    ☐ High risk medications (not anticoagulants) long-term use [V58.69AK]

  ▽ **Diabetic Labs-Microalbumin (Dx: Diabetes)**

Fig. 6.3 Screenshot of the pre-physical lab orders

cooperative, interested and in general open to change and innovation, and his support staff was well organized and well trained.

A meeting was held with all of the providers who worked at the pilot site. Starting with Fallon Clinic's recommended screening tests as a baseline they devised a reasonable list of tests by age, gender, medications and illnesses. The BPAs were created which then would make a particular order show or not show based on patient-specific information. In addition, since certain labs could be ordered based on different diagnoses, a hierarchy of importance had to be devised such that the most serious diagnosis would be chosen. For example, it would be more appropriate to order a glucose associated with the diagnosis of "diabetes" in a diabetic rather than "screening for diabetes". Worse still would be to order both tests at the same time or reorder a test that had recently been ordered or performed.

Once these lists and order sets were completed, they had to be tested with multiple scenarios and patients to check for issues and errors. For example, to avoid duplication of ordering, one diagnosis for electrolyte ordering had to cancel out another so that if a patient had hypertension, diabetes and took a diuretic, only one test was ordered and it was associated with the appropriate diagnosis.

The order set and workflow then underwent usability testing by the front desk staff to ensure that end users would understand the process with minimal training. Initial reviews were favorable and staff in the call center that had used the prior process began referring to the order set as "the easy button". However, three modifications were made. First, additional logic was developed to better accommodate the complex Medicare rules around glucose testing and BMI measurements. Second, additional training was provided for situations when the primary provider was not assigned correctly, as this was the trigger for what order set was shown to what department. Finally, a short instructional handout was created to leave with the staff for reference. The end result of this iterative development process was a highly efficient and effective tool for ordering the appropriate tests prior to physicals.

After the list was created, a complete order set was built and tested with all the potential orders. The billing and compliance department was consulted to review the diagnoses and associations for accuracy with no adjustments needed. The legal department was involved next to review any risk issues with the workflows. Their major concerns were addressed by requiring all orders to be cosigned by the appointment provider.

The lab ordering process was then implemented at the pilot site. Each order was cosigned by the appointment provider, but a copy was also sent to the physician champion/builder to review for accuracy of the computer logic. Very few errors were noted, but those that occurred were rapidly corrected.

Spreading the Innovation. After 6 weeks of testing, the process was deemed sound and ready for dissemination to the rest of Fallon Clinic. A short instruction manual was created for providers and secretarial staff to keep on hand if any questions arose. Each office manager and office physician leader was approached and engaged in a discussion. Finally, a live demonstration that explained the rationale, the development process, and the robust design elements behind the order set were given to each office so that providers could feel comfortable that the correct orders would be obtained. The site chiefs were then tasked with creating consensus within their own offices and submitting a list of requested testing. Once a list was submitted, a new order set was created and implemented in the office.

Improving the Documentation Process

As a reminder, the initial process of trying to create standard templates for all visits failed due to the inability to customize at both patient and physician levels.

Brainstorming. In order to rethink how to best leverage the EHR for more automated and personalized documentation options, a brainstorming session was held with all interested parties. This included PCIS management and implementation members, providers and MAs from the pilot site, providers and MAs from the office that recently implemented the process, training staff, IT personnel and the physicians responsible for creating much of the EHR documentation tools. A cross-section of both highly skilled IT users and some less skilled users were included to obtain all perspectives. Several clusters of differing opinions were identified, which grouped the providers into distinguishable subsets. One group wanted no templates at all, another wanted templates on physicals only, yet another wanted templates on physicals and acute visits but did not want MA's documenting any information. A final group wanted templates on all encounters and were comfortable with MA's starting documentation, but only for certain chief complaints.

A New EHR Tool. The Fallon Clinic EHR had a function called SmartLinks, which was used to automatically pull specific pieces of information into a note. This could range from a simple task, such as pulling in the patient's name or gender, to more complex tasks, such as bringing in all of the diagnoses and associated orders from a particular visit. However, it was not sufficient to address the customization issues being brought up by the brainstorming team.

Fortunately, around the time when the team was working through this process, a newer version of the SmartLink functionality was released. This new "conditional SmartLink" functionality allowed the EHR to used *if/then/else logic* to pull in different information based upon patient or situation-specific circumstances. The optimization team realized that with conditional links based on provider preferences, the correct template could automatically be presented to the MA within the documentation section of the chart. In other words, this new tool could pick *the right list for the right provider* and would require no memorization, no picking from lists, and no decision making by the MAs. The MA could even be notified whether, depending on the provider, they should complete any questions or not.

Since the conditional SmartLink used logic based on patient criteria, one could create rules based upon the age, sex, account type, coverage type or chief complaint of the patient. For example, one could say if the patient's sex is "female" with complaint of "abdominal pain", then show template X, but if "male" and "abdominal pain", show template Y. Rules could also be created based on the department, specialty, name or type of provider or on any combination of factors. And on top of all that, rules could be created based on actions performed at the visit (e.g. procedure completed, medications written) or prior visits (e.g. immunizations given, last physical date). In fact, virtually anything the computer knows about the patient now could be used to leverage how the documentation tools appear to the provider.

Prototype, Pilot and Spread. In the following week, a test scenario was created demonstrating the process. The concept was approved and a complete set of notes was created over the ensuing weeks. They were then released into the pilot site and subsequently became the model for PCIS documentation. Providers were given the option of choosing from the following options: Did they want their MAs to start templates for them or not; and did they want their MAs to do any documentation in these templates or not. Thus, providers were allowed to choose the personalized process that fits their style of practice best. And the MA's no longer require extensive training on how to choose or fill in templates, since they know they can now just complete whatever appears before them.

Results

Better Pre-physical Lab Ordering

Office Efficiency. The call center handles all initial phone calls for eight offices (six PCP and two Urgent Care) and performs various duties, including initial triage, scheduling, initiating prescription refills and generating letters and forms. In four of these offices they also order pre-physical labs. The prior pre-physical lab ordering process was a difficult, frustrating and cumbersome. The pre-physical order set is designed to be accurate and easy to use by secretaries as only the correct options are presented. The result is a process which saves a significant amount of time as the secretary does not need to look through the chart or review protocols for ordering. The new process has reduced the length of each physical scheduling contact by 80 % (5–1 min per call). Since physical scheduling and lab ordering constituting approximately 5 % of call contacts, this increase in efficiency has reduced the overall call center work equivalent by 0.5 FTE out of a total 10 FTEs.

Therefore, as the call center expands to cover more offices, they will not need to increase staffing as much as initially anticipated. If the call center were to cover the entire organization in the same manner, 2–3 FTE's could be saved as a result of this process. Perhaps the most telling response to this project was from the director of the call center:

> How helpful your "invention" is to the call center staff! It's not often someone says "let me help you with your most difficult task" – and then does! I really appreciate your partnership.

Quality. The process of defining pre-visit labs also impacts quality in a number of ways. First, by ensuring that all needed labs are ordered, the compliance with quality metrics such as pay-for-performance and HEDIS measures has improved. Preliminary data in the pilot site has shown an increase in anticonvulsant monitoring rates from 66 to 80 % and Chlamydia screening has improved from 88 to 92 %. The remainder of testing was already above 90 % compliance, so additional quality improvements are not anticipated.

Second, the system helps eliminates the ordering of tests which are not needed. One specific example was the ordering of urinalysis in smokers to screen for blood. Review of the literature by the Quality Management department found no guidelines recommending this test and no evidence it reduced the rate of bladder cancer morbidity or mortality and so it was not included in the order sets logic. On the other hand, the legal department found examples in the literature where medical liability was increased because this test was done as part of a screening panel, and a slight abnormality did not get a robust workup. In other words, if the patient ever developed cancer, the provider might be held liable for a missed diagnosis, even if not related in any way. Of note, several offices have requested this test be added to the screening list, but rescinded their requests after reviewing the lack of efficacy coupled with the increased legal risk involved.

Cost Savings. In addition to decreasing unnecessary tests, the system also decreases duplicate test ordering because it scans for recently completed tests done anywhere in the system. For example, a patient could be seen in other departments and have blood work drawn there, and then schedule a physical and have the same test repeated, even though the previous test was normal. Another common scenario is the young patient with normal cholesterol levels who has it redrawn every year despite little chance of a significant change. An informal review of orders suggests there is the potential for a 20 % reduction in testing rates with the appropriate protocols in place.

Patient Satisfaction. The office visit itself has become more useful and efficient for the patient when lab results are available at the time of their visit. Results of tests can be discussed, questions can be answered, and changes in therapy initiated at the time of the visit rather than waiting for results to be available and having to reach the patient by phone or other methods. A nurse talking about this workflow noted:

> I can honestly say the pre-physical order set has made an impact on patient satisfaction, as well as decreased some of our call volume. Prior to having the option to schedule labs prior to a physical, the labs were ordered at the time of the physical exam. If patients preferred to have their labs prior to the appointment, they would have to call our office and request their labs to be ordered. This would require a message to the PCP who would then decide which labs were needed. This resulted in 2–3 calls to and from the patient.

Physician Efficiency and Satisfaction. In addition to improving the patient's workflow, the physician's overall work time and effort is reduced and work satisfaction is improved. For example, for a typical internal medicine physician with 63 appointments during a week, 24 of those visits would previously have resulted in messages to the physician for lab ordering, then 24 nurse messages and finally 24 letters or phone calls to the patient. All of these were eliminated with the pre-physical order set. Not surprisingly, one physician commented on this efficiency gain:

> Before the pre-physical lab order set the process to have labs ordered was haphazard. It took up provider time and energy to review each request for lab orders. Often patients were told to wait till the appointment when the doctor would order what was needed which was not as satisfying for the patients or doctor who wanted to talk about the results during the appointment. Also the process of standardizing the orders forced the providers to think about their ordering habits. Overall, it has been a great step forward for us.

Another physician pointed out the benefits of having a system checking for accuracy:

> This is so much less frustrating for me. With the old process, I was constantly finding mistakes and had to open each order and check. With the new system, every time I think there is a mistake it turns out I am the one who is wrong. I feel very confident now the computer

is better at checking the chart than me. I very rarely have to add or delete anything and I have only had to send 2 patients back to the lab in the last 6 months. Because I have everything I need at the office visit, don't have to order my own labs and don't have to send extra lab letters, I have cut out at least 15 messages a day from my workload.

Of course, there are some providers who continue to want their own lists and have difficulty accepting the inevitable compromises associated with a group decision and they are allowed to opt out of pre-physical lab ordering. But it is significant that even in the relatively early stage of this new innovation, there were only 3 physicians out of 70 have chosen not to participate.

Better Documentation Tools

The use of the conditional documentation tools and links has allowed for much more robust, versatile, and customizable documentation options resulting in both improved efficiency and better quality of care.

Physician Efficiency and Satisfaction. The physicians are able to continue to document in a style that is to their liking but still benefits from work the MA completes, while taking advantage of templates that are designed with quality measures and billing rules in mind.

Medical Assistant (MA) Efficiency and Satisfaction. The MA's workflow has improved as they do not need to remember each provider's personal preference and they are now able to easily cover each other and float to other sites in order to satisfy staffing needs. The system knows and gives them the note template the provider wants.

Coding and Billing Improvements. The BPAs were leveraged to ease billing difficulties by showing or hiding options based on the qualities of the patient. For example, the system can check the insurance status of a patient, note that the patient has Medicare and is in for a physical, and direct the provider to the specific billing and documentation options needed in this situation. This improves the speed and accuracy of billing and reduces the administrative burden of already stressed providers.

Other Benefits. Conditional tools have also been used to provide more versatile lab letters, after visit summaries and meaningful use topics. For example this method was used in the documentation of smoking status for all patients age 13 or over in order to meet the Federal Meaningful Use program. It was desirable to have the question be present in the documentation template to remind the providers to ask and document; however, having the question in an ear pain template for a 2 year-old was clearly unfavorable. The different templates could be created for every chief complaint based-upon age, but that seemed like a labor-intensive solution to what should be a simple problem. By using the conditional link patients under age 13 do not have a question about smoking status in the template, but if 13 or older they do.

This process has also been used to customize the content of the after visit summary (AVS). For example, a traditional workflow for vaccines is that an MA has to find and provide a patient with an up to date vaccine information sheet (VIS) after a vaccine is given. With the new system, if an order for a particular vaccine was placed in the EHR, the correct VIS would automatically print as part of the AVS, thus saving time and ensuring up to date information.

Lessons Learned

Balancing Standardization vs. Individualization. One common problem was the *inability to force standardization*. As every provider and every individual office operates differently it is important to recognize that while some of these differences can and should be eliminated to create standard processes, there are others that need to remain individualized. A large misstep encountered was failing to account for site-to-site and provider-to-provider variations. In the case of lab ordering, this was addressed by breaking the organization into groups that could make unified decisions. For documentation, the EHR did allow for more individual customization when needed.

Getting Physicians to Trust in the System. It is essential to develop trust in the process among physicians and staff. Doctors don't pay attention to details about computer and workflow processes in which they are not invested. The EHR team still gets complaints about the order set not working. One internal medicine physician recently complained that an electrolyte panel and CBC wasn't being ordered on his patients and assumed "something was wrong with the order set". In fact, his group had asked only for a screening hematocrit and the patient in question had an electrolyte panel at urgent care the previous week, so none was needed. He blamed the computer rather than checking what should and should not have been ordered.

It is imperative that physicians feel comfortable and trust that the order set is reliable. In order to foster this trust, extensive testing is required to assure a robust and accurate setup. The logic is very complicated and confusing given the many scenarios. Therefore, it is very important to have an invested individual who understands the process onsite to monitor the initial phases and to check for logical errors.

Garbage In, Garbage Out. Many times an "error" reported by a provider actually is due to inaccuracies in the patient chart, not an error in the conditional order set. In other words, if the medication list or problem list is not correct, then incorrect orders will be suggested. Therefore, when the IT support staff is contacted and the problem is identified as a lack of correct information, this scenario is used as an opportunity to educate on the need to maintain an accurate and up-to-date problem and medication list. The provider involved is contacted directly, usually by a physician on the IT support team, and good EHR practices are reviewed and the reasons for the "error" discussed. Proper workflows are reinforced in the office as a whole by the optimization team when needed.

Fortunately, this represents a good alignment of good chart documentation matched to physician efficiency gains. So as providers increasingly rely on these types of clinical decision support tools to improve their efficiency, they have a strong incentive to keep their records highly accurate. This is good for everyone!

Focus on the Most Common and Highest Risk Areas. Despite the extensive logic and effort expended, the lab ordering process has limitations that can frustrate physicians. There is a virtually unlimited list of diagnoses that may need lab monitoring that is simply too long to be accommodated in an order set. Including more than 30 combinations of tests would create a slow, unwieldy and difficult to maintain and validate order set. Therefore, only the most common or highest risk issues are included.

Timing can be an Important Confounding Factor. One limitation for the lab order set is the inability to look into the future. It can only review the chart at the moment the order set is opened. This becomes an issue if the physical appointment is made many months in the future. For example, if an annual physical is made 1 year in advance and the yearly tests have just been completed, the order set will not suggest any testing. In these cases, a manual process must be set up to review the schedule and run the program closer to the scheduled appointment time. Hopefully as the rules and logic of the EHR become more advanced it will be possible to better address this situation.

A Multidisciplinary Team needs to be Involved. If a team does not have all interested parties engaged in a solution, there is a high likelihood that after the process is designed and implemented others will demand that changes be made. This leads to provider and staff frustration as well as decreased probability of long-term success. Thus, it is essential to have a team with complementary skills and interests willing to share and problem solve together. A multidisciplinary team that includes providers, office staff, compliance, billing, utilization management, and IT staff needs to be involved from the beginning of any major project. Multiple individuals with complementary skills must have the opportunity to interact, as innovation is more successful as a *collaborative process*.

Working with the Right Physicians. Physicians who are on the front line of patient care need to be involved in all aspects of the EHR roll-out and optimization. Only through seeing patients on a daily basis and using the tools can one fully understand the implications of how the system works. To harness the power of the EHR and streamline workflows, providers who maintain a clinical practice and use the product must be included in all aspects of the rollout and post go-live optimization.

Additionally, these physician/IT members must be given the security to make appropriate rapid changes without a burdensome process. They must be trained and facile in the available tools. Many organizations are very reluctant to give physicians the security to build in the EHR. It is essential for an interested subgroup of users to have access and training in all the tools to allow customization in a timely manner without excessive bureaucracy. Only through having this access can the physicians truly understand what can be done and how best to get the system to do what is necessary to develop an effective and efficient workflow.

The Future

The pre-physical order set was designed for testing prior to an annual physical, which accounts for approximately 30 % of primary care office visits at the Fallon Clinic. However, this concept can easily be expanded to other scenarios such as chronic disease management or specialty care. For example, the Cardiology Department is working on an Amiodarone pre-visit order set, since they may need several labs such as thyroid hormone levels and liver enzyme levels, as well as other tests such as CXR and EKG at certain intervals.

The conditional documentation process continues to be a work in process. The new Medicare Wellness exams were not considered in the original rules for physical documentation and will require an additional layer of if/then logic. Some physicians are still dissatisfied with the documentation templates so comments and suggestions are being gathered for further refinements.

Finally, the use of conditional SmartLinks will be expanding to other documentation areas over the coming year. For virtually any procedure in which a handout or post-procedure information is given to the patient after the procedure is performed, the information could be automatically included into the AVS. For example, this process is currently in development for topical fluoride application in pediatric patients, dermatological procedures and wound repairs.

Conclusion

For many established providers the transition to an EHR is a difficult process. Simply giving providers and their staff the electronic system and converting the paper workflows to an electronic format is not enough. If we are going to truly improve the quality of care that is provided and ease the overwhelming burden that healthcare providers currently face, new innovative workflows that truly harness the power of what a computer can do are necessary.

As we continue into the era of Accountable Care Organizations, Pay for Performance, physician shortages, cost containment requirements and widespread EHR adoption, it is vital that the EHRs that we use work in more sophisticated ways to leverage already known and documented information to improve the patient and provider experience. Providers of medical care in an EHR environment are now required by "meaningful use", HITECH and CMS to gather what would previously have been considered extraneous information for the care of our patients. It is time for physicians (and patients) to finally receive tangible benefits from the work such as easier ordering, easier documentation, fewer messages, more efficient appointments, lower cost of care, and higher quality time with the patient.

Fallon Clinic has set three overlying goals to guide any large projects and endeavors over the next few years: (1) Become the employer and delivery system of choice by improving satisfaction and engagement of our patients and employees. (2) Improve the ability to succeed under a value-based reimbursement system by the efficient use of health care resources resulting in total medical care cost that is 20 % less than "market cost" and a 90 % attainment of pay-for-performance funding and (3) Increase the capacity of patients that can be cared for at Fallon Clinic.

In order to accomplish these lofty and aggressive goals it will be essential to make the best possible use of the technology available. The EHR cannot simply be thought of as a replacement for paper, but rather a critical tool to help in the creation of a completely new model of care delivery. More innovations, such as the pre-physical lab ordering process and conditional documentation tools, will need to be developed. Only through truly utilizing the full power of the EHR will organizations such as the Fallon Clinic achieve seemingly unreachable goals, allowing the US healthcare system to thrive during these challenging times.

Chapter 7
"All or None" Bundle Philosophy

Thomas R. Graf

Barbara finally got her husband to go to the doctor. Well, it wasn't just her really; it was Tina from the doctor's office. She sent a birthday card, and then called. "Hi Ray. We've missed you! It's been 2 years since your last visit to Dr. Jim."

"I'm actually fine, and feeling great." Ray rolled his eyes wondering how he was going to get out of this.

"That's really good, but we need to keep you that way. You're behind on a few tests including your cholesterol and blood work. It's also time for a colonoscopy. Let's book them, and then can I talk to Barbara? We need to set up some work for her too." Ray smiled at that. At least it wasn't only him this time.

"Hi Barbara. Dr Jim would like you to see Angie our physician assistant to work on getting your blood sugar under control. Angie can see you at the same time your husband is coming if that is convenient."

"That would be great. I saw my blood sugar test results last night online, and am kind of concerned." Her comprehensive diabetes score had not changed in months; she had her flu shot for the year, and her pneumonia shot. She had gotten her blood pressure under good control about 6 months ago with the addition of exercise and a new medicine, and her blood work was up to date.

So there they were, 2 weeks later, sitting in exam rooms in the office. Barbara was looking over her diabetes report card but then started thinking how amazing it was that the dual appointment was even happening. Not too long ago it seemed everything was a surprise and last minute. Now, everyone at Dr. Jim's office was so proactive. I like this new world, she thought.

T.R. Graf, M.D.
Community Practice Service Line, Geisinger Health System,
Community Practice Service Ling,
100 North Academy Ave, Danville, PA 17822-2412, USA
e-mail: trgraf@geisinger.edu

L. Berkowitz, C. McCarthy (eds.),
Innovation with Information Technologies in Healthcare, Health Informatics,
DOI 10.1007/978-1-4471-4327-7_7, © Springer-Verlag London 2013

Background

Geisinger Health System is a physician-led organization, grounded in the concepts of group practice and the interdisciplinary approach to patient care, as well as a commitment to educational and research programs. The Geisinger system is a vertically integrated organization based in central Pennsylvania, composed of a 1,000 physician medical group, four acute care hospital campuses, an inpatient drug rehabilitation center, and a 300,000 member health plan. Leveraging of this integrated system has allowed for a plethora of innovations focused on creating patient value and health. Geisinger has embedded a culture of innovation throughout the organization, led by the Community Practice Service Line.

The Innovation

Geisinger's innovations use healthcare information technology (HIT) systems to eliminate, shift, or automate as much of the workflow as possible. Additionally, Geisinger has committed to using an "All or None Bundle Philosophy" to measure the success of their program. This methodology looks at the percentage of patients that have received every element of recommended care rather than the percentage of patients that achieve any particular measure. This encapsulates the patient centered view as well as creates a great deal of cognitive dissonance as the all or none bundle score is often quite low, driving systematic changes in care delivery.

For example, determining what health maintenance activities are due for a patient was something that physicians or nurses might have originally used precious time to do at each visit. However, having the computer determine what is due and then having call-center staff contact the patient to update this information and schedule their required tests before an office visit could provide a more efficient and higher quality experience. Success would be measured by what percent of the time all their activities were completed.

In the new model of primary care, physician-directed teams work to provide all aspects of care in a consistent and reliable manner. The redesign is incorporated into the standard workflow using charting tools, checklists, reminders, and alerts.

Reason for This Innovation

The innovation story began with a leadership commitment in 2004 to re-engineering care to provide greater value for the five major parties in healthcare: patients, providers, hospitals, payers, and purchasers of care. Geisinger's leaders realized that this redesign would have to integrate HIT into clinical care, involve the patient and family, ensure total accountability through aligned incentives, and reduce variability through care redesign and performance feedback to improve patient outcomes, thereby decreasing costs. The underlying cause for the change was the realization by the operational leaders that (1) the status quo was untenable in the long term, (2) the quality of care provided was far from optimal, and (3) improving quality would likely drive lower cost. The ability to leverage the relationship with the Geisinger Health Plan was key, it created an environment where the optimal care of the patient was foremost, and only once this was determined, was the payment mechanism discussed.

Why This Innovation Succeeded

Organizational Culture

"Make my hospital right, make it the best," was the charge Abigail Geisinger gave Harold Foss, the first superintendent of the George F. Geisinger Memorial Hospital nearly 100 years ago, and those words continue to drive the performance of every team member. Despite the tremendous growth of the system and the evolution from a hospital centered organization to one focused on caring for populations as close to home as possible, the goal of being the best continues. Geisinger continues to use this sentiment to develop a truly patient- centered, value-driven culture which leverages HIT to accelerate theses changes.

Organizational Structure

The Community Practice Service Line, the 200 providers and nearly 40 sites outside of the main hospital locations, made up of Family Physicians, Internal Medicine Physicians, Medicine-Pediatric Physicians, and Pediatricians caring for over 300,000 patients in central and northeast Pennsylvania and, comprising nearly a third of the medical group, led the system in technology supported value re-engineering. Moving from an HMO-like "doc on every corner" approach to the current hub and spoke model allows for a concentration of critical mass to deploy advanced resources close to patients' homes. Regional hubs supported by small community centers have technology such as advanced imagery and subspecialty physician outreach. This deployment of tertiary level services overcomes some of the geographic challenges of rural Pennsylvania. Shared technology provides the integrating function to allow timely responses despite intermittent presence. The greatest strength of the Community Practice Service Line is the training and ability of the middle level physician leaders. Charged with leading 20–30 providers over two to five sites, the ability to understand data and translate it into clinical meaning and make the operational changes necessary to change the outcome is critical to the ongoing success of Geisinger.

Geisinger's franchise-like departmental substructure utilizes paired physician and administrative leadership at all levels (site, region, and service line) and is supported by unified goals, frequent shared decision-making meetings, and a high performance culture to drive outcomes for cost, quality, and experience. Additionally, providing compensation to all team members around shared goals is used to increase team cohesion, focus attention on important initiatives, and reward the adopters of the new model.

Shared Strategy

Each site is regionally integrated with community or Geisinger resources but unified by shared strategies and tactical approaches. These unifying strategies are designed to create a meaningful difference for our patients. Strategies have migrated over time from Advanced Access, Care Systems, Professional Reputation, and Transparency to our current strategies that maintain a focus on Systems of Care and Professional Reputation but also now include "System-ness" and Automation.

HIT Involvement

The HIT focus of the Automation strategy and the key role played by HIT in the Systems of Care emphasize how integral HIT has been to Geisinger's success. These principles and strategies, as well as a culture embracing data and feedback of meaningful and actionable information, coupled with physician and administrative leadership skilled in the translation of this into programmatic evolutions has allowed Geisinger to rapidly develop innovations, deploy innovations to all CPSL sites, and continually refine these innovations. Because the physicians are fully embedded in the local communities and because of a commitment to provide the best care as close to home as possible, unique value is created for patients and families.

Innovating at Geisinger

Any change process requires timely measurement and feedback of performance data. Primary care redesign initiatives use accurate clinical information from the patient record, claims data, and survey results to measure their success. Claims-based information is often the easiest to report, but developing accurate clinical information from the patient chart in the form of patient registries is a powerful tool to improve population management.

Using these techniques and principles, the care for the Geisinger population was redesigned. In determining the best means to manage the 220,000 adult patients preventive care needs across the 200 providers, it became clear that an office based approach would be ineffective. Additionally, the concept of having every team member working at the top of their license, dictated that the EHR be the prime driver of this process. Creating and environment where prevention is managed in an entirely automated fashion took nearly a year. Now however, each patient is enrolled in a proactive outreach effort for up to 5 years by their physician and from there automation takes over. All needed testing is ordered by the EHR via protocols agreed to upon enrollment by the physician. An auto-dialer efficiently connects the patients by phone with access center representatives. These representatives, through advanced HIT functionality, know who has been reached, why they have been called, what testing in what order needs to be completed, and they can arrange everything in the proper order ending with a physician visit. This results in a maximally productive visit for the patients and physicians.

Additionally, all necessary chronic disease care is integrated into this process. Ongoing chronic disease care is managed by "just in time" alerts to the various team members to support their performance in coordinating testing and appointments (phone room and front desk staff), process measurement and education management (nursing staff), and complex medical decision-making and patient relationships (provider staff). This redesign resulted in highly efficient offices with improved staff and patient satisfaction.

Finally, innovation projects are tracked by quality measures which address the Institute of Medicine's six aims for improving health care: making healthcare more safe, effective, patient-centered, timely, efficient, and equitable [1]. In addition, more recent quality literature has emphasized the need for high reliability in health care, highlighting the importance of leadership, safety culture, and robust process improvement [2]. Additionally, measures of quality for a program should attempt to include an evaluation of the ability of the program to provide recommended care, of patient and provider satisfaction with the program, and of patient clinical and functional outcomes.

Workflow Redesign Philosophy

When redesigning workflows, three principals were always adhered to:

1. Perform work outside of an office encounter when possible
2. Distribute tasks so that people are working at "the top of their license"
3. Improve the efficiency and reliability of work done using tools in the Electronic Health Record (EHR)

All or None Bundle Philosophy

Geisinger has committed to using patient-centered measures with patient-specific goals and an "all-or-none" methodology to comprehensively deliver all evidence-supported care to each patient. All-or-none care measures that bundle a host of related care processes and outcomes offer a new approach to clinical process improvement. The all-or-none bundle measures the percentage of patients who achieve all of the recommended measures, rather than an average or composite of the individual measures. Performance, according to Nolan and Berwick [3], is improved by the all-or-none measurement system in three ways

1. More closely reflecting the interests and likely desires of patients
2. Fostering a systems perspective encouraging concern with all aspects of the team care
3. Offering a more sensitive scale for assessing improvements.

Results

Improving quality while providing more efficient, less wasteful care, increases the value for all. Contrary to the prevailing view in the 1990s, that it was necessary to choose high quality or low cost, there are now many examples of high-quality and low-cost care across the country [4]. Redesigned models of care often eliminate waste therefore reducing cost and improving quality. Measuring the quality of care provided is essential for demonstrating high-value health care and for demonstrating that the new model of care is not cutting cost to the detriment of the patient.

Disease Related Bundles

Targeted alerts for complex medical-decision-making increases the completeness of care and overcomes clinical inertia. Improving the completeness of visits reduces rework and allows targeting visit frequency by patient disease severity while ensuring all patients health improves. Patients with good control are seen less frequently, thus allowing poorly controlled patients to be seen more often. Non-MD resources are deployed proactively to manage all non-MD work, anything not involving complex medical-decision-making or patient relationships, thus creating more time and ability to maximize physician resources. In other words, physicians and nurses benefitted from the improved workflows and electronic tools embedded in the EHR, allowing better flow and also faster and more complete documentation. Similar patient-oriented views bring patients a complete picture of their care and prompt them to play a more active role.

As an example, Geisinger redesigned the approach to managing patients with diabetes in 2005 to include a nine-component all-or-none diabetes bundle [5] as shown in Table 7.1. This redesigned process led to more reliable and accountable team-based service. The all-or-none bundle score and all nine process and intermediate outcomes improved within the first year of implementation and consistently

Table 7.1 Bundles for diabetes and coronary artery disease

Diabetes	A1C every 6 months
	A1C<7.0 % or 7–8 %
	LDL every 12 months
	LDL <100 mg/dl or <70 mg/dl if high risk
	Microalbumin screening
	B/P <130/80 mmHg
	Documentation of non-smoker
	Pneumococcal vaccine
	Influenza vaccine
CAD	LDL<100 or <70 if high risk
	ACE/ARB in LVSD, DM, HTN
	BMI measured
	BP <140/90
	Antiplatelet therapy
	Beta blocker use S/P MI
	Documented non-smokers
	Pneumococcal vaccination
	Influenza vaccination

Table 7.2 Improving diabetes care for 24,791 patients

	3/06 (%)	3/07 (%)	6/10 (%)	6/11 (%)
Diabetes bundle percentage	2.4	7.2	12.8	12.6
% Influenza vaccination	57	73	75	77
% Pneumococcal vaccination	59	83	84	83
% Microalbumin result	58	87	79	78
% HgbA1c at goal	33	37	51	50
% LDL at goal	50	52	53	55
% BP <130/80	39	44	54	56
% Documented non-smokers	74	84	85	85

thereafter [6]. Since deployment of the bundle, we have seen a 500 % improvement in the comprehensive diabetes scores (see Table 7.2). The power of the "All or None" bundle is clearly seen. Starting with just 2.4 % of the patients receiving every element of agreed upon care, the first elements to improve are the process measures. In the first year significant improvements are realized in immunizations, microproteinuria testing etc. In the out years, improvement in the "All or None" bundle can only be achieved by increasing the intermediate outcome scores such as cholesterol control, blood pressure control, and blood sugar control. A parallel system was then developed for coronary artery disease (see Table 7.1), leveraging all the same tools with similar impact for physicians, nurses and patients. Comprehensive CAD scores improved 300 % in 3 years (see Table 7.3). Similar to the diabetes bundle, the process measure scores improve first, with vaccination rates and moving to the control measures as time progresses. Measurement and management of weight assumed an intermediate improvement position related to culture and resources. Blood pressure

Table 7.3 Improving CAD care for 15,440 patients

	9/06 (%)	3/07 (%)	6/10 (%)	6/11 (%)
CAD bundle percentage	8	11	21	23
% LDL<100 or <70 if high risk	38	37	49	52
% ACE/ARB in LVSD, DM, HTN	65	66	76	77
% BMI measures	79	86	99	99
% BP<140/90	74	74	78	80
% Antiplatelet therapy	89	91	92	93
% Beta blocker use S/P MI	97	97	97	97
% Document non-smokers	86	86	87	87
% Pneumococcal vaccination	80	80	86	86
% Influenza vaccination	60	74	79	79

control and antiplatelet agent use showed progressive modest improvement as a result of the system of care approach with each team member supporting improved patient care.

Geisinger has now added bundles for hypertension, chronic kidney disease, and osteoporosis, as well as ten acute care bundles such as CABG, Prenatal Care, and PCI. These exhibit the same kinds of improvements with initial gains in the process measures followed by intermediate outcome improvements. The acute bundles have led to reduction in morbidity, mortality, and total cost of care.

Wellness Related Bundles

Moving from disease-oriented bundles to a wellness related bundle necessitated the development of new skills, tools and HIT supports. Geisinger's automated "Happy Birthday" program married advanced EHR capabilities with an auto dialer and specially trained schedulers to create an effective out of office approach to creating wellness. This begins with a letter, and 10 % of patients respond to this. For those that do not, the auto dialer engages. All of the patients with identified care gaps are included based on the all or none bundles devised to optimize care. Patient response to the message, 'Happy Birthday, this is Geisinger and we care about your health. To minimize your chances of significant health problems down the road, national experts recommend that you receive the following care…,' has been overwhelmingly positive. This not only manages prevention, but also lifts that work out of office encounters and creates more effective encounters in the office. The impact of these quality improvements allowed Geisinger Community Practice Service Line (CPSL) to earn 6 % of their total revenue from P4P programs. The comprehensive approach to preventive care allows the Geisinger physicians to broadly improve care regardless of insurance coverage of individual patients. Progressive improvements of the preventive care bundle are achieved (see Table 7.4) as these are essentially all process measures. The challenge of this bundle is the ongoing, repetitive nature of

Table 7.4 Improving preventive care for 219,289 patients		11/07 (%)	6/11 (%)
	Adult prevention bundle	9.2	31
	Breast cancer screening (q 2 40–49, q 1 50–74)	46	61
	Cervical cancer screening (q 3 year Age 21–64)	64	71
	Colon cancer screening (age 50–84)	44	66
	Prostate cancer discussion (age 50–74)	72	77
	Lipid screening (every 5 year M >35, F >45)	75	87
	Diabetes screening (every 3 year > 45)	85	90
	Obesity screening (BMI in epic)	77	97
	Documented non-smokers	75	79
	Tetanus diphtheria immunization (every 10 year)	35	71
	Pneumococcal immunization (once age >65)	84	87
	Influenza immunization (yearly age >50)	47	60
	Chlamydia screening (yearly age 18–25)	22	37
	Osteoporosis screening (every 3 year age >65)	52	73
	Alcohol intake assessment	84	91

the measures (i.e. annual performance) and the growth in the managed patient population, in this case 10 % over 3 years.

Lessons Learned

Where to Focus When Redesigning Care

Geisinger's leaders wanted a new system of care that would consistently deliver all necessary care while avoiding care that did not create value for patients. It was clear that to do this, physicians must be given the time and support to focus their attention on the critical physician tasks. These physician level tasks are: complex medical decision-making and patient relationships. To do this, one must subdivide the population, determine the most appropriate intervention and the optimal means to deliver that intervention. Often maximized HIT is the best intervention. The second critical element is to reliably and proactively provide that intervention. This requires the creation of optimized workflows and incorporating them into a highly reliable care process.

Enabling traditional techniques through HIT, such as guideline development, provider and staff education, accurate clinical measurement, timely feedback of data, and patient/family engagement education, is as important as developing newer techniques including the development of accountable team responsibilities and EHR alerts and reminders that rely on HIT for implementation. The commitment to a population of patients involves the use of disease registries to pull patients into care when needed, in addition to addressing all necessary elements of care when patients are seen. Care in settings outside of the traditional face-to-face encounter should be a part of any redesign, including phone and electronic communication.

Finding the Right Metrics

Determining metrics for a quality program involves an analysis of available data sources, accuracy of the data, timeliness of the data, and reporting capabilities. A combination of process measures (such as diabetic foot examination rate), intermediate outcomes (blood pressure control), or patient outcomes (myocardial infarction rate) are often included. Geisinger used a multidisciplinary multi-specialty steering committee to perform a comprehensive literature review and reach consensus on a balanced set of measures. In combination, the metrics should create a complete picture of the comprehensive disease control and the process to deliver this. Development of the current Geisinger approach involved a rapid cycle learning iterative process to generate value.

Challenges with Expanding to Wellness

One of the greatest challenges encountered was the move from the disease-oriented bundles to a prevention-oriented bundle. The operational impact of moving from a 15 to 25,000 patient disease bundle to a bundle with over 200,000 adult patients was not fully appreciated. Additionally, the work for the preventive bundle, unlike the previous bundles, was disproportionately distributed to the nurses. This combination meant that essentially every patient encounter needed additional support from nurses which created a dramatic flow disruption across CPSL. These disruptions necessitated the development of the out of office approach to managing wellness. The solution was to leverage technology coupled with two specially trained non-clinical staff to manage the prevention bundle. The automation created to drive this bundle lifted vast amounts of low value work from the office and created the infrastructure to reliably deliver superior care to every patient, every time. The two staff members are used to create a high value connection with patients and ensure appropriate translation.

Need for Patient Specific Goals

Adjustment of specific bundle metrics by allowing patient centered goals was critical to success. For instance, moving from targeting a blood sugar control goal of HbA1C <7 % for all patients to allowing the physician/patient team to determine medically appropriate control targets (e.g. elderly cardiac patients with a goal of 7–8). This created better care and better physician engagement with the process. The physician/patient team sets individual goals by altering patient specific diagnoses in the EHR, while the determination of the appropriate goals can be time consuming, the recording of the decision requires minimal manipulation of the EHR.

Coordinating Multiple Bundles

Appropriately coordinating inter-bundle interactions was another critical factor. For instance, patients with both diabetes and CAD had disparate LDL goals in each bundle. Creating the ability to report a consistent target for every patient was necessary for true patient value. So if a patient's LDL target on one bundle is <70 and for the other bundle is <100, the patient specific target becomes <70 for *both* bundles. This was a programmatic change instituted at the request of the physicians after review and endorsement by the multidisciplinary, multispecialty oversight group for each bundle.

Future Plans

Geisinger's CPSL has deployed all of the current bundles across all of their 200 providers. They have recently added 70,000 patients with hypertension and are adding patient engagement and shared decision making skills to drive not only comprehensive hypertension control but also improved control in all the other bundles as well.

The next frontier they are tackling is the ability to allow patient entered data and capture patient preferences via the patient portal and via in-office touch screens. This will in turn allow these data points to be used in real time to improve and personalize care during the index encounter.

Additionally, they will incorporate advanced algorithms into the EHR to bring subspecialty knowledge and evidence based guidelines into the primary care exam room to support the physician and patient team. This will involve a high quality rules engine which will determine expert recommendation standards for clinical situations. These recommendations will then be individualized to the patient by a clinical decision support engine fueled by both EHR information and patient entered data. Finally, advanced visual display techniques and scripting cues will be used to assist the primary care physician in engaging their patients.

Conclusion

This journey has been invigorating for the physicians and the other medical professionals involved and has resulted in meaningful health improvements for Geisinger's patients. Leveraging the unique contributions of team members, patients and the electronic health record has created an exciting place to both care for patients and receive care as a patient. Geisinger has demonstrated consistent improvement in process and intermediate outcomes as well as professional and patient experience measures. Emerging internal evidence indicates that these care innovations have additionally improved patient end outcomes, such as reduced heart attack and stroke rates. Health information technology has been a critical tool in this process and accelerates virtually every improvement in the system.

References

1. Committee on the Quality of Healthcare in America, Institute of Medicine. Crossing the quality chasm: a new health system for the 21st century. Washington, D.C.: National Academies Press; 2001.
2. Chassin MR, Loeb JM. The ongoing quality improvement journey: next stop, high reliability. Health Aff. 2011;30(4):559–68.
3. Nolan T, Berwick D. All-or-none measurement raises the bar on performance. JAMA. 2006;295:1168–9.
4. Fisher E, Goodman D, Skinner J, Bronner K. Health care spending, quality and outcomes. Dartmouth Institute for Health Policy and Clinical Practice. 2009. http://www.dartmouthatlas.org/downloads/reports/Spending_Brief_022709.pdf. Accessed on 30 June 2011.
5. Bloom FJ, Graf T, Anderer T, Stewart WF. Redesign of a diabetes system of care using an all-or- none diabetes bundle to build teamwork and improve intermediate outcomes. Diabetes Spectr. 2010;23(3):165–9.
6. Weber V, Bloom FJ, Pierdon S, Wood C. Employing the electronic health record to improve diabetes care: a multifaceted intervention in an integrated delivery system. J Gen Intern Med. 2008;23(4):379–82.

Chapter 8
Automatically Getting Better

David C. Stockwell and Brian R. Jacobs

Isabelle was nervous walking into the emergency room with her 3-year old Stephan. She had heard a few years ago that there were many problems at hospitals with people making mistakes. Between being frightened of hospitals and that, she started not feeling good herself. "Hi, can I help you?" asked the ER receptionist.

"My son Stephan has been really sick the past week. His cough has gotten much worse in the last day. He sounds awful." Moments later, Isabelle and Stephan were resting comfortably in an intake room, when the ER doctor knocked at the door. "Isabelle? Hi I'm Doctor Richardson. You can call me John. So what's going on with Stephan here?"

Isabelle shares the details of Stephan's cough, and ends with "John to be frank. I have to say I'm nervous being here. I've heard so many horror stories about mistakes in hospitals."

"Well, I can appreciate that, and glad you shared that with me. What I can tell you is this. Several years ago here at Children's National, we created a system to detect errors. Since then we've eliminated most of the errors in the system. We are proud at just how safe our system is, and we're recognized as a leader in safety. We're here to help Stephan get better in the safest way possible."

"I had no idea! That makes me feel better, so now let's try to make Stephan feel better too. Thank you, John." Just knowing that there was a system to prevent all those things she was hearing about, really did make her feel safer.

D.C. Stockwell, M.D., M.B.A. (✉) • B.R. Jacobs, M.D., M.S.
Pediatric Intensive Care Unit, Children's National Medical Center,
Critical Care Medicine, 111 Michigan Ave., NW, Suite M4800,
Washington, DC 20010, USA
e-mail: dstockwell@childrensnational.org; bjacobs@childrensnational.org

L. Berkowitz, C. McCarthy (eds.),
Innovation with Information Technologies in Healthcare, Health Informatics,
DOI 10.1007/978-1-4471-4327-7_8, © Springer-Verlag London 2013

Background

Children's National is a 303 bed urban free standing children's hospital in Washington, D.C.. With its long history of innovation, Children's National implemented computerized physician order entry (CPOE), the electronic medication administration record, electronic results retrieval and digital radiology with full adoption in 2005. In 2008, full nursing and physician electronic documentation was implemented in the inpatient units and Emergency Department.

The Innovation

The Children's National informatics and technology team built an electronic reporting tool which identifies adverse events occurring throughout their hospital based upon queries of their electronic health record (EHR) system, such as abnormal lab data (e.g. low glucose) or antidote medications prescribed in the event of a medical problem (e.g. Naloxone). This daily report, termed the Automated Adverse Event Detection (AAED), is monitored by a nurse who analyzes each abnormal item to determine its level of harm and whether it was preventable. The appropriate physicians and managers then study this information to determine how they can improve their processes and avoid similar adverse events in the future. The review team may include the clinicians involved with the event as well as "trigger-specific experts" (e.g. hypoglycemia cases are reviewed with endocrinologists, naloxone adverse events are reviewed with pain medicine experts). Table 8.1 shows all current adverse event triggers, as well as the trigger-specific experts whom might be involved in their review.

	Adverse event trigger	Trigger specific experts
Table 8.1 Electronic event triggers which are part of the Automated Adverse Event Detection program	Naloxone	Sedation Committee and ICU Leadership
	Flumazenil	Sedation Committee and ICU Leadership
	Glucose <50 mg/dL	Endocrinology and Neonatology
	Protamine	Anticoagulation Task Force
	PTT >100 s	Anticoagulation Task Force
	INR >4.0	Anticoagulation Task Force
	Anti factor Xa >1.5	Anticoagulation Task Force
	Creatinine doubling	Nephrology
		Radiology (contrast cases)
	Bilirubin >25 mg/dL	Neonatology
	Digibind	Cardiology
	Hyaluronidase	Pharmacy and Nursing
	Transfers to the ICU	PICU, NICU and CICU Leadership

Reason for This Innovation

In 2007, Children's National engaged in an initiative to increase the detection of errors and adverse events by creating an automated process that leveraged their EHR system. As hospitals strive to deliver safe and effective care, it is no surprise that they first need to understand the scope and type of adverse events in their own institutions. Having this data allows hospitals to more easily comprehend and prioritize these events, as well as improve and innovate on how to solve them. Unfortunately, this data is not often easy to obtain.

While all hospitals use voluntary reporting from its employees and physicians as a mechanism to identify the adverse event, it is well established that voluntary reporting does not deliver more than a fraction of the true rates of adverse events that occur (Cullen et al. [1]) Limiting factors may include:

- *Culture.* An organization needs to have the appropriate non-punitive culture to have optimal reporting.
- *Time Constraints.* Voluntary reporting requires a certain amount of time and effort to complete. Clinicians often find it difficult to complete another task in an already burdensome workload environment.
- *Lack of Transparency.* Clinicians want to feel their actions result in changes, but the process and actions that result from voluntary reporting are often not visible to the reporting provider.
- *Intuitive and Efficient Reporting Tools.* Ideally integrated into the clinician workflow and requiring minimal data entry.

Why This Innovation Succeeded

As Children's National had been using an EHR for quite some time, they recognized that the possibility existed to query the record electronically for potential and actual errors and adverse events. Since errors and adverse events were not usually recorded as such, a proxy for these events needed to be defined. Children's National realized that within any EHR there are structured data elements (triggers) that have a reasonable likelihood of representing an error or an adverse event. Examples include:

- Lab Values, such as abnormal glucose, potassium, creatinine, platelets and prothrombin time.
- Use of certain antidotes, such as naloxone which indicates that the clinical team assessed the patient as potentially overmedicated by an opioid medication.

Choosing Triggers. The initial assessment of triggers appropriate for pediatrics involves combining literature review of existing reports with real world clinical experience. For example, the creation of a low glucose alert in the Neonatal Intensive Care Unit required a review of the evidence surrounding adverse events related to neonatal hypoglycemia and clinical discussion with Neonatology experts to determine a glucose threshold which would have clinical significance and a high signal to noise ratio.

Technical Development. Specific EHR queries were developed to allow reports to be generated for each trigger. The logic behind each trigger was developed at Children's National and then translated into EHR query language in partnership with the EHR vendor.

Education. Most clinicians were not experienced with receiving this degree of detailed adverse event data. Therefore much of the first few weeks of the program were focused on helping clinicians understand the accuracy and reliability of the data, the automated adverse event detection methodology and the potential utility of the initiative. The approach varied from email communication announcing the program's goals and processes to personal communication with the services which had concerning findings. These communications were a crucial step that helped ensure stakeholder acceptance and increased the clinicians' ability to embrace the feedback they were receiving. It also has helped to solidify the appropriate safety culture and highlighted the need to pay attention to every patient outcome that can be monitored using this methodology.

Event Investigation. A full time nurse analyst utilizing the EHR-integrated AAED tool investigates each AAED Program trigger within 24-h of its occurrence (Fig. 8.1 and Table 8.2). The nurse analyst first identifies if there has been a true adverse event by reviewing the clinical record. Second, the nurse analyst determines if this event was preventable or non-preventable. Finally, the nurse analyst assigns a level of harm associated with the event. If the preventable or non-preventable event represents a significant level of harm, the hospital's Safety Department is immediately notified. Several of the AAED Program triggers also get immediately reported to the respective clinical leaders so that the opportunity to improve care is passed to the team caring for the patient. The investigator also prepares reports for each inpatient unit in the hospital with a summary of their adverse events for the previous month, the individualized trending of certain areas of concern for each unit, and any areas of improvement.

Clinical Integration. This innovation has been well integrated into the fabric of clinical activity at Children's National. A key component for its success has been providing adverse event information to the clinical leaders and then ensuring they receive adequate feedback about any intervention that they made. The data that is given to these clinicians helps them assess the potential risks present in their environment, and then their investigations facilitate their understanding of the problem while ongoing data collection allows them to test changes made to their processes. The ongoing iterative nature of the program has allowed many victories and the program has highlighted their successes hospital-wide.

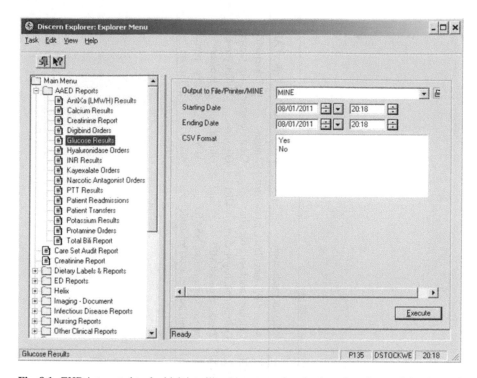

Fig. 8.1 EHR-integrated tool which is utilized in automating the detection of potential and actual adverse event triggers

Spreading the Innovation. *Prioritizing Dissemination.* The rapid spread of this innovation was partly due to identifying which of the hospital's units would most benefit from these improvement efforts and focusing attention on them. This was accomplished by the Steering Committee triaging the findings and studying those inpatient units that had a higher number of adverse events and/or a high severity of events. Themes were sought and identified. These themes of adverse events drove targeting of specific units.

The Power of Collaboration. Reports were disseminated to Unit Managers electronically and resulted in a breakthrough for collaboration on quality improvement initiatives. For example, several triggers identified areas that needed improvement with existing protocols and order sets. Most representative of such a trigger was the identification of hypoglycemia events in neonates receiving insulin to treat hyperglycemia. This insulin protocol was found to be challenging, however there were clear improvements that could be designed and implemented within this protocol. These findings were only apparent once the adverse events were identified and the clinicians were queried as to why they were occurring. Adoption was facilitated by unit-level participation in monthly organizational AAED Steering Committee meetings. Several of the Unit Managers participate in this Steering Committee to help guide the AAED Program and contribute to adverse event prevention efforts.

Table 8.2 Sample summary report for the creatinine trigger

MRN	Admit DX	Trigger value	Base value	Unit	Relevant medications	Renal issues	Type of AE
XXXXXX	Meningitis, resp failure, seizures	1.2	0.5	PICU	Acyclovir, vanco, lasix, phenobarb	Anuria	Preventable
XXXXXX	Prematurity, resp Distr, congen renal anom	2.5	0.8	NICU	Calcitrol, amikacin, bactrim	Creat elevation	Non prevent
XXXXXX	ALL, pancreatitis	2.4	0.9	PICU	Ceftriaxone, flagyl, contrast MRI	Oliguria	Non prevent
XXXXXX	Cerebral glioblastoma	1.4	0.5	PICU	Zantac, contrast MRI	Oliguria	Prevent
XXXXXX	HIV, pharyngitis	1.8	0.8	PICU	Vanco, lasix, zantac, NSAID	ATN	Non prevent
XXXXXX	Congenital heart disease	1.2	0.2	CICU	Gent, aspirin, acetazolamide	Anuria	Prevent

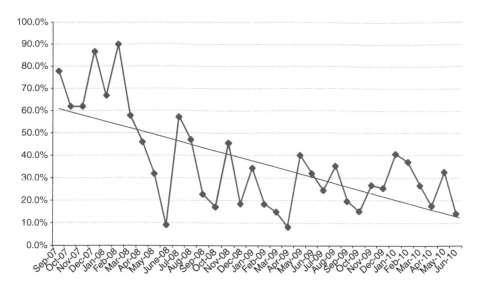

Fig. 8.2 Rate of preventable adverse events over time since implementing the AAED program at Children's National Medical Center

National Spread. Once the benefits of this program were identified locally, other organizations were recruited to join a national collaborative of 26 children's hospitals called the AAED Collaborative. The goal of this Collaborative is to share the findings of each program and allow for experiences and learning to be rapidly spread across multiple organizations. This invaluable group fosters innovation at a fast pace as learning is reviewed and compared monthly between organizations. The Collaborative discusses each trigger and findings from each institution are compared. Since the Collaborative uses similar triggers it helps to facilitate discussions and comparisons.

Results

During the first 3 years of the AAED program, 7,457 triggers have been investigated at Children's National, of which 1,681 (22.5 %) were identified as adverse events. Of those 1,681 adverse events, 487 (29 %) were deemed preventable. More importantly, the hospital has noted a decrease in the overall rate of preventable adverse events, which can be represented in several ways. First, the chance that a patient will experience any recognized adverse event during their hospitalization at Children's National has fallen from 90 to 30 % of all admissions (Fig. 8.2). Second, the overall number of adverse events occurring per hospitalization has decreased from 1.4 per admission to 0.8 per admission.

It is believed that these improvements were largely due to the increased focus on adverse events resulting in workflow changes, as well as the fact that the unit leaders then received additional feedback about the changes made. Some specific examples of how this program benefited patients include:

- *Hypoglycemia.* Once the AAED Program began, it became clear there was a significant rate of hypoglycemia (i.e. glucose values under 50 mg/dL) occurring in the hospital. The AAED program identified the Neonatal Intensive Care Unit (NICU) as the primary unit with hypoglycemia events and further study found that continuous insulin infusion was the principle medication associated with this hypoglycemia. Once this issue was understood, awareness was raised and a partnership was established with the NICU Care Delivery Team so that interventions were put in place, resulting in a dramatic reduction in the incidence of neonatal hypoglycemia. The results of this initiative were presented and published to allow other organizations to realize the benefits of such initiatives [2]. In addition to the hypoglycemia events in the NICU, the AAED Program has detected and addressed hypoglycemia in the Child and Adolescent Psychiatry Unit as well as in hospitalized Cystic Fibrosis patients.
- *Hyperkalemia.* Iatrogenic hyperkalemia was identified in two common patient scenarios and then addressed via a clinical decision support solution that nearly eradicated the occurrence of this problem. In one scenario, clinicians commonly added potassium supplements for patients while they were also being administered potassium wasting medications. It was not uncommon for potassium supplementation to continue after the potassium wasting medications were discontinued. This resulted in periodic episodes of iatrogenic hyperkalemia. Identification of this scenario allowed for decision support to be built which encouraged clinicians to discontinue both medications simultaneously.
- *Anticoagulation.* The use of anticoagulant medications in children is fraught with potential risks and the AAED Program provided an invaluable monitoring system for identifying potential problems. For example, it was identified that the systemic anticoagulation protocol was challenging to follow. The work resulted in the development of a more efficient and intuitive protocol.
- *Renal Injury.* Renal injury was identified when a patient's serum creatinine doubled in a set time frame. Clinical teams would be alerted in near real-time to potential renal injury, allowing for earlier intervention and treatment. For example, after being notified of a creatinine change, the unit-based pharmacist would suggest renal-based dosing for appropriate nephrotoxic medications.
- *Reversal Agents.* By studying when the narcotic antidotes naloxone and flumazenil were used, the AAED Program identified opportunities for improvement with procedural sedation as well as with Patient Controlled Analgesia (PCA) prescribing and administration.
- *Patient Deterioration.* As well as watching for abnormal labs and medication use, the AAED program also has a trigger for all patients transferred to any of the intensive care units from lower acuity patient care areas. By using these reports, the organization developed improved acute care admission criteria and improved the monitoring system for the Rapid Response Team. Information regarding

patients transferred to one of the ICUs is shared with ICU leadership who now perform 100 % review of these events.

Lessons Learned

Several lessons have emerged as a result of this program.

- *Clinical Leadership and Partnerships.* Close collaboration with clinical leadership is crucial to the success of any program of this type, especially when there were unexpected findings. For example, the scope of neonatal hypoglycemia was much greater than anticipated. Partnering with the clinical leaders of the respective units allowed for a productive program as it helped to identify a problem, design and implement appropriate interventions, and then monitor the impact of these interventions.
- *Constant Clinician Involvement.* Early clinician feedback has been instrumental to the success of this program and will continue since the data and investigations represent the work that occurs on their units, and if it is not providing value to them then the product will not succeed. Clinicians now actively request the data and eagerly participate in the improvement efforts. Since this started as a grass roots program with just a few people, incorporating these clinical leaders as early as possible has increased the appetite for data derived from this program and also helped it to evolve at a more rapid pace. Once that process was well delineated and implemented, the AAED Program grew quickly, expanding to every corner of the hospital as clinical leaders realized the data could enhanced their ability to improve care.
- *Better Understanding of the Scope of Adverse Events.* The use of the AAED system greatly increased awareness of previously unrecognized adverse events. In fact, of the aforementioned 1,681 adverse events identified, only 57 (3.3 %) of these events were also documented via the Children's National web-enabled voluntary incident reporting system.
- *Creating a Fair System.* Clinicians wanted assurance that the identification of adverse events was fair and reliable. Therefore, it was stressed that this was a consistent process of evaluating each trigger in a fully objective way. Additionally, the process for classifying the errors and adverse events was a transparent system which allowed for more effective classification of events as preventable or non-preventable as well as an appropriate determination of harm level. This consistency and transparency were important in enhancing the reliability of the data as well as in ensuring the validity of the results provided to clinicians.
- *The Importance of Piloting.* Piloting the program in a test environment is useful prior to widespread dissemination. For example, the hypoglycemia trigger identified this issue across multiple patient care units. Rather than intervening in all units, the AAED Program focused on what they considered to be the greatest priority unit (NICU) with in depth investigation, intervention, design,

implementation and subsequent follow up and feedback. With success in this unit, the methodology could then be moved to secondary units.

- *Addressing Technical Barriers.* Implementing electronic queries into the EHR requires resources and patience. AAED methodology is typically not plug and play but rather requires organization-specific localization of the query tools and diligence to ensure that the queries are performing as anticipated.
- *Required Staffing.* Each investigation takes approximately 10–15 min per trigger to complete. Organizations can expect to generate at least 200–300 trigger events per month, depending on the size of their trigger library. Therefore, initial efforts generally require a few hours each day to investigate. Dedicated resources need to be available to perform this analysis.

Future Plans

At a local level there are plans to further expand the AAED Program. The first step is to increase the size of the trigger library and enhance the depth of reporting and analysis. This will allow an even better understanding of errors and adverse events as well as provide the opportunity to decrease the rate of such events. It will also necessitate an increase in the number of resources available for investigation. A second step is to allow online reporting so clinicians can view their data in real time, as well as construct unique reports on their own. This is expected to improve the clinician's use of the AAED Program data as well as increase participation in the program.

On a national front, future plans are to increase the size and scope of the nation-wide collaborative and increase the number of AAED Program triggers that each hospital is utilizing. This will lead to enhanced discussions regarding national findings, along with the most appropriate interventions to reduce the incidence and impact of errors and adverse events in children.

Conclusion

As a result of this innovative AAED Program, Children's National has experienced significant value by increasing adverse event detection resulting in widespread process improvements which have improved quality and decreased costs for patients. Automated detection of adverse events is both cost-effective and synergistic with voluntary event reporting. Organizations who currently utilize the EHR or plan to in the future can achieve significant safety value by carefully designing and implementing such a detection system. Significant triggers may now be compared across institutions to provide greater meaning and innovative solutions.

References

1. Cullen DJ, et al. The incident reporting system does not detect adverse drug events: a problem for quality improvement. Jt Comm J Qual Improv. 1995;21:541.
2. Dickerman MJ, Jacobs BR, Vinodrao H, Stockwell DC. Recognizing hypoglycemia in children through automated adverse-event detection. Pediatrics. 2011;127:e1035–41.

Section II
Meet You at 01100101

The answer is out there my dear patient, and it's looking for you, and it will find you if you want it to.

We love Facebook and Twitter. We like SMS and email. Phone is ok. Driving to an office can be iffy. The world around us is changing. How we communicate has become both increasingly simple and mind-bogglingly complex. It is faster and easier, but the modalities can be overwhelming. And the healthcare space seems to be the last of big industry to come to this digital party. With concerns about HIPAA, poorly aligned incentive systems, and fragmented data infrastructures, the digital experience is just finding its groove in healthcare.

This section thus explores the expanding options that make getting and giving care easier, quicker, and a bit more twenty-first century. As computer, webcam, and internet prices lower their sophistication, ease of use, and ubiquity rise, all conspiring to allow for a whole new high-definition world to emerge. One where data flows fast, where that slight crease across the forehead on the HDTV is an indicator that a patient is puzzled, where your weight and blood pressure are tweeted and tracked, where the distance between patient and provider no longer matters and where your language of choice is never a barrier to care. 01100101 is indeed a good place to be.

In this section we explore a "whole lotta'tele": televisit, teleconsult, telemonitoring and teletranslation. Places like Partners Healthcare, Group Health, the Veterans Health Administration, Indiana's Memorial Health System and the California HealthCare Foundation explain how they better connect patients and their providers. We end with Via Christi's twisty ride of making ePharmacist a reality. Who knew that part of the innovation was partnering with the legislature?

The key concept is clearly "tele". You should exit this section wondering, imagining and scheming on what products and services can be broken from the tyranny of four clinical walls to build interactions that are easier, smarter, and more responsive to your clinicians and patients.

Chapter 9
The Connected Patient

Jonathan S. Wald

"Well, he said I could email him. Here goes." mutters Barbara hesitantly. At her visit with Dr. Baker last week he increased her dose of Avapro, and mentioned that her A1-something was a little high. That concerned her. And then on her daily walk she started feeling a little dizzy. Could it be the A1-thing? The Avapro? Normally she would wait until her next visit mostly because she hates the back and forth phone tag. While in the waiting room last week she noticed the "Patient Gateway" poster. Then Dr. Baker mentioned it to her and she signed up as soon as she got home.

Barbara entered her logon and password into the Patient Gateway; the layout felt familiar to her from the other websites she used. She giggled thinking about the first time she used her bank's site; she felt so clumsy back then. But her daughter, the digital whiz, taught her the tips and tricks of web navigation. This was easy compared to that!

"Hmmm. What am I trying to ask him? I'm going to poke around first."

Barbara clicks on her medications, finds her new dose of Avapro, and then clicks on the medications side effects to learn a little more. "It says mild dizziness may occur." She clicks over to the Labs, and notices a test called A1C. "That's what he was talking about!" she exclaims, very satisfied with her sleuth skills. She read more about A1C, and notes that her results really are not that high. She points her cursor to the Mail Center, and begins to type:

"Dear Dr. Baker: Wanted to let you know that I immediately changed my dose of Avapro as you told me to a week ago. While walking this morning I felt dizzy. It didn't stop until I sat down and rested. Any thoughts on this? I did a little reading on the Patient Gateway and noticed that this could be a side effect. I also read a little more about A1C; and would like more information about what to do. –Barbara"

J.S. Wald, MD, MPH, FACMI
Director, Patient-Centered Technologies Center for the Advancement of Health IT,
RTI International,
1440 Main Street, Suite 310, Waltham, MA, USA
e-mail: wald.jon@gmail.com

L. Berkowitz, C. McCarthy (eds.),
Innovation with Information Technologies in Healthcare, Health Informatics,
DOI 10.1007/978-1-4471-4327-7_9, © Springer-Verlag London 2013

That night, as Barbara settles in after a long day at work, she notices a message from the Mail Center. She clicks through and is astonished to see that Dr. Baker already responded. "Are you kidding!?!? This is great! Now let's see what he has to say", she says smiling. She thinks she is going to like the Patient Gateway very much. "It's easier than banking."

Background

Partners HealthCare was founded in 1994 by Brigham and Women's Hospital and Massachusetts General Hospital. Partners is an non-profit integrated health care system that includes primary care and specialty physicians, community hospitals, the two founding academic medical centers, specialty facilities, community health centers, and other health-related entities.

The Innovation

Partners Healthcare's Patient Gateway (PG) system was one of the earliest patient portals implemented in the US. It offers patients the ability to view their medical information ("Health Record"), access relevant medical reference services ("Health Library"), and communicate with their physicians ("Mail Center") (Fig. 9.1).

In addition to this patient portal, there were two other important portals for different user groups that are part of Patient Gateway. A *support portal* was created for staff to configure practice settings in preparation for a practice "go-live" and to track and manage any patient enrollment requests submitted using online web

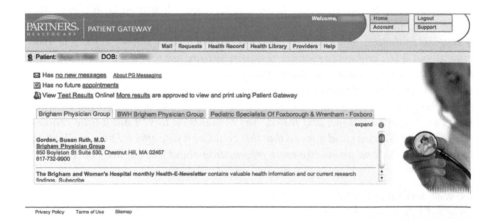

Fig. 9.1 Patient Gateway home page, including the menu options for Mail Center, Health Record, and Health Library

forms. A *practice portal* featuring message and workflow tools was created for physicians and office staff to manage incoming patient requests, create outgoing responses, set out-of-office and other automated responses, and modify web page text displayed in the patient portal.

To complement these three primary portals, an analytic dashboard was also created for metrics and reports. Individual practices were encouraged to monitor the number of patient enrollments each week, as well as the number of inbound patient requests by request type (e.g., appointment, prescription, referral, registration, or general message requests). Additional tools and sub-portals were set up, as needed, for research.

Reason for This Innovation

The idea of using the internet to connect patients directly with electronic health record (EHR) systems and to communicate with their doctors electronically surfaced in the late 1990s – as email and EHRs became more widely used in a number of hospitals and clinics. In 1999, when Partners HealthCare leadership asked what would happen if patients could directly connect with their EHR information using the internet, the Patient Gateway (PG) project was started. The recommendations presented to senior leadership in 2001 were to provide three types of "service" to patients securely via the internet that would enhance and extend services being offered to patients without the internet – communication, chart information, and medical reference information services [1].

In addition to the executive vision to embark on this project for clinical reasons, another critical driver of the Patient Gateway project was research. Funding from the Agency for Healthcare Research and Quality (AHRQ) received during 2002–2005, matched by in-kind contributions from Partners, fueled patient portal adoption, software development, and evaluation, including a number of peer-reviewed publications. New interactive tools for patients were developed and tested, including a care-planning tool to help patients with diabetes to self-report changes in their status, how they used their medications, and their agenda for the upcoming visit (Figs. 9.2 and 9.3) [2, 3].

How This Innovation Succeeded

The Patient Gateway project required a multi-disciplinary team having clinical, research, informatics, and software-development expertise. The early work led to a feasibility pilot in 2002 with a small number of practices and several hundred patients. Since patient data was involved, software development was accompanied by a review of corporate health information management policies, state and federal requirements for privacy and security, information technology protections, and practice communication policies.

ALLERGIES:

Current Allergies:

Penicillins Reaction(s): Unknown	I am unsure if this information is correct.	MD Open

DIABETES CARE:

Goals:

Blood sugar control	Is satisified; Wants to discuss medications; Wants to discuss HbA1c testing	MD Open
Cholesterol control	***Would like to improve; Wants to discuss medications; Wants to discuss cholesterol testing	MD Open
Blood pressure control	***Would like to improve; Wants to discuss medications; Wants to discuss blood pressure monitoring	MD Open

Referrals & Self-Care:

Eye care	Doesn't want to discuss; Doesn't wabt a referral;	MD Open
Foot care	Would like to discuss; Doesn't want a referral;	MD Open
Nutrition	Doesn't want to discuss; Doesn't want a referral to a nutritionist;	MD Open
Exercise program	Doesn't want to discuss; Doesn't want a specific exercise program;	MD Open
Smoking cessation	Doesn't want to discuss; Doesn't want a referral;	MD Open
Daily aspirin	Would like to discuss; Not allergic to aspirin; Doesn't take aspirin	MD Open

Fig. 9.2 Diabetes care plan self-reported by a patient (*right-hand column*) using Patient Gateway in 2006 as part of a research study (JS Wald, unpublished data)

MEDICATIONS:

Current Medications:

Ceftin (CEFUROXIME AXETIL) 500 MG by mouth twice a day	*** No longer taking (Stopped By Other, Don't Know). It was no longer needed; Don't know if PCP is aware of change;	MD Open
Gemfibrozil 600 MG (600MG TABLET take 1) by mouth twice a day	Taken as listed. *** Concerns: Yes. I'm not sure this medication is helping; Also: No trouble taking this; Not having side effects from this; I take this medication for: Cholesterol. No refill requested;	MD Open
Indocin 25 MG by mouth three times daily	*** No longer taking (Stopped By Other-Don't recall, Don't Know). It was no longer needed; Don't know if PCP is aware of change;	MD Open
Lisinopril 10 MG by mouth every day; Refills: 3	Taken as listed. Also: No trouble taking this; Not having side effects from this; I feel this medication is helping; I take this medication for: High Blood Pressure. No refill requested;	MD Done
Metformin 500 MG (500MG TABLET take 1) by mouth twice a day, one tab with breakfast for first week, then add one tab with dinner; Refills: 3	*** Changed (Changed By Other - Marcy Bergeron). Form - tablet; Strength - 500 mg tablet; Dose - 250 mg; Frequency - Twice a day Taken Regularly; Don't know if PCP is aware of change; Also: Not having side effects from this; I fell this medication is helping; I take this medication for: Diabetes. No refill requested;	MD Open

ALLERGIES:

Current Allergies:

Penicillins Reaction(s): Unknown	I am unsure if this information is correct.	MD Open

Fig. 9.3 Medications and allergy review as self-reported by a patient (*right-hand column*) using Patient Gateway in 2006 as part of a research study (JS Wald, unpublished data)

The initial project was exploratory in nature and raised many questions. People *excited* by the idea asked what would draw patients to use Patient Gateway. Would they look at chart information even if they had difficulty understanding the jargon and abbreviations? Would they send electronic messages when they should be picking up the phone or calling 9-1-1? Would using the portal create so many questions they'd need reassurance from their doctor? And, there were fears – worries that a security breach was inevitable, and that physicians and staff would be overburdened by having "one more thing" to do – especially since communicating by email with the patient wouldn't be reimbursed.

Calling the early work a "pilot" led to further questions. Was it going to be turned off after a certain period of time, or continued? What kind of resources would be needed to support and maintain the system if it remained on? Questions, such as the 5-year projected cost for the project and who should pay, were not easy to answer. The PG team needed and obtained support from senior IT leadership to proceed without charging physicians or patients, and assurances that patient needs, in addition to physician and staff needs, would be prioritized as the system evolved. The pilot went "live" in 2002 with a plan to continue providing patients with uninterrupted services, given successful projects at several other early adopter organizations. Organizational leadership was critical, as highlighted in interviews of senior leaders about patient-centered care [4].

Metrics to track the use of Patient Gateway were important for management and practice leadership. At first, metrics were used to establish baseline measurements, since no one knew how many enrollments or how much patient portal use to expect when the project began. Patient enrollments averaged 100 per month during the first year, advancing to 1,000 per month starting in year two as PG adoption expanded from 3 to 15 primary care practices, and as recruitment of patients for an AHRQ-sponsored research study began. Different practices had very different enrollment patterns, as shown for four representative primary care practices in Fig. 9.4. The reasons for variation included differences in: leadership concerns, marketing methods, service orientation, and practice incentives. These practice-driven factors were found to strongly influence the pace of patient enrollments, in addition to patient-specific influences such as age, race, socio-economic status, frequency of use of technology, and frequency of contact with physicians [5].

In 2005 an independent research firm was contracted to conduct surveys on patient and provider experiences and attitudes about PG. For the patient perspective, 300 telephone interviews were conducted among non-users, users, and registered (but never activated) users. Internal data showed that regular users (5+ logins in the last 6 months) reported the highest satisfaction with PG and the highest value in communicating with their doctor's office, receiving chart information, and placing trust in use of the system. Occasional (1–4 logins in the last 6 months) or non-current (0 logins in the last 6 months) users had lower scores in each area. Most patients reported they signed up because PG sounded convenient – like an efficient way to receive information and communicate with the practice. Some patients cited specific benefits they anticipated – like communicating more easily with their doctor or checking information in their medical record. The patient survey also identified

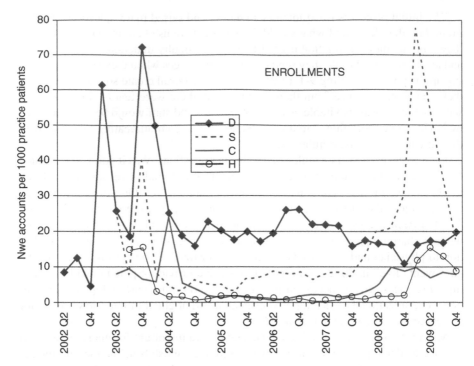

Fig. 9.4 Variations in patient enrollment at four primary care physician practices – downtown (*D*), suburban (S), on-campus (*C*), and community health center (*H*) (*Source*: Wald [5])

reasons for low satisfaction among some users. The most consistent reason was "poor response/communication from the practice". Patient requests that were unanswered or slow in being answered strongly discouraged patients from using and trusting Patient Gateway.

The results of the survey pointed to specific areas for development and improvement. Patient access by system assignment of a username and password was cumbersome and needed to be streamlined. Patients wanted to be able to select or modify their username. They also wanted more information and greater transparency in general within the 'View Health Record' feature. They reported that requesting a prescription took too many clicks. Some patients requested the ability to edit their medication list, if it was wrong, or see their doctor's schedule online. Collecting feedback from patients who used PG (at different levels) and those who did not offered invaluable information to system designers and developers.

Research interviews with practice staff were also revealing. Staff reported that the patient portal improved their ability to prioritize work tasks and be proactive with patients through the use of patient messaging tools. Staff felt they could refill prescriptions and book routine appointments more efficiently, provided a sufficient *number* of patients were enrolled in PG and had activated their account, the final step in verifying identity. Implementation staff used this information to devise better ways of quickly enrolling patients as practices went live. For example, some practices began collecting patient email addresses several months before the system was ready. Then, once the PG system was live, a "blast" email went out to invite those patients to sign up. Practices that were most effective in engaging patients to use PG used on-going marketing efforts through a variety of channels, including direct conversations, automated telephone scripts mentioning the Patient Gateway website, and quick email replies when patients used PG.

Multi-browser capabilities were introduced in early 2008, and in early 2010, the online enrollment process was enhanced significantly through the use of knowledge-based authentication (KBA), which allowed a patient who enrolled online to immediately activate their Patient Gateway account – a step that previously required them to wait several business days for a mailed password. Finally, patients could "instantly" begin using rich functionality in Patient Gateway – this was a big step forward.

Until KBA was introduced, internal usage reports showed that fully one-third of all patients who completed enrollment for PG, never activated their account. This meant that one-third of the enrollment workload for staff was wasted, and that physicians and staff could not communicate online with one-third of the patients whose names were listed as "users". Not only did the use of KBA reduce staff workload by eliminating 70 % of all online requests for enrollment from their work queue, it also promoted a high rate of account activation – over 98 % of new accounts – giving more patients a chance to try using PG features, and giving practices much higher reliability in reaching PG patients when using broadcast messages and sharing information from the EHR.

Results

Adoption. By late 2011, over 2,500 providers had offered the Patient Gateway to more than 200,000 patients, with new enrollments exceeding 6,000 patients per month. Practice reports helped practice leadership track their progress in using a variety of marketing activities ranging from automated telephone messages to direct mailings to encourage patients to enroll. A few words of introduction from a trusted physician or staff member were often the most effective way to interest a patient in signing up for PG. In 2008, summer contests were held to challenge staff members to sign up 300 patients in 8 weeks – with great success in some practices (Fig. 9.5).

Patient Benefits. For the patient, the benefits of Patient Gateway range from simple efficiencies to more complex and indirect value. Patients are *delighted* at how easily they can look at lab results, medication lists, radiology reports, immunizations, appointments, and other information that in the past was easily lost or misplaced, or required a time-consuming phone call (or "telephone tag") with the doctor's office to obtain. Having even basic information through Patient Gateway provides value in many different ways, depending on the context and use of the information. In a 2005 internal telephone survey of 100 regular users of Patient

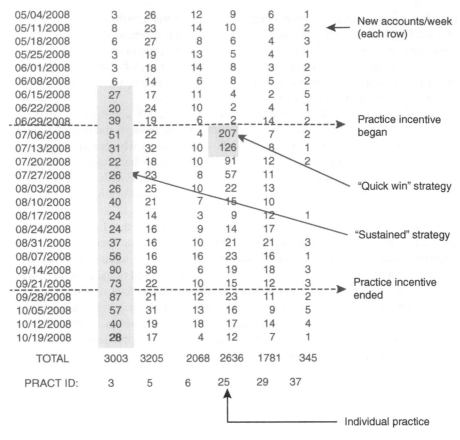

05/04/2008	3	26	12	9	6	1
05/11/2008	8	23	14	10	8	2
05/18/2008	6	27	8	6	4	3
05/25/2008	3	19	13	5	4	1
06/01/2008	3	18	14	8	3	2
06/08/2008	6	14	6	8	5	2
06/15/2008	27	17	11	4	2	5
06/22/2008	20	24	10	2	4	1
06/29/2008	39	19	6	2	14	2
07/06/2008	51	22	4	207	7	2
07/13/2008	31	32	10	126	8	1
07/20/2008	22	18	10	91	12	2
07/27/2008	26	23	8	57	11	
08/03/2008	26	25	10	22	13	
08/10/2008	40	21	7	15	10	
08/17/2008	24	14	3	9	12	1
08/24/2008	24	16	9	14	17	
08/31/2008	37	16	10	21	21	3
08/07/2008	56	16	16	23	16	1
09/14/2008	90	38	6	19	18	3
09/21/2008	73	22	10	15	12	3
09/28/2008	87	21	12	23	11	2
10/05/2008	57	31	13	16	9	5
10/12/2008	40	19	18	17	14	4
10/19/2008	28	17	4	12	7	1
TOTAL	3003	3205	2068	2636	1781	345
PRACT ID:	3	5	6	25	29	37

New accounts/week (each row)

Practice incentive began

"Quick win" strategy

"Sustained" strategy

Practice incentive ended

Individual practice

Fig. 9.5 Increased patient enrollment during a practice "contest" to add 300 new patients over a 12-week period (JS Wald, unpublished data)

Gateway, 84 % felt it was a safe and secure way to access personal medical information and communicate with their doctor, 76 % felt PG was a good and reliable source of information on medical conditions and diseases, and 81 % reported that the breadth of things they can do on the website satisfied their needs. Positive patient feedback peaked with the Lab Results feature, as represented by this typical patient message received in May 2006: "Fantastic improvement. Being able to see my labs is very important to me. Thanks."

In many cases, the information simply helps the patient *to understand*. Engaging in health activities is a constant learning process, and patients need both trusted sources of information as well as cognitive strategies and supports for learning and remembering what's important. For example, so much information is covered during an office visit – with as much as 62 % lost to recall [6] – that the patient portal serves a critical role as a simple memory aid for the patient, family members, and any caregivers authorized by the patient to access their information. By linking reference information to the patient's chart information, Patient Gateway supports a patient who is trying to make a decision or take action – to deal with a new symptom, learn about a condition, consider a new medication, or discuss their overall health status with a loved one. Speed is important – the patient portal helps the patient find many different kinds of information - fast! Patients and caregivers place a high value on having the right information at just the right time to support their actions. Internal analysis of 1,093 Results Letters sent electronically to Patient Gateway users from their provider in 2009 showed they were read quickly: 72 % on the same day, 85 % within 1 day, and 95 % within 5 days.

Physician and Staff Benefits. Patient Gateway also directly serves physicians and office staff by helping them to communicate effectively with patients. Physicians and staff can easily send specific recommendations, clinical reminders, informational bulletins, and follow-up after procedures and office visits to patients using Patient Gateway. The more patients they enroll, the more valuable the tool becomes. Many patients report feeling greater trust and a stronger connection with their doctor using a patient portal, according to multiple surveys [7, 8]. Patient portals also play a prominent role in helping physician offices to satisfy Meaningful Use criteria since they provide a secure means for providing patients with timely access to chart data such as lab results and problem lists, offering tailored patient education materials, and supporting electronic data extracts [9].

Quality Benefits. In many cases, small details of care can make a big difference such as fixing an inaccurate medication dose or noticing that a lab test should have been performed. Patient Gateway allows a "second or third set of eyes" to notice whether information is accurate, complete, and considered during a medical decision. Stories abound of patients who play a pivotal role in the quality of their medical care, such as by reading the details of their own radiology report and noticing incidental findings their primary care physician missed [10, 11], or correcting medication information in their record, which is often inaccurate [12]. A patient's family member receiving only vague information from the patient about their last doctor's appointment can learn (with permission) from the patient portal about details of the visit and how to support the patient in understanding what their doctor has recommended.

Specialized interactive pre-visit tools for patients have great promise for improving care. In 2005, as part of an AHRQ-sponsored research study of patient portals and quality of care, 2027 consented patients were offered a new electronic journal (eJournal) module of Patient Gateway. Three weeks before a scheduled office visit, each patient was prompted to review information from their doctor's chart including medications, allergies, diabetes results, family history, and health monitoring data (e.g. cholesterol, Pap smear, pneumovax, etc.). By study protocol, patients received some but not all medical chart topics. Seventy-one percent of 1,052 patients submitted medication information concerning 4,935 medications (a mean of 6.6 medications per patient), adding new details for their physician 98 % of the time. Forty-eight patients with diabetes submitted 419 diabetes-related updates (mean of 8.7 items per patient), communicating new status information to their physician 84 % of the time. Many patients reported benefits from using the eJournal: 75 % would complete one again if offered; 67 % would recommend eJournals to a friend; 58 % felt

their provider had more accurate information about them; and 56 % felt more prepared for the visit. About one-third felt their communication improved during the
visit and felt more satisfied with the visit – an important finding for practices striv-
ing to improve patient satisfaction [13].

Efficiency Benefits. Many patients and doctor's offices that use Patient Gateway
gain efficiency. Getting questions answered is faster and simpler with Patient
Gateway compared to using the telephone because it is non-interruptive (asynchronous) communication that fits into the workflow of clinical and administrative staff.
Required information in prescription refill and appointment request forms ensure
that practice staff receives more fully completed requests from patients, which
require less time and fewer call-backs to manage. Automatic replies and templates
allow staff to rapidly respond to messages from patients. And unlike phone calls,
everyone – especially the patient – can re-read a message at any time, since the Mail
Center automatically creates permanent documentation of the message exchange.
Physicians especially appreciate when clinical advice and patient information from
messages can be quickly saved as a "progress note" in the EHR in much less time
than a phone call. Efficiency gains are not guaranteed, however – they are very sensitive to workflow and volume. Patient Gateway requests and messages take longer
to handle if not streamlined into a staff's workflow, and even quick handling of a
message will not improve efficiency noticeably unless many messages are managed
that way.

The medical practice also uses Patient Gateway to streamline operations and
improve service. Flu shot reminders and other practice information, such as the
addition of a new specialist or holiday hours, can be posted and broadcast to patients
easily. The more patients are signed up, the more quickly lab test results and doctor
letters are received. Some practices have stopped mailing certain follow-up letters if
they see that the patient viewed the online copy, and tracking reports allow doctors
to know whether an important communication, such as a follow-up recommendation for another mammogram, was read. As more patient requests are submitted
online, telephones and staff time are freed for use by patients without access to
Patient Gateway and for issues that are better discussed by phone.

Lessons Learned

Our experience with an EHR-connected patient portal offered many lessons about
innovation among physician groups, practice staff, and patients.

Physician hopes and concerns. Early in the project, physician groups volun-
teering to become early adopters of the Patient Gateway shared their hopes and
concerns (Table 9.1).

Physician buy-in. Physician hopes reflected their genuine interest in providing
better service, better communication, and more transparent information. Their concerns, overall, reflected their uncertainty about having to take more time to support

Table 9.1 Physician hopes and concerns commonly shared during pre-implementation Patient Gateway discussions

Feature	Physician hopes and concerns
Lab Results	*Hope:* Patients would love having quick access to lab results and other chart information without always having to contact practice physicians or staff.
	Concern: Patients would feel anxious receiving "news" from the computer instead of their doctor.
	Resolution: Physician concerns typically fade quickly with experience sharing lab results electronically, since a very tiny fraction of patients are dissatisfied with this feature, and they can simply opt out of using it.
Mail Center	*Hope:* Patients would communicate simple requests more easily to staff and physicians, and receive quick responses. Physicians and staff would find it efficient to use web mail with patients.
	Concern: A large volume of patient requests would consume the time of busy staff and physicians. Some patients would send lengthy or inappropriate (e.g., time urgent) messages via web mail, creating liability.
	Resolution: Once physicians realize that it is rare to receive inappropriate messages, their concerns diminish greatly.
Health Library	*Hope:* Patients would more easily answer basic questions about their lab results and other health concerns.
	Concern: Self-service information might not agree with physician advice tailored for a specific patient, leading to patient confusion.
	Resolution: Physician concerns subside when they realize that patient information sources and physician recommendations often do not exactly agree, but the Health Library tool has no noticeable impact.
Access	*Hope:* All my patients will sign up!
	Concern: Many of my patients will not sign up – because they do not use computers, or are non-English speaking.
	Resolution: Physicians are in a unique position to introduce the patient portal and state its value to non-users. Physicians who do this routinely are best able to maximize the number of their patients who *do* sign up, as well as identify the biggest limitations that patients experience – and ask system designers to address them when possible.

patients in using PG without reimbursement or a reduction in other types of their work. Additionally, concerned or fearful physicians were less likely to talk about PG with their patients, encourage their staff to educate patients about it, or use it spontaneously with patients. Even though the physician was not essential to initial configuration and go-live of the system, their enthusiasm was crucial for subsequent marketing and adoption by patients.

Marketing approach. The PG team learned that a good strategy for marketing PG to patients was for their physician to tell them about it personally. "Got email? Got Internet? Get Patient Gateway." was quick and effective. Hearing about PG from staff or a trusted friend or family member also worked well, as did automated telephone prompts that advised callers to visit www.patientgateway.org to sign up. Among physicians who already used their own personal email with their patients, adding an "auto-signature" that included information about Patient Gateway was also easy to do and effective.

Whole-practice adoption. Adoption of PG by the entire physician practice was critical for increased patient adoption. In some cases, only one or two physicians in a practice initially wanted to offer PG to their patients, and the others did not. Whenever this was done, it created additional challenges. As a communication tool, the PG system routes patient requests to appropriate staff who handle prescription requests, appointment requests, messages from patients, lab results, etc. If only certain staff in the practice used PG and others did not, it was difficult for messages to be handled efficiently and reliably using PG. Selective physician adoption also created marketing challenges, since posters in the waiting room, information cards at the front desk, and other types of marketing were aimed at all patients, rather than targeted to specific patients of participating physicians within a practice. If a practice insisted on starting the adoption of PG with one or two physicians, the implementation team would usually agree to a time-limited pilot period of 1–2 months, followed by a decision to adopt fully or turn the system off. This allowed practice leaders to experiment with workflows and marketing activities before launching full use of the patient portal.

Transparent data is more trusted. Transparent patient information turned out to be powerful motivation to improve chart data quality. As one practice prepared to go-live they insisted that the patient medication list should *not* be shown to the patient via PG – a big surprise considering that patients already knew the medications they were taking (or…were supposed to!) and physicians had asked for this feature for their patients. The practice physicians who objected explained that the medication information they kept up to date was in the *progress notes*, rather than in the EHR medication list. Since PG displayed the medication list (not the progress note information) to the patient, it would be wrong. Concerned about causing patient confusion or distrust if they displayed an empty or outdated medication list, physicians asked to turn off that feature. A few months after go-live, having had time to correct the inaccurate medication lists, the feature was turned on. Having patients view EHR data using PG was a strong motivator to physicians and staff to maintain accurate, high quality, medication lists.

Value for each patient. We learned that there were many, many different reasons that patients used Patient Gateway, and identifying the needs of patient subgroups was important. While all patients appreciated having lab results available, cancer patients asked for the specific tumor markers to be released, based on their treatment protocol. Patients taking few medications found the renewal request forms to be satisfactory, whereas patients renewing multiple medications found them to be cumbersome because they looped through pharmacy information repeatedly, with each medication. Sometimes lab results were missing for the patient – because their doctor's office used a non-Partners laboratory that did not feed results into the data repository connected to Patient Gateway. Some patients already emailed their doctor directly, and did not feel that communicating via PG provided any advantages to them.

Spontaneous patient feedback and survey data showed strong enthusiasm for Patient Gateway, and some concerns, too. Patients asked for additional chart information such as echocardiograms that were in the EHR but not shown in PG. Some asked to download their chart data so they could maintain their own electronic copy and use it as they wished. And they asked for access to PG on the Macintosh computer or using web browsers besides Microsoft's Internet Explorer.

Appropriate patient use of messaging. An important observation – counter to many physicians' expectations – was that the volume of electronic messages received from patients was low. This was repeated (the physician fears, and the actual low volume) as practice after practice adopted Patient Gateway. Only 50 % of patients with an activated PG account *ever* used the messaging feature. Patients who sent a message using Patient Gateway often expressed lots of respect and appreciation when they did hear back from their doctor. This clearly signaled that for patients, PG is a relationship tool. They use it to maintain their connection with the doctor's office and with their doctor, specifically. And their trust in using PG is likely linked strongly to their overall trust in the reliability of the information and communication they receive from their doctor's office.

User needs. Just as patients have different clinical needs, their preferences in using technology to address those needs also varied. Some felt strongly that the system must support patient-entered data such as observations about their symptoms, their treatment regimens, and discrepancies they found in their EHR data, whereas others showed little or no interest in these kinds of tools. Some patients had no interest in using Patient Gateway. Rather than try to satisfy all people equally, the PG team learned that it's important to do certain things very well, especially to support people (patients, doctors, staff) in their performance of care activities.

Product oversight. The team responsible for managing the development and adoption of Patient Gateway was constantly learning new things. An early focus was making sure that the enrollment process was simple for patients and support staff. Shaving clicks and steps from the process made it simpler, reduced the number of support issues generated by patients, and improved product maintenance and troubleshooting.

Service. Practice leaders also understood that even if the product functioned correctly, the patient would have a bad experience if practice staff did not handle patient messages consistently and efficiently. A number of mechanisms were created to set consistent expectations with patients and practice staff, alike. Patients were advised that messages were only received and processed during business hours – not on weekends or holidays. Staff were shown how to monitor message "aging" and use out-of-office settings to help avoid missed messages and frustrated patients.

Embargo periods for lab results. Lab results policies were discussed among an expert panel of clinicians to set embargo periods (the days until a lab result was shared online with the patient). It was often difficult to reach agreement among primary care, specialist, and sub-specialist physicians about the embargo period. We often advised the group to select the smallest time period possible in support of greater access and transparency, knowing that some patients might become anxious from seeing results too soon, while others would be frustrated with too much delay. Many lab results were released immediately, about one-third had a 2-business-day delay, some were actively blocked from release (e.g., genetic tests), and a small number were held for 30 days (e.g., Lyme titers requiring special interpretation and

Table 9.2 Product management hopes and concerns before Patient Gateway, an EHR-Connected Patient Portal, had achieved widespread adoption

Feature	Product management hopes and concerns
Enrollment	*Hope:* The enrollment process will be secure, yet simple and self-evident to first-time users, creating few support requests and satisfying patients.
	Concern: Too many patient support issues will overwhelm support staff and frustrate new enrollees.
	Resolution: Careful usage and support data identified steps in the process that caused confusion or led to abandonment. Changes in the enrollment process were evaluated by measuring account activation rates. Eventually, a new "Get Access Now" online authentication method proved extremely effective at improving activation rates.
Mail Center	*Hope:* Staff will respond quickly to patient messages, reinforcing their trust in using the system instead of phoning the practice.
	Concern: Staff will not respond to messages in a timely way, leading to patient frustration, reduced staff buy-in, and lower adoption.
	Resolution: Dashboards were created to help monitor message response latency and notify staff if service levels were not being met. Most issues were resolved with additional staff training.
Lab Results	*Hope:* Patient access to chart data will improve understanding and communication between patients and providers.
	Concern: Policies will overly delay patient online access to lab results, reducing the value to patients and physicians.
	Resolution: Lab result release policies were generally made consistent with other health systems offering similar features.
Workflow	*Hope:* The use of Patient Gateway by practice staff and physicians will support their workflow as they use the ambulatory EHR.
	Concern: Given variations in workflow, some users will not find the Patient Gateway tools – especially the messaging component – easy to use.
	Resolution: Optimizing workflow is an ongoing process – difficult for some physicians and staff, and easy for others. Addressing practice-to-patient communication and information sharing is an important area, no matter what technology is used.

consultation). Other types of information followed specific policies, such as an embargo period of 5 business days for most radiology reports. Over time, there is pressure for embargo periods to shorten as patients demand greater access, health care reform regulations and incentives reward data sharing, and increased electronic exchange of data lowers access barriers.

Product management focus. The PG team, including analysts, developers, implementation staff, and support staff identified a number of areas of potential concern before go-live with Patient Gateway, as shown in Table 9.2. A large number of decisions had to be made early in the project, ranging from establishing new enrollment procedures, to lab result embargo policies, to policies for staff monitoring of patient requests. Coordinating the approach to identifying and addressing these challenges required a strong product management approach – in which business requirements, user priorities, support team observations, and product plans were surfaced and shared across the team, frequently. Often, a software enhancement request identified the need for better training rather than changes to the software. Or, a patient support issue pointed to something that was confusing on the website and could be easily changed. Very often, contributions from technical staff to the support team, or implementation staff to the design team, proved critical in understanding and addressing an issue, and highlighted the continuous learning taking place across team members, users, and managers (Table 9.2).

Access policies. Over time, access policies for PG have evolved. During enrollment, a patient must identify a practice and a physician (from the list of available practices and physicians) to start using PG. However, since physicians sometimes leave practices, and patients sometimes transfer their care elsewhere, there are times when patients are still accessing PG even though they no longer receive care at a Partners practice. Should these registrations be continued? If so, would it make sense to allow any patient with a medical record to use PG, even if they don't have a provider currently? As additional features are added, such as access to financial data, the individuals who should be granted access to Patient Gateway are likely to broaden. It's important for access policies and other product policies to be reviewed and updated as PG use extends over time and new issues surface.

Trust. Overall, the introduction of PG involves changes to people, processes, and technologies. We've learned that getting patients connected and having them *stay* connected requires meaningful interactions with information and people they access using the system. Trust in the system by provider and patients was critical to its success - ans requires close attention. If the tools, processes and security are unreliable, trust in the system will fracture. Orchestrating priorities among multiple stakeholders is critical. Also, as the functionality and use of Patient Gateway matures, there is greater need for direct patient involvement in its governance.

Future Plans

With Internet use in the United States exceeding 85 % of all Americans, consumer and medical adoption of smart phones and mobile technologies accelerating dramatically, and health IT becoming mainstream, patient-centered tools and approaches to care are becoming a core component of healthcare for both patients and medical professionals [4].

Patient portal information will grow to include physician progress notes, all laboratory test results, digital copies of scanned reports from anywhere in the hospital or physician practice, and volumes of administrative data, insurer and benefits management data, and financial information. Much of the shared data will benefit patients through greater transparency, but unintended consequences will also rise. Medical claim billing codes offer a good example of this challenge: the same code used for "rule out cancer" is also used for "patient has cancer". The challenge of secondary use of data will grow as more data sources become available to patients and clinicians alike. Addressing digital divide issues to allow access for all will continue as a priority [16].

New services will emerge, similar to other consumer systems. For example, patients will have care reminder emails to help them with their daily routine (e.g. medication reminders) and periodic care (e.g. upcoming vaccines, visits, follow-up referrals, etc.). Third-party applications offering more options will challenge "monolithic" patient portal systems, providing greater choice to patients and greater advantage to systems that can offer interfaces to data services, security services, and communication services. Patient-generated data through environmental sensors (e.g., location in the home), wearable and portable devices for capturing physiologic and subjective data directly from patients, and real-time analysis tools available for individual or patient community use will impact patient self-management and care delivered by health professionals. Greater data sharing and exchange will accelerate interest in standards development, lowering the cost and complexity of critical systems interfaces and improving the quality of automated decision aids.

Future research will focus on more sophisticated tailoring of information and decision support for patients, based on a combination of patient clinical data from multiple sources, physician practice data, actuarial and predictive data, and other factors such as patient/family preferences and cost. Models for patient behavior and motivation will continue to shape technology, which will become more and more "persuasive" [14], leading to improvements in the way a patient receives, interprets, and acts upon information relating to a health concern. Spoken words, videos, and tailored descriptions, along with more sophisticated tools to adapt to an individual's level of health literacy will be critical [15].

Expanded patient-sourced, community-sourced, and crowd-sourced information and tools will enable patients to examine patient portal data for errors or safety risks, complete symptom checklists, provide family medical history, assess pain, and manage home regimens for prevention, exercise, and nutrition. With patient self-management capabilities strengthened through information transparency and timely communication, physicians will work more effectively with better-informed patients and caregivers. Errors that result from medication discrepancies or communication missteps will be easier to avoid or correct quickly – especially during patient-care "handoffs" such as hospital discharges that are known to be error-prone today.

Advanced features and services will also create integration challenges: how will the patient and their family find one tool, or just a few tools, to perform the activities they find most relevant? Simplifying various communication, data capture, social interaction, and care management tasks through useful and usable applications on mobile and other platforms makes this consideration a critical one for the future as well.

Conclusion

A patient portal provides a platform for supporting the way each patient, physician, and organization improves communication, information sharing, and decision-making. Like any multifunction tool, its use and impact vary based on the task, the decisions, and the differing roles and skills of its users. An individual patient using a patient portal can improve their ability to remember, to organize, to follow through, and to manage health-related tasks. A health team, including all its individual stakeholders – patients, caregivers, physicians, nurses, etc. – can reduce delays and errors due to missing information and poor communication, substantially improving their effectiveness.

The benefits of using a patient portal – savings in time, reduced delays, greater access to key pieces of information, more robust communication – are accomplished through improvements in the underlying processes of care, whether provided by others or by the patients, themselves. Patient questions don't require weeks to get answered (if not forgotten entirely); using email, they are answered without delay. Concerns about lab test results, medication side effects, and whether a diagnosis is confirmed are identified more easily because chart information is transparent to patients and their stakeholders. Physicians can encourage their patients to prepare for a visit or follow-up more effectively after a visit by encouraging use of the patient portal, and can maintain contact to reinforce patient engagement. In aggregate, many small changes in doctor-patient interactions and patient learning create improvements in both the experience of care and the quality of care for patients – changes that may be missed using typical metrics such as patient portal access or message counts. Even those who access their patient portal infrequently feel strongly it's a service they don't want to lose.

Patient portals offer substantial tools for patients to fully engage as partners in their own care – placing not just professionals, but patients, in the innovation driver's seat. They provide a big step toward the mantra of *'nothing about me without me'* developed by a group of visionary patients and stakeholders in 2001 [17]. By addressing two critical barriers – timely patient access to information, and simple ways to communicate across key individuals, the patient portal offers a substantial step forward in providing not just information for patients and their stakeholders, but information that is "actionable".

References

1. Wald JS, Pedraza LA, Reilly CA, et al. Requirements development for a patient computing system. Proc AMIA Symp. 2001;731–735.
2. Grant RW, Wald JS, Poon EG, et al. Design and implementation of a web-based patient portal linked to an ambulatory care electronic health record: patient gateway for diabetes collaborative care. Diabetes Technol Ther. 2006;8:576–86.
3. Grant RW, Wald JS, Schnipper JL, et al. Practice-linked online personal health records for type 2 diabetes: a randomized controlled trial. Arch Int Med. 2008;168(16):1776–82.
4. Luxford K, Safran DG, Delbanco T. Promoting patient-centered care: a qualitative study of facilitators and barriers in healthcare organizations with a reputation for improving the patient experience. Int J Qual Health Care. 2011;23(5):510–5.
5. Wald JS. Variations in patient portal adoption in four primary care practices. AMIA Annu Symp Proc. 2010;2010:837–41.
6. Aspden P. Preventing medication errors. Institute of medicine report from the committee on identifying and preventing medication errors. Washington, DC: National Academies Press; 2007. p. 182.

7. Westin AF. Markle foundation report: Americans overwhelmingly believe electronic personal health records could improve their health. 2008 Report from a nationwide survey conducted by knowledge networks and developed by Alan F. Westin, Professor at Columbia University. At: http://www.markle.org/sites/default/files/ResearchBrief-200806.pdf. Accessed on 15 Aug 2011.

8. Undem T, et al. Consumers and health information technology: a national survey. California HealthCare Foundation, 2010. At: http://www.chcf.org/publications/2010/04/consumers-and-health-information-technology-a-national-survey. Accessed on 15 Aug 2011.

9. Blumenthal D, Tavenner M. The meaningful use regulation for electronic health records. N Eng J Med. 2010;363:501–4.

10. Cohen ES, editor. The empowered patient: How to get the diagnosis right, buy the cheapest drugs, beat your insurance company, and get the best medical care every time. New York: Ballantine Books; 2010. p. 65.

11. CNN news video from June 5, 2008 spotlighting Doug Smith, a Vanderbilt Medical Center patient, using their patient portal, MyHealthAtVanderbilt. At: http://www.youtube.com/watch?v=gKX1xtXgdzA. Accessed on 15 Aug. 2011.

12. Kaboli PJ, McClimon BJ, Hoth AB, et al. Assessing the accuracy of computerized medication histories. Am J Manag Care. 2004;10(2):872–7.

13. Wald JS, Businger A, Gandhi TK, Grant RW, Poon EG, Schnipper JL, Volk LA, Middleton B. Implementing practice-linked previsit electronic journals in primary care: patient and physician use and satisfaction. JAMIA. 2010;17(5):502–6.

14. Fogg BJ. A behavior model for persuasive design. Presented at a conference, Persuasive '09 26–29 Apr, Claremont. 2009 ACM ISBN 978-1-60558-376-1/09/04.

15. U.S. Department of Health and Human Services, Office of Disease Prevention and Health Promotion. National action plan to improve health literacy. Washington, DC: Author; 2010.

16. Yamin CK, Emani S, Williams DH, et al. The digital divide in adoption and use of a personal health record. Arch Int Med. 2011;171(6):568–74.

17. Delbanco T, Berwick DM, Boufford JI, et al. Healthcare in a land called peoplepower: nothing about me without me. Health Expect. 2001;4:144–50.

Chapter 10
The Virtual Consult

Erin DeMarce Leff, Marc Mora, Gwendolyn B. O'Keefe, Tim Scearce, and James Hereford

Fourteen-year-old Cindy was running hard for the ball at lacrosse practice when she crashed into a teammate and fell to the ground with a thump. "Mom!" she screams. Cindy's mom, Barbara, seeing her injured daughter splayed out on the field, comes running to her aid, and quickly realizes that the Urgent Care Clinic is in their immediate future. "Oh, not again," she sighs to herself. Barbara and her family seem to be repeat customers these days.

While sitting in the waiting room, Barbara starts thinking about all the "personal time off" that she doesn't have, and starts wondering how her family is going to manage.

E.D. Leff, B.A., M.B.A.
Specialty Services, Group Health Cooperative,
320 Westlake Ave N # 100, Seattle, WA 98124-1590, USA
e-mail: leff.e@ghc.org

M. Mora, M.D.
Consultative Specialty Services, Group Health Medical Centers,
201 16th Avenue East, D634, Seattle, WA 98112, USA
e-mail: mora.mw@ghc.org

G.B. O'Keefe, M.D. (✉)
Group Health Permanente, Quality and Informatics,
320 Westlake Avenue N. Suite 100, Seattle, WA 98109, USA
e-mail: okeefe.g@ghc.org

T. Scearce, M.D.
Department of Neurology, Group Health Permanente,
Group Health Cooperative, Medical Informatics,
320 Westlake Ave. N. Suite 100, Seattle, WA 98109-5233, USA
e-mail: scearce.t@ghc.org

J. Hereford, M.S. Mathematics
Palo Alto Medical Foundation, 2350 W. El Camino Real, Mountain View, CA 94040, USA
e-mail: herefoj@pamf.org

L. Berkowitz, C. McCarthy (eds.),
Innovation with Information Technologies in Healthcare, Health Informatics,
DOI 10.1007/978-1-4471-4327-7_10, © Springer-Verlag London 2013

In Dr. Albert's exam room, Barbara is becoming increasingly nervous. "Barbara, since Cindy is such an active athlete, seeing an orthopedist would be recommended. I can get you an appointment for tomorrow, if that's ok."

"I can't take Cindy to the orthopedist – I can't take anyone to any more visits until after school gets out!" yelps Barbara as she bursts into tears.

Feeling terrible, Dr. Albert remembers another option, "How about we do a Virtual Consult? We can get an expert opinion without the need for a face-to-face visit or you missing any more work." He sends a secure EMR message with his questions to the Orthopedist, with a link to the patients' chart. Within 30 min, he has a response to his question clearly documented as a "virtual" encounter. The Orthopedist reviewed the x-rays and Dr. Albert's exam, and is confident that he can describe the plan of care so that Dr. Albert and the family can follow it without Cindy needing to see him in person.

"Thank you for making this easy," says a more relaxed Barbara. "I had visions of days more of missed work. Sorry for breaking down earlier."

"When do I get to play again?" asks Cindy without looking up from her texting.

Background

Group Health Cooperative is a consumer-governed integrated delivery system established in 1947 that provides care and coverage for over 600,000 members in 26 locations across the state of Washington. Group Health employs approximately 1,200 physicians and other care providers. The Epic electronic medical record (EMR) system was implemented in 2003 with a shared patient record, secure messaging, and patient portal as an integral part of the record from the very first day.

The Innovation

In 2010, Group Health modified their EMR system to allow for "Virtual Consults," which involve asynchronous communication between physicians, either between Primary Care and a Specialist, or between Specialists. The intended use is for medical questions about ongoing or new clinical concerns and for fully documenting care that does not require a face-to-face interaction between the patient and the consulted physician. The response to the initial consult request happens quickly (often within 1–2 h, but always within 24 h), is formally documented in the medical record, and is recognized by the corporate entity and incentivized. See Fig. 10.1 as an example of a virtual consult completed by Neurology for a headache patient. Figure 10.2 then shows the "dummy" level of service (LOS) assigned by the provider completing the consult, which allows for reporting and relative value unit (RVU) assignment for service compensation. This internal assignment allows clinical and operational leaders to track the "value" of the intervention in a way that

Reason for consultation: Dr. Smith posed the following question: "I have a 35 year old woman with migraines and now daily headaches for two months. She is using Excedrin migraine every day. Head CT scan is normal. What recommendations do you have? Should I refer her to see you?"

The virtual consult is provided based on my review of the clinical question as formulated by the clinician named above. I am providing advice based on general principles of medicine as well as information provided to me in the clinical question above and focused review of the electronic medical record.

Assessment: Probable rebound headaches due to overuse of OTC pain medication
What to do now: Begin weaning off Excedrin, suggest that patient begin keeping a headache journal to track occurrences and symptoms
What to do next: Follow up via secure message, see in clinic in 2 weeks, sooner if symptoms worsen
When to refer to specialty: If headaches do not improve after 6-8 weeks, please re-consult virtually or we would be happy to see her for a consultation in Neurology.

Tim Scearce, MD
CSC Neurology

Fig. 10.1   Example of a virtual consult completed by neurology for a headache patient

Fig. 10.2   The "dummy" level of service (LOS) assigned by the provider completing the consult, which allows for reporting and RVU assignment

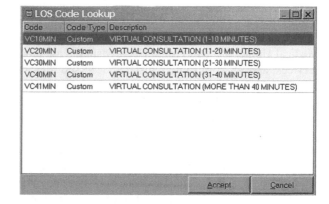

allows Group Health's prepaid model of care to compare and contrast performance relative to volume or RVU based models of care. For instance, in measuring a provider's total productivity to compare with industry norms, one could add the visit based RVUs to the "dummy" RVUs for virtual care to obtain a total measure of productivity.

Reason for This Innovation

Shared patient care is a pillar of Group Health's integrated group practice, so part of the early EMR configuration was to create consult "pools" for the majority of specialties. Primary care doctors could send messages to these pools and a specialist responsible for that pool that day would respond. As a result, routine use of messaging between Primary Care physicians and specialists for asynchronous consultation became a common occurrence. However, almost all of this virtual care was undocumented and, therefore, not valued from a business perspective. Additionally, this type of care was often not taken into account during subsequent clinical encounters.

During this same period, Group Health recognized that the current healthcare system was unsustainable and was particularly hard on primary care physicians, due to increasing clinical demands coupled with EMR-related inefficiencies. So in 2008, Group Health invested $10 million dollars in the development of a Medical Home system, which was rolled out across all of Group Health's clinics in 2009 and 2010.

The overall Medical Home project increased the total number of primary care providers, who are salaried in Group Health's model. The time they could spend with each patient per visit was increased, and time was allowed in the day for virtual visits with patients instead of making them come to the office. Group Health's focus is on total cost of care, or a value based model, rather than in visit volumes to drive revenues. Investments were targeted toward primary-care-population based management strategies and virtual care that resulted in a positive return on investment to Group Health overall in the first year due to decreased ER visits and hospitalizations [1].

Due to the focus on increasing patients' adoption of online services as part of the Medical Home, 65 % of Group Health patients are now registered to utilize online services, and 95 % of those registered accessed their online account during 2011. Therefore, it has becoming increasingly common for primary care physicians to do virtual visits with their patients. Meanwhile, specialists observed that a critical part of the Medical Home involved their provision of virtual advice to both patients and primary care physicians via the shared EMR system. Specialists thus clamored for similar standardization and reimbursement of this work they were already doing. Recognition of this by both Specialty leadership and executive leaders led to the decision to develop a standard virtual consult encounter within the EMR. The goal was to create a single solution that would help close both clinical and business practices gaps related to the less standardized messaging system that was in place. Implementation of virtual consults represented the next logical step in the journey to improve integration and communication in the multispecialty group and create additional alternatives to the direct office visit.

Why This Innovation Succeeded

The success of this innovation was due to multiple factors.

Value based Reimbursement. The most important factor was likely Group Health's structure for physician employment - which is that all physicians are employed in a salaried status by the Medical Group. In addition, the linkage of coverage through provision of insurance in a capitated reimbursement model allowed for more focus on the overall care of the patient, rather than on episodic face-to-face visits. Specifically, as part of Group Health's model of integrated care and insurance coverage, physicians are not penalized by a loss of revenue when they provide care that avoids an office visit. Additionally, management recognized the need for time for completion of virtual work and allocated it to occur in the daily schedule.

Lean Process Methodology. Group Health's Medical Home processes were all developed using Lean process improvement techniques and monitoring. The workflow for the Virtual Consult was just as important as the creation of the encounter, and involved collaboration between Primary Care and Specialty. The workflow was developed by a cross functional group that included specialty and primary care users, IT and informatics leaders, local clinic mangers, and was led by a physician champion. Lean Process Improvement methodology was utilized for both technology and workflow development in a Rapid Process Improvement Workshop (RPIW) held with formal and informal leaders from both Primary Care and Specialty. The design process, which involved these frontline staff and leaders, led to agreements established **between** the groups that were critical to development of trust and initiating use of the encounter.

The usual RPIW format involves process walks of current state, design of a future state and immediate test and feedback. In order to incorporate the technology, this format had to be modified to allow for the technical work that needed to be done but could not be completed real-time during the RPIW. Modeled after an earlier prototype, the technical framework would allow the workshop participants to see the possibilities and still be able to fine-tune the specific design, working with the system analysts during the workshop.

This empowered the teams to be able to visualize barriers and devise methods to overcome them. The Lean process of first designing the workflow with the people who do the work, and second adding in the technology component, sped up the design and acceptance of the model. Primary care physicians did not have to change their previous workflows with respect to how they requested input from specialists – they continued to send messages to the same Specialty pool and work was divided up based on that Specialty's workplan. This made implementation much easier.

Physician Scheduling. Physicians are allocated time during the day to complete their virtual consult work. This varied by specialty, but typically blocks of appointment time that had been used for face-to-face visits were set aside for virtual consult. In some areas this is also used as part of the on-call regimen as team leaders were encouraged and empowered to identify how they wanted to allocate their virtual consult time in a way that worked within the flow of the clinic and their schedules.

Executive Sponsorship was very important to the success of the project, given the anticipated political challenges. Initial executive sponsorship came from the Executive Vice President (EVP) for the Medical Group, and from the EVP for the IT organization. They ensured that resources were allocated for this work both from the IT teams and the clinical practice teams, as well as providing Lean consultant resources and support, a commodity that was in demand from multiple areas in the enterprise. The Medical Director for Specialty was also a highly supportive driver for this work. Having a project championed by a Specialist was somewhat new for the organization, which had previously been focused on Primary Care improvement. The Specialty groups clearly relished the devotion of resources and attention to their departments. Corporate sponsorship was important in providing the compensated time for specialists including Orthopedic surgeons and others to engage in the design work without adverse financial impact.

Engagement of Primary Care leadership was equally important in working through the agreements in expectations between their department and Specialty. For

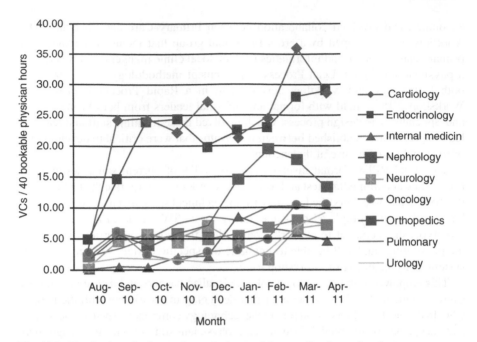

Fig. 10.3 Distribution of volume of consults by specialty over first 9 months of use

example, Primary Care leadership felt it was very important not to change the existing workflow for primary care physicians, which became a key factor in the final design. As this requirement had an impact on the actual steps the Specialist needs to take when creating this encounter (added some "clicks"), it was crucial that the Specialty groups supported this requirement.

The combined leadership from all of the areas and their commitment to working through the difficulties that arose led to the ultimate success of the initiative.

Results

Results for the Virtual Consults included the following:

- **Volume and Distribution**. Group Health is now averaging about 1,500 virtual consults a month. The two most frequent virtual consults are with the Endocrine and Cardiology departments, far ahead of other departments (Fig. 10.3). They currently perform between 25 and 30 virtual consults for every 40 h of appointment time in their respective departments; the most active physician is an Endocrinologist who does over 100 virtual visits per month. Nephrology is a close third with 15–20 virtual consults per 40 h of appointment time. Meanwhile, the average primary care physician sends 3–4 virtual consults a month. Of course, the average volume continues to increase over time, as this project was just implemented in the past year. Every specialty has experimented and begun to incorporate the improvement into practice. Monthly reporting at the specialty and individual clinician level is provided to each department.

- **Affect on Access**. Preliminary data suggests that in high-utilization clinics, for every virtual specialty consult performed in 40 h of appointment time, the wait time for that clinic was reduced by an average of 1.3 days [2]. These preliminary findings remain to be verified, as more specialty clinics increase their volume of virtual consults. As expected, access has not improved uniformly across all specialties, as demand patterns and other issues are different. It is also difficult to separate out the true effect of this work from other work occurring at the same time to improve access.

- **Cost Savings**. Work has not yet been done to measure cost savings to the organization, but it is assumed that there is a significant savings in avoiding use of bricks-and-mortar facilities when it is not necessary. Additionally, patients save on co-pays (the typical co-pay is at least $20 a visit for a Specialist), as well as travel time and work loss related to face-to-face visits. Future work may involve quantifying this effect for reporting the benefits of this model to employer purchasers of Group Health insurance.

- **Patient Satisfaction**. Anecdotal evidence suggests that patient satisfaction has improved due to patients' ability to get questions answered more quickly and without extra visits. In fact, there are numerous stories of virtual requests being answered while the patient is still in the primary care clinic, thus creating greatly satisfied patients, who are impressed with the integrated level of care provided by Group Health.

- **Primary Care Satisfaction**. Virtual Consults have been widely utilized by Primary Care providers who use them to receive input on patient care questions. Providers value this ability for easy consultation and view it as a positive aspect of working in an integrated system. A primary care physician, who has been with Group Health for 36 years, said "Patients are saved a visit and are pleased I'm talking to a specialist about their care. Virtual consults are one of the best things that have been developed between Primary Care and Specialty." Primary care leadership considers the availability of virtual consults to be a powerful recruiting tool for primary care providers.

- **Specialist Satisfaction**. Specialists appreciate these virtual consults since they result in a decrease of unnecessary visits as well as preparation via pre-visit testing for patients they feel should be seen. Additionally, by appropriately focusing the work of the specialist on those patients most likely to benefit from an in-person office visit, the specialist is seeing a more complicated and interesting patient population. Finally, a number of specialists have commented that they appreciate being able to educate providers in real time. The Neurology Service Line Chief noted that this is a chief benefit of the virtual consult, commenting "This work helps to educate Primary Care physicians 'in the moment', and provides education for other caregivers as well when they see the documented information for the patient's problem."

Lessons Learned

This change in the care of patients across a broadly representative primary and specialty care delivery system was successful and helped to contribute to the development of the organization's leadership and implementation skills. A great deal was learned including:

- **Promoting Adoption and Utilization**. Despite Group Health's employed physician model, utilization of the virtual consult was not mandated. It was expected that the adoption would vary by provider and by specialty. The cognitive specialties have been quick to adopt this process. One endocrinologist has topped 1,000 virtual encounters with PCPs and other specialists in less than a year since roll out. Consultations originate primarily from PCPs, but it likely specialty physicians may originate more consultants in the future as they increasingly adopt and are engaged in providing this service to PCPs. Finally, correlation has not been done specifically between departments with long wait times and demand for virtual consultation. This may be another area of investigation in the future.
- **Incentives**. Once the work was rolled out across Specialty in 2010, leadership then incorporated incentives into the operating agreement between the overall corporate goals and the medical group for 2011 to further incent adoption. The targets, generating 1,000 virtual consults a month or 12,000 a year, were set for the Consultative Specialty division overall, but not for individual providers or specialties. The effect was to message the importance of this work as a "strategic differentiator," develop regular monitoring at the individual, team, service line, and division level, and to ensure that the progress toward goals and success of this innovation was regularly included in leadership communications. The financial benefit or incentive revenue accrues at the medical group corporate level and not at the individual or division level. These incentives and attention by leadership resulted in a strong "pull" of this work into the teams, who see it as a way to improve quality and care, and as a way to track the non RVU based work they do that contributes to organizational success.
- **Resistance**. There continue to be areas of resistance to this new work with certain specialties or with individual providers. As expected, the conversations usually revolve around the need for time to be allocated to do "virtual" care. Many specialties now have incorporated a "dummy" RVU incentive value to this work, which then roles up to annual reporting on productivity and is used to set team and service line targets which are aligned with the Group Health's care model. The root causes for the resistance to adoption appear to fall into three main areas. First, some specialties do not appear to lend themselves as easily to this form of virtual documentation, such as general surgery and ophthalmology, which require more hands on work. The second root cause is the "tyranny" of competing priorities. In the absence of dedicated time, some clinicians have found it difficult to incorporate this innovation into their work flow. And finally, problems with the local chief-clinician leadership's messaging, understanding, and modeling of this work in the teams has contributed to slower than anticipated adoption: physician leadership matters and the roll out of this work made gaps in local

.virtualconsult

Reson for consultation:***posed the following question:"***"

This virtual consult is provided based on my review of the clinical question as formulated by the clinician named above. I am providing advice based on general principles of medicine as well as information provided to me in the clinical question above and a focused review of the electronic medical record.

Assessment:***
What to do now***
What to do next***
When to refer to specialty***

Fig. 10.4 The standard disclaimer language developed by the legal department and automatically included in all virtual consult documentation

leadership teams more visible. Specialty leadership found a strong correlation between strong effective local leaders and success in this work.

- **Non-Standardized Answers**. Because consult-pool requests are answered by various members of the specific Specialty, conflicting information can be given when the question is repeated. Virtual consults have made this issue of "variation" in practice styles within teams more visible, as the conversations and recommendations normally made within the exam room are now widely visible to referring and consulting clinicians. It is hoped that with the greater visibility of the advice and recommendations from specialty physicians, that this will promote more effective conversations about how teams care for patients in a consistent and evidence-based way

- **Importance of Early IT Involvement**. There was a great deal of learning about how to best incorporate technology changes into the process of redesigning workflows using the Lean methodology. The initial phases of work did not include information technology analysts during many of the improvement workshops, which led to misunderstandings of possible IT changes to support process development that were subsequently discovered not to be feasible when fully explored. The process improvement piece then benefitted tremendously from getting the IT and informatics team involved up front. These benefits included greatly reduced rework, allowing the IT analysts to truly understand the intent of the work, and humanizing the IT staff to the clinicians and vice versa. This and subsequent partnerships have led to the current good partnerships and working relationships between the IT, Clinical and operational teams. Once designed, the IT technical changes then allowed the clinical leaders to focus on the "adaptive" changes required to ensure implementation and a meaningful change that impacted patients.

- **Legal Issues**. Physicians had significant concerns about how legally to provide documentation in the chart without a face-to-face visit. Group Health's Risk Management group reviewed the procedure and provided excellent guidance. They clarified that the formal documentation of a virtual consult was actually both better care and provided superior legal evidence as all aspects of a case were so clearly documented. Additionally, they provided standard disclaimer language for use in the body of the note (Fig. 10.4)

- **EMR Usage Issues**. The drive to standardize work and processes through Lean methodologies exposed previously unrecognized gaps in physicians' abilities to use the EMR, despite it having been long established in our system. When rolling out the Virtual Consult, communication trainers discovered that some Specialists had not been participating in the previous work with Specialty pools and did not know how to access them, making informal refresher training necessary.

Future Plans

Primary Care physicians are now increasingly interested in partnering with Specialty to optimize the process as well as to increase visibility of this work to patients. The leadership team plans to continue messaging on how this work links to the organizational strategic plan and has incorporated ongoing performance monitoring into the leadership structure in Specialty Care. The focus in the intermediate future is to increase the visibility of the value of this work for patients, such as by making it visible in the future in the patient portal, while also analyzing the variation in team and individual performance. As an integrated system, Group Health is committed to pulling patients closer to the process. Group Health envisions patients potentially having access to the outcomes of the discussion and potentially contributing to it in new ways. As patients and their families want increasing access to information and involvement in developing their care plans, virtual consults will allow Group Health to meet those needs in exciting new ways.

Conclusion

Formally documenting the clinical conversations between physicians is not new to medicine. Case conferences in fields such as Oncology have long employed joint review of cases to determine clinical management. What has not existed is the documentation of this in the medical record and a routine and expected valuation of this type of care across the broad spectrum of specialties.

Group Health has been able to leverage the functionality of the EMR with a small customization to make it easier to communicate between physicians, often in near real time. The combined improvement of workflow and process redesign, agreements between Primary Care and Specialty for "rules of the road" and inclusion of technology specialists in the up-front design, all contributed to a very successful intervention that enables truly patient-centered care in a cost effective manner. This type of work will carry organizations like Group Health into the future of new healthcare models aimed at patient-centered and cost-effective care.

References

1. Reid R, et al. Patient-centered medical home demonstration: a prospective, quasi-experimental, before and after evaluation. Am J Manag Care. 2009;15(9):e71–87.
2. Chase D. Impact of virtual consults on patient access to specialty care. Unpublished thesis. 16 (2011)

Chapter 11
TeleVisit Keeps IT Local

Ajay Sood, Katherine S. Thweatt, Stacey Hirth, Sharon A. Watts,
Renée H. Lawrence, Julie K. Johnson, and David Aron

"Ah! Silvio, it drives me crazy that you won't keep your appointments! Is it really so hard to get yourself out there?!" Barbara is not pleased. Her brother-in-law, Silvio, is 2-years younger than her husband Ray and no better off. Both have diabetes,

Disclaimer
The opinions expressed are solely those of the authors and do not necessarily represent the views of the Department of Veterans Affairs or any other organization.

A. Sood, M.D. (✉)
Department of Endocrinology, Medicine, Louis Stokes Veterans Medical Center,
University Hospital Case Medical Center, Cleveland, OH 44106, USA
e-mail: ajay.sood@va.gov

K.S. Thweatt, M.A., Ed.D.
Research, Department of Communication Studies,
Louis Stokes Cleveland VA Medical Center, West Virginia Wesleyan College,
10701 East BLVD Mailstop 151W, Cleveland, OH 44106, USA
e-mail: katherine.thweatt@va.gov

S. Hirth, B.A.
Department of Education, Louis Stokes Cleveland Department of Veterans Affairs
Medical Center, 14(W) 10701 East Boulevard, Cleveland, OH 44106, USA
e-mail: stacey.hirth@va.gov

S.A. Watts, DNP, MSN, BSN • R.H. Lawrence, Ph.D.
Medical Service Office, Louis Stokes Cleveland Department of Veterans Affairs
Medical Center, 111(W)10701 East Boulevard, Cleveland, OH 44106, USA
e-mail: sharon.watts@va.gov; renee.lawrence2@va.gov

J.K. Johnson, MSPH, Ph.D.
Faculty of Medicine, University of New South Wales,
AGSM Building 105, Sydney, NSW, Australia
e-mail: j.johnson@unsw.edu.au

D. Aron, M.D., M.S.
Louis Stokes Cleveland, Department of Veterans Affairs Medical Center,
Case Western Reserve University, 10701 East Boulevard, Cleveland, OH 44106, USA
e-mail: david.aron@va.gov

L. Berkowitz, C. McCarthy (eds.),
Innovation with Information Technologies in Healthcare, Health Informatics,
DOI 10.1007/978-1-4471-4327-7_11, © Springer-Verlag London 2013

and both were told that their blood sugar is uncontrolled. "You two are like peas in a pod. What will it take to get you to take this seriously? Tamika, your diabetes nurse, wants you to call her about rescheduling."

"Barbara. I want to, but it's so hard. The specialist the VA doc wants me to see is a hundred miles away. I would lose a day's pay to go. I can't afford it." Silvio is a veteran and receives his health care at the local VA's outpatient clinic. That has always been convenient, but the specialist is just too far away. "Look I will call right now to see what I can get locally...ok?"

"Fine... but put Tamika on speakerphone. I want to know what's going on." Barbara feels bad. She didn't realize about his loss of a day's pay. But he is one of the family and needs someone to stay on top of things since he lives on his own.

Silvio calls Tamika and is surprised to hear that there are indeed other options. "Silvio, can I arrange an appointment for you with the specialist using videoconferencing as part our normal visit?" At first Silvio was confused, "You mean, I can see the specialist without driving a hundred miles?" "That is exactly what I mean," said Tamika smiling, sensing a breakthrough with Silvio.

Two weeks later, Silvio and Barbara were in a conference room at his primary care physician's office. Silvio was excited, despite the fact that he was meeting with a new health care provider. As he was checked in, Tamika measured Silvio's weight, pulse rate and blood pressure. She downloaded the blood glucose readings from Silvio's glucose meter. Silvio and Barbara sat in front of a flat screen monitor with a camera mounted on the top. The image of the diabetes specialist flashed on the screen who greeted them with a warm 'good morning'. Silvio whispered to Tamika sitting next to him, 'Can he see us too?" Tamika smiled and nodded.

After the visit, Silvio and Barbara were in the car headed back to Barbara's place. "Wow. That was so much easier than I thought it would be. I really like that he had all my health information. I can't wait to try the new treatment!" Silvio was obviously pleased. But Barbara was especially pleased; she had not seen Silvio so interested in his health before. "If only Ray could get a video specialist too," she murmured. One thing at a time.

Background

The Veterans Health Administration (VHA) is a government-run health care system, which is national in scope and cares for over eight million veterans across the United States. VHA is a leader in health information technology, supporting a broad range of patient care. Factors that have promoted or facilitated success include openness to innovation, a research program linked to operations, adoption of best practices regardless of their origin, and a system-wide electronic health record. This Computerized Patient Record System (CPRS) has been a one of the important pillars contributing to the successful transformation of the Veterans Healthcare Administration.

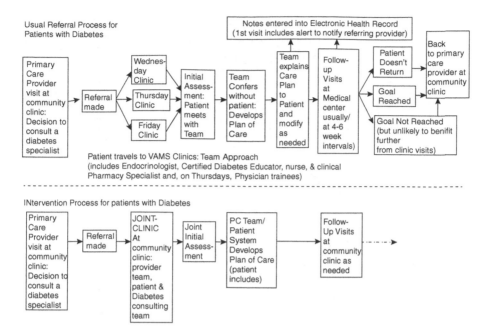

Fig. 11.1 Comparison of usual and new referral-consultation processes for diabetes. (*PCP* primary care provider, *CPRS* Computerized Patient Record System, i.e., the VA's electronic medical record, *CDE* Certified Diabetes Educator, *CBOC* Community-based Outpatient Clinic)

The Innovation

The Diabetes Telemedicine Clinic at the Cleveland VHA facility provides real-time specialty consultation and continuing education for patients with diabetes mellitus and their healthcare providers in community clinics known as community-based outpatient clinics (CBOCs). Specifically, a patient at a CBOC is able to use a locally based videoconferencing system to have a virtual visit with an endocrinologist located at the Cleveland VHA's main campus (VAMC). Figure 11.1 compares the usual face to face referral process with the new referral process, which uses a tele-health system to enable a virtual consult with a specialist. In the usual process, a decision is made by the primary care provider in the community clinic that referral for a diabetes consultation is required. An electronic consultation is sent and reviewed at the medical center. If approved, the patient is then scheduled into one of three different clinics that provide specialty care for diabetes. The patient travels to Cleveland and is seen by a diabetes team. This team confers outside the exam room and develops a plan of care. This is explained to the patient, and a progress note is written in the electronic health record. The patient is told to follow up as needed in the specialty clinic or the primary care clinic. On the other hand, the process for the teleconsultation clinic is much simpler. The virtual visit includes not only the remote diabetes specialist and diabetes nurse, but also the locally based community clinic nurse and

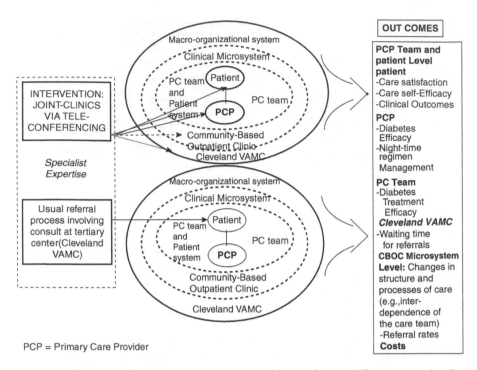

Fig. 11.2 Conceptual framework portraying points of impact for two different approaches for delivery of specialist expertise

sometimes even the primary care provider. Figure 11.2 shows the conceptual framework portraying points of impact for the two different approaches to consultation.

In addition to the use of telehealth technology, another unique aspect of this model has been the active involvement of the community clinic's diabetes nurse, who is present with the patient during the entire virtual consult. Nurses not only facilitate the consultation, but also take an active role in the subsequent management of diabetes for the patient in concert with the primary care provider. During the subsequent care, the endocrinology specialist actively provides any needed specialty recommendations to the diabetes nurse. This model affords the diabetes nurses continuing medical education because of frequent interaction with the specialist on difficult-to-manage cases.

On the day of the virtual visit, the diabetes nurse case manager starts the process by checking in the patient. The case manager measures the blood pressure, pulse, body weight, downloads the patient glucose meter data, then faxes the downloaded glucose readings and patient blood glucose logs to the central Cleveland main facility. Interoperability issues prevent uploading the readings directly into the patient's electronic medical record at the clinic at this time, but it is being explored.

At the Cleveland VA's main facility, an endocrinologist reviews the patient records online from the electronic medical record. He then dials into the conference room where both the patient and the diabetes nurse case manager are using the videoconference equipment.

The endocrinologist at the central clinic initiates the interaction with patient, as he would do in the regular diabetes clinic. The case manager then fills in some details, including the problems that the patient has been facing. The endocrinologist does not conduct a physical examination. However all these patients have a primary care provider, and have had a physical examination conducted during prior visits with the primary care providers. The diabetes nurse can examine the injection sites and the feet during the telemedicine interaction.

At the end of the consultation, two sets of recommendations are negotiated with the patient. The first set of recommendations will be for the patient, such as changes in medications, laboratory tests and lifestyle modifications. The second set of recommendations is for the diabetes nurse as she/he continues to follow the patient over the next few months. This may include suggestions on how to change the doses of medication with respect to changes in blood glucose levels, when and which type of insulin should be started, and how and when to monitor the patient.

The patient then returns to the diabetes nurse with his blood glucose log after a few days for review of his blood glucose control. At that time, the diabetes nurse may suggest changes to the treatment based on the patient's blood glucose. The diabetes nurse reschedules the patient in the diabetes telemedicine clinic if the glycemic control or glycated hemoglobin (HbA1c) does not improve. Based on the clinical situation, the endocrinologist may also decide to reschedule the patient for follow up in the telemedicine clinic.

After the telemedicine consultation, the endocrinologist types a clinic note into the EMR, which is accessible to the diabetes nurse and the patient's primary care health provider. At the primary care clinic, the diabetes nurse goes over the immediate changes to be made in the management of the disease with the patient. At that time, he/she also addresses any other issues requiring reinforcement, such as insulin injection technique, rotation of sites, education regarding hypoglycemia, foot care, and finally, provides the patient with written home instructions.

For the next several weeks or months, the patient follows up with the diabetes nurse at the primary care clinic. The nurse continues to titrate the doses of the medication as per the protocol discussed during the telemedicine clinic appointment. This plan requires the primary care provider authorization, which he performs by reviewing and cosigning the note and prescribing medications if a new prescription is required. If the nurse wants to do anything different from the approved protocol, she has easy accessibility to the primary care provider to discuss the changes. The diabetes nurse can also request that any decisions be reviewed by the endocrinologist or can reschedule the patient for another telemedicine clinic appointment at any time.

Reason for This Innovation

Patients, primary care staff, ambulatory clinic administrators and the remote diabetes specialists all recognized a need to improve the care of their patients with diabetes mellitus and were looking for developing newer models for improving delivery

Table 11.1 Spectrum of specialist input in patient care

Model of specialist expertise input	Specialist-PCP interaction	Specialist-patient interaction	Formal (note in chart by specialist) vs informal	Intensity of specialist involvement
Transfer of care to specialist	Minimal if any	Direct	Formal	++++++
Co-management	Direct via phone/chart	Direct	Formal	+++++
Consultation in person	Direct via phone/chart	Direct	Formal	++++
Tele-consultation	Direct via phone/chart	Direct	Formal	++++
Tele-conference case discussions	Direct	Indirect	Formal/ Informal	+++
E-consult	Direct via chart	Indirect	Formal	++
Curbside consult	Direct	Indirect	Informal	+
Decision support	Indirect (e.g., guidelines)	none	none	None

of medical care. Table 11.1 shows the spectrum of means by which specialist input can be brought to a patient's care. Some of the major reasons for moving forward with this innovation included the following:

Distance Decreases Visits and Increases Costs. The Cleveland VA Medical Center (VAMC) currently serves veterans in northeast Ohio for inpatient and outpatient care. Primary care for these patients is provided by community-based outpatient clinics (CBOCs), which are located anywhere from 7 miles to 108 miles away from the main campus, with an average distance of almost 55 miles. Many specialty services are not provided at the CBOCs, such as an endocrinologist for patients with poorly controlled diabetes mellitus. Not surprisingly, the distance prevents some patients from seeing centrally-located specialists. In addition, when patients do travel to see the specialist, the VA reimburses travel expenses or pays for local out-of-system specialists, thus incurring additional expense.

Diabetes Significance is Increasing. Unfortunately, despite a three-fold increase in the number of VHA diabetes specialty clinics, demand exceeds supply. The Cleveland VAMC provided service to 54,000 veterans in 2000 and to 90,000 in 2006. This increase was particularly noteworthy in that the rate of diabetes in the VHA population is over 20 %, significantly higher than the overall US population rate of 8.3 %. (2011 National Diabetes Fact Sheet; www.cdc.gov/diabetes/pubs/factsheet11.htm accessed April 17, 2011) [1]. Additionally, the Cleveland VAMC found that their difficult-to-manage diabetes cases were increasing.

Communication Issues. An interview with a local nurse illuminates the importance of good and robust communication between CBOCs and the centralized specialists and the problems of simply sending patients to a distant clinic without having closer coordination of care. She said, "I don't think communication is as clearly defined as it should be. I think that we rely on the record because it's transmittable and you can just throw a signature on it and send it to somebody else. But I don't know that is always communication. That's sharing information, but communication goes further than that, I think. Communication is a piece that makes the care for the patient come together . . . I think we need more accessibility to the providers at Wade Park as far as talking with them, education from them."

Research Opportunities. The VA's preferred approach to research in healthcare delivery is to link research to local operational needs that have broader implications. Thus, a good project meets two major criteria: (1) the issue needs to lend itself to a research study (e.g. it will generate new knowledge using a rigorous approach), and (2) the issue should address a local need common to other settings. The local need for this innovation was to provide more convenient consultation for patients and education for providers in community clinics. While it was more convenient for patients living in the catchment area of the Cleveland VA Medical Center – Northeast Ohio, it had even greater potential for VA medical centers that serve large geographic area [12].

This project was thus viewed as a way to increase the capacity for consultations, and it turns out the research dollars provided the incentive for top management to pay for additional specialist time. One risk of this approach is that the research project brings resources that disappear when the research funding ends. However, using an approach that balances research rigor and operational relevance allows for the potential to make the business case to continue the project. In fact, this is exactly what happened in Cleveland.

Why This Innovation Succeeded

The potential benefits of a telehealth program were clear: reduce waiting times, expand specialist access without a concomitant increase in resources, and eliminate the need to travel for specialty care. However, there were several factors that helped the VHA system be successful in this endeavor.

Previous Telemedicine Experience. The VHA has implemented many innovations to provide specialist expertise. For example, asynchronous e-consults via shared access to the electronic health record provide a more informed consultation, may substitute for routine in person consultations and facilitate appropriate evaluation prior to specialty referral [15]. Another example is the VA Specialty Care Access Network (VA SCAN), which provides teleconference case discussions between specialist teams and primary care providers in CBOCs. This mode of care delivery, based on the project ECHO model developed at the University of New Mexico (http://echo.unm.edu/), has demonstrated improvement in process and outcome measures equivalent to direct referral of patients to specialists [20, 21].

Understanding the Spectrum of Tele-Specialty Options. The VHA leaders recognize that the needs for specialist expertise vary, ranging from decision support to transfer of care from the primary care team to the specialist team. This spectrum can be conceptualized according to several dimensions (see Table 11.1), including intensity of specialist involvement; direct vs. indirect interaction between specialist and primary care provider; formal vs. informal consultation; and direct vs. indirect interaction between specialist and patient.

The envisioned solution for this situation thus needed to do more than simply solve the immediate access problem (i.e. patients being seen by a specialist), it also had to address the increasing demand and complexity of caring for patients with diabetes by involving and empowering CBOC staff. Teleconferencing technology was seen as the answer because it could minimize the time spent by specialists and/or patients in travel and maximize the time they are available for consultation [4, 16]. In other words, it avoids the need for physical proximity, while potentially offering the same benefits in communication. Most previous telemedicine studies involving diabetes used direct data download/transfer, telephone follow-up calls to patients (usually from nurses), educational videoconferencing to patients, or other mechanisms of electronic communication (phone, fax, e-mail, or web-based) between specialists and PCPs. The methodology of the clinic described here is different and innovative.

The Shared EMR: The VHA has been a leader in the successful implementation of IT, supporting a broad range of patient care and administrative functions [17, 18]. Most VAs are nearly 100 % electronic using the Computerized Patient Record System (CPRS), which supports multiple features, such as order entry, laboratory and other results, and digitized radiographs. One study concluded that as a result of the implementation of these systems, the VA is one of the few national, health IT–enabled, integrated delivery systems in the United States [7].

A key component that facilitated the development of the teleconsultation project was that the VA system has a single electronic medical record (EMR) shared across the system. The specialist team and PCP teams thus have direct access to the same EMR during the consultation. In addition, the IT-friendly environment allows for quicker and easier IT-based innovations. For example, among the IT projects at the Cleveland VAMC was the development of a Clinical Diabetes Registry, which was instrumental in collecting data for the teleconsultation project (see Fig. 11.3) [11].

Space and Connectivity: A comfortable room with excellent video conferencing equipment was a key element of the innovation. This included sound, lighting, comfortable chairs, and most importantly access to the EHR. For a successful videoconference encounter the light conditions where the health care providers and patients are located have to be optimum for a good picture quality on the video. Similarly good quality of sound is essential for error-free communication. The appearance of the room from where the specialist carries out the videoconference should be as professional in its appearance as any outpatient clinic room. Placement of the video screen for easy and comfortable viewing is important. Similarly the placement of the camera should be such that the patient should perceive that the physician is looking at the patient through the screen and not at an angle away from the patient.

Importance of local Diabetes Nurse Experts. A trained Diabetes Nurse or Case Manager were required at the community clinics to assist with the teleconsults as well as perform long-term titration of the diabetic medications [19]. In general, there was one diabetes-trained nurse per community clinic to serve as a resource for all the diabetes patients in the clinic. Community clinics range in size from about 3,000 and 12,000 primary care patients of whom about 700–2,800 have diabetes, of which a smaller subset would require specialty consults. But these tele-consults were often done just once, with the bulk of the follow-up work being performed by

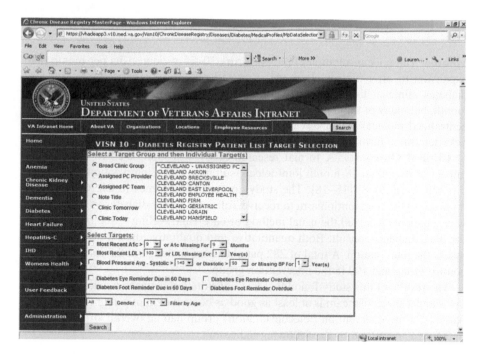

Fig. 11.3 Home page of the Cleveland VA–VISN 10 diabetes registry

the local diabetes nurses. After the initial tele-consult, the patient would be seen again by the nurse within 1 week to 3 months, depending on the clinical requirements of an individual patient. The patient would then only repeat the tele-consultation if the specialist thought it would be necessary or if the diabetes nurse manager thought that the treatment was not leading to the expected improvement.

Health Care Administrators: The support of health care administrators was recognized to be a crucial part of this innovation's success. In the VHA system, the central health facility and the primary care centers fall under the same overall health administration, so administrative issues regarding coordinating the availability of site and personnel were easier to manage once the administration realized the importance of the diabetes telemedicine clinic. Continuing support from the administration has been vital to the success of this venture.

Clinical Leadership: Both the Chief of the division of Endocrinology and the Chief of Medicine in the institute were very supportive of the project. Having executive sponsorship from both primary care and the specialties is always critical for these types of innovations.

Moving a Research Project into Operational Use. When the funded research intervention period ended, there were requests and even demands that the teleconsultation program be continued and extended to the CBOCs that served as controls. Word of its value had spread. Having seen the value of the project, top management ensured that the necessary resources would be provided. Teleconsultation was opened to all Cleveland-based CBOCs and became part of usual care by the end of 2008.

Results

Volume. The teleconsultation clinic performs 20–25 patient visits per month, and expansion to offer more slots is under considered. By comparison, the standard diabetes clinic at the centralized medical center sees about 60–70 patients per month, but many of these patients receive primary care or other specialty care at the centralized medical center already. More formal research is being undertaken to help determine further statistics about the clinic statistics.

Clinical Outcomes. A formal research study was completed to evaluate the impact of the initial 18-month joint teleconsultation clinic intervention (Nov. 2006 through April 2008) [15–18]. The study compared outcomes in five CBOCs randomized to the intervention arm to receive Teleconsults for diabetes vs. six CBOCs where patients received the usual method of care via traveling to the main campus for their diabetes consult. Both quantitative and qualitative data were collected to assess the intervention. A total of 282 patients were included in the study: 83 in the control group and 199 in the intervention group.

The results of this study found that tele-consultation between a patient with diabetes and a specialist team is at least as good as consultation in person. Specifically, patients in the intervention (teleconsultation) group had an overall similar clinical outcome as measured by the following indicators:

- Glycated hemoglobin (HbA1c), a measure of blood glucose control (both had a mild improvement)
- Low-density lipoprotein cholesterol levels (no significant change)
- Serum creatinine levels (no significant change)
- Systolic blood pressure (slightly better in the intervention versus control)

Patient Satisfaction. The research project also studied patient and provider satisfaction. Not surprisingly, the results from patient questionnaires indicated that Telemedicine Consultation was as good or better than usual consultation from a patient's perspective. Perceptions of ease of communication with the specialist were the same in both groups. Patients in the teleconsultation group responded positively to a question about whether the specialist was able to understand their situation more often than those in the usual care group. The proportion of patients who were very satisfied with the consultation was actually greater in the teleconsultation group. Finally, in the teleconsultation group, 99.3 % agreed that telemedicine made it easier to get medical care and <2 % would have preferred to see the specialist in person.

Provider Satisfaction. The primary care providers appreciated that their patients received care in a timely fashion, had help from the diabetes nurse case manager and had a specialist in caring for a time-intensive disease. A quote from a primary care provider best summarizes their feelings: "[Teleconsultation] has been an excellent change. It's a win-win situation for providers and for patients."

Meanwhile, the diabetes nurses were pleased to receive support from the endocrine specialists. The nursing interaction in this clinic with an endocrinologist helped them to improve and gain new diabetes knowledge, thus serving as continuing education. The endocrinologists liked this model because it freed up time which could then be spent in dealing with their more difficult patients. Endocrine time savings were due to the fact that the follow-up for the titration of medications and some of the monitoring could now be performed by the diabetes nurse managers. In addition, it obviated the occasional need for them to travel the CBOCs for various reasons. Finally, Health administrators like this arrangement as a higher number of patients with diabetes mellitus that lived far from the tertiary care center received specialized care more efficiently and effectively.

Process Improvements. The research project also performed qualitative assessments to compare the processes associated with telemedicine consultations. Semistructured interviews were conducted at two points during the project. During the *pre-intervention phase* of the project, interviews were conducted with diabetes team members at the Community Based Outpatient Clinic (CBOC). These interviews provided the baseline data. After the *intervention phase*, semi-structured interviews were repeated at participating CBOCs.

The results of these qualitative interviews indicated that there were many positive changes in practice that resulted from the telemedicine intervention. Specifically, five major themes emerged from the interviews: Changes in Referral Process, Communication of the Care Team, Alignment of Role and Training, Patient Focused Care, and Patient Care / Compliance with Care Plan. These are discussed below and selected verbatim comments are included from a variety of participants.

Changes in Referral Process: Prior to the intervention, the process for consultation required that the patient always go to Cleveland for the visit. Travel was a significant issue and placed a burden on the patients. Providers commented on the travel burden as a negative aspect of usual care: "I would say less than 10 % of our patients would be willing to be referred to Wade Park because of the distance. It's just really a cumbersome situation." [Nurse] The lack of desire for travel to Wade Park to see a specialist also had the potential to lead to fragmented care for the patient, who would choose a local, non VA-affiliated specialist, and then come to the CBOC for medication. The diabetes telemedicine clinic made it easier for patient and primary care providers to have a specialist consultation.

Communication within the Care Team. Prior to the introduction of tele-consults, interviewees reported that communication was problematic due to the segregated nature of the care. In other words, they did not feel like they were truly acting as a team. So with use of the synchronous tele-consult, all the team members (physicians, nurses, patient) could finally be in the same virtual room and thus be able to have a full conversation amongst themselves. The result was felt to be quicker and more effective discussions about patient care and management.

Alignment of Role and Training. In addition to the telemedicine consultation for diabetic patients, another change in the Cleveland VA Health system was that each CBOC had to have a nurse (usually a certified diabetes educator) to handle most of the more complicated diabetes patients. This was an improvement from the baseline, where not all CBOCs had a diabetes nurse, or diabetes nurse staffing was inconsistent.

In the interviews, once PCP noted "At one time we did not have a diabetic case manager here and really, it was hard. It was very heavy before we got a case manager. Because the patients need to be seen more than once every 3 months. If you start seeing them more than once every 3 months, your schedule is so bogged down doing something that should be done by somebody who is not paid as much money, you know, instead of me being the diabetic educator."

Since the telemedicine intervention, the PCPs more regularly refer diabetic patients to the diabetes nurse case managers. These nurses teach glucose monitoring classes, diabetes classes, and see their own panel of patients. The nurses meet with patients monthly, bi-weekly, or weekly as necessary to review blood sugar numbers and to titrate medications in a timely fashion. The diabetes nurses sit in on the teleconference appointments along with the patient and are responsible for follow-up care, teaching, etc. as necessary. Diabetes nurses reported increased satisfaction associated with having a greater role in caring for patients. Primary care physicians also expressed satisfaction in being able to "hand over" diabetic patients that needed more attention to the nurses. And of course, these nurses could also make the decision to request a telemedicine consultation.

Patient-Focused Care. The telemedicine intervention introduced more patient-focused care. Care is provided in a setting familiar to the patient and results in better engagement on the part of the patient given the inclusion of the patient as part of the team. "It means more to the patient to hear it from the specialist. I could have been telling them for years about what they need to do, but as soon as they hear it from the specialist on the teleconsult, it means something." [PCP] "The patients seem to like the teleconsult! It's me, the patient, the NP, and the physician. Four people focused on the patient – the patient feels like they are getting a lot of attention." [Nurse]

Patient Care /Compliance with Care Plan. In the post-intervention interviews, providers related stories that support the use of the telemedicine consultations. "Telemedicine works well for a lot of our patients. I schedule patients for telemedicine if they are a 'good candidate.' Compliance has a lot to do with who would be a good candidate. Patients who take a more active role in their care are good candidates." [Nurse Coordinator] It is important to note that patients with non-adherence are also seen and an attempt is made to come up with best possible management solutions for them.

Lessons Learned

Patient Identification. The types of diabetic patients initially scheduled into the telemedicine clinic fell into three categories: (1) Patients referred to an endocrine specialist by their primary health care provider (physician, physician assistant, nurse practitioner), (2) Patients under the care of the diabetes nurse case manager at the CBOC who felt that additional input was required from the diabetes specialist, and (3) Patients who were identified by the diabetes telemedicine clinic coordinator to have poor blood glucose control as evidence by a high HbA1c on review of the electronic health database.

Currently, the clinic coordinator is no longer actively identifying patients from the EHR database due to a few reasons. First, it was found that the first two categories generated enough referrals to fill the schedule of the Telemedicine Diabetes clinic. Second, while the initial research paid for someone to actually identify the patients with a high HbA1c, that funding was not continued. Rather, it was felt that it was most appropriate to train the diabetes nurse managers to actively recognize these patients and refer them at the point of care of seeing them in the clinic.

Scheduling Visits. Coordinating the schedules of different health personnel to be on the videoconference at the same time can be challenging. Coordinating with different clinics at different sites can be complex, requiring more effort than the usual scheduling in the routine clinics. This was recognized and supported by the administration. However, in the future it would be useful to create software to better coordinate and assimilate teleconsultation scheduling into the general scheduling of the outpatient clinics for the whole facility.

Diabetic Nurse Volume. Most of the sites already had enough diabetes nurses for their caseload, but they did have to free up some time to be available for the teleconsultations. Fortunately, this did not require much time since each primary clinic was only on the tele-consult schedule during a two-hour time period every 6 weeks (i.e. an average of under 30 min a week).

The Physical Exam. One main drawback of a telemedicine clinic consultation is the inability for the specialists to directly examine the patient. However, there were two solutions to this problem. First, the diabetes nurse managers are able to do focused examinations, such as review of the feet and of the insulin injection sites. Second, if a clinical situation required a more robust physical examination, the patient would be referred by the nurse to the primary health care provider for a quick consultation, often done on the same day.

Data Sharing. It was clear that new patient data had to be quickly transmitted to the specialist at the start of a teleconsultation. Typical nurse collected data, including vitals and medications, were entered into the EMR at the start of the visit, thus allowing the specialists to have immediate access. However, there was occasional non-computerized data which also needed to be transmitted, such as when patients would bring in their home blood glucose log sheets. Instead of entering each data point manually into the EHR, it was found that faxing them was as effective and much quicker. In the future, the ideal solution will be to have home monitoring machines which interface directly with the EHR.

Importance of local Diabetes Nurse Experts. As described previously, the long-term titration of medications requires a trained Diabetes Nurse or Case Manager in the off-site clinics [19], which illustrates another important factor in how specialist expertise can be integrated into primary care.

Importance of a well aligned reimbursement system. Since the VA health system is self-insured, it was easier to create a return on investment in better managing diabetic patients. However in a more typical non-capitated environment, a payment mechanism would have to be worked out with the health insurance companies. Hopefully, as payment structures evolve, (e.g. accountable care organizations) there may be more incentives for this type of system.

Future Plans

Expanding to other disease states. Having accomplished successful implementation of this model for patients with diabetes mellitus, it would be useful to spread this model to management of other diseases. For example, in the field of endocrinology, management of hypothyroidism and hypogonadism could easily lend itself to this model. Other chronic diseases such as hypertension, heart failure, asthma and pain may also be managed using this model. And it should be pointed out that teleconsultation clinics for pain management and mental health issues are also being carried out in other areas of the VA health system.

Expanding to the patient with multiple or complex management problems. As this model is translated to the care of other chronic diseases, it may become easier to coordinate care for patients with multiple or complex management issues. In this model, all the changes in a patient's care for all their diseases would be routed through the primary care provider, who would monitor results and confer with specialists when needed. A key question will then be how often the patient actually needs to be seen by the specialist or whether the review of the case by the specialist along with the primary care team is sufficient. To further explore this concept, the VA is sponsoring a project where multiple health care providers log on to do a videoconference with a specialist while one of them presents a case with difficult management issue. Current examples to date include cases for diabetes mellitus, pain management, congestive heart failure and hepatitis C.

Conclusion

What started as a research project to study the impact of the use of videoconferencing to deliver care for patients with diabetes mellitus in the VHA system in the Cleveland facility network has evolved into a robust and real-world telemedicine diabetes clinic which serves the needs of patients from less accessible rural areas. At the same time, this clinic empowers primary care providers with more specialist access, while increasing their knowledge with regard to the management of diabetes mellitus. Additionally, it appears to decrease cost to the VA health system by preventing travel expense, optimizing utilization of health resources and preventing diabetic complications via delivering better care to a wider population. This has been a win-win situation for patients, primary care providers, specialists and health administrators.

Acknowledgement We gratefully acknowledge the contribution of Susan R. Kirsh, MD, who has played a key role in the process of conceptualizing how specialist expertise can be integrated into primary care (Fig. 11.4).

Disclosures: This work was supported by VA HSR&D QUERI Program and VA HSR&D Grant IIR 03-254.

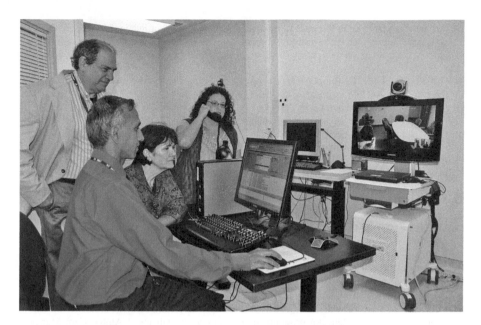

Fig. 11.4 The diabetes specialist teleconsultation team (from *left* to *right*: David Aron, M.D. – endocrinologist and project director; Ajay Sood, M.D. – endocrinologist; Sharon Watts, DNP, RN-C, CDE – diabetes nurse practitioner; and Stacey Hirth, B.A. – teleconsultation coordinator)

References

1. Pogach L, Aron D. Quality of diabetes care (current levels, distribution, and trends) and challenges in measuring quality of care. In: Moran S, Gregg E, Williams D, Cowie C, Narayan K, editors. Diabetes and public health: from data to policy. New York: Oxford University Press; 2009.
2. Bailey J, Black M, Wilkin D. Specialist outreach clinics in general practice. Br Med J. 1994;308(6936):1083–6.
3. Bowling A, Stramer K, Dickinson E, Windsor J, Bond M. Evaluation of specialists' outreach clinics in general practice in England: process and acceptability to patients, specialist, and general practitioners. J Epidemiol Community Health. 1997;51(52):61.
4. Powell J. Systematic review of outreach clinics in primary care in the UK. J Health Serv Res Policy. 2002;7(3):177–83.
5. Black M, Leese B, Gosden T, Mead N. Specialist outreach clinics in general practice: what do they offer? Br J Gen Pract. 1997;47:558–61.
6. Black M, Gosden T, Leese B, Mead N. The costs and benefits of specialist outreach clinics in general practice in two specialties. Manchester, England: National Primary Care Research and Development Centre, University of Manchester; 1996.
7. Byrne C, Mercincavage L, Pan E, Vincent A. The value from investments in health information technology at the U.S. department. Health Aff. 2010;29(4):629–38.
8. Nazi K, Hogan T, Wagner T, McInnes D, Smith B, et al. Embracing a health services research perspective on personal health records: lessons learned from the VA My HealtheVet system. J Gen Intern Med. 2009;25 Suppl 1:S62–7.

9. Darkins A, Ryan P, Kobb R, Foster L, Edmonson E, et al. Care coordination/home telehealth: the systematic implementation of health informatics, home telehealth, and disease management to support the care of veteran patients with chronic conditions. Telemed e-Health. 2008;14(10):1118–26.
10. Hill RD, Luptak MK, Rupper RW. Review of veterans health administration telemedicine interventions. Am J Manag Care. 2010;16(12 Suppl HIT):e302–10.
11. Kern E, Beischel S, Stanlnaker R, Aron D, et al. Building a diabetes registry from the Veterans Health Administration's computerized patient record system. Diabetes Sci Tech. 2008;2:7–14.
12. Greenhalgh T, Robert G, Macfarlane F, Bate P, Kyriakidou O. Diffusion of innovations in service organizations: systematic review and recommendations. Milbank Q. 2004;82(4):581–629.
13. Batalden P, Nelson E, Edwards W, Godfrey M, Mohr J. Microsystems in health care: part 9. Developing small clinical units to attain peak performance. Jt Comm J Qual Patient Saf. 2003;29(11):575–85.
14. Nelson E, Batalden P, Huber T, et al. Microsystems in health care: Part 1. Learning from high-performing front-line clinical units. J Qual Improv J Comm. 2002;28(9):472–93.
15. Verhoeven F, Tanja-Dijkstra K, Nijland N, Eysenbach G, Gemert-Pijnen L. Asynchronous and synchronous teleconsultation for diabetes care: a systematic literature review. J Diabetes Sci Technol. 2010;4(3):666–84.
16. Weinstock RS, Teresi JA, Goland R, et al. Glycemic control and health disparities in older ethnically diverse underserved adults with diabetes: five-year results from the informatics for diabetes education and telemedicine (IDEATel) study. Diabetes Care. 2011;34(2):274–9.
17. Chumbler N, Vogel W, Garel M, Qin H, Kobb R, Ryan P. Health services utilization of a care coordination/ home-telehealth program for veterans with diabetes. J Ambul Care Manage. 2005;28(3):230–40.
18. Hopp F, Hogan M, Woodbridge P, Lowery J. The use of telehealth for diabetes management: a qualitative study of telehealth provider perceptions. Implement Sci. 2007;2:14.
19. Watts SA, Lawrence RH, Kern E. Diabetes nurse case management training program: enhancing care consistent with the chronic care and patient-centered medical home models. Clin Diabetes. 2011;29(1):25–33.
20. Arora S, Geppert CMA, Kalishman S, et al. Academic health center management of chronic diseases through knowledge networks: project ECHO. Acad Med. 2007;82(2):154–60.
21. Arora S, Kalishman S, Thornton K, et al. Expanding access to hepatitis C virus treatment—extension for community healthcare outcomes (ECHO) project: disruptive innovation in specialty care. Hepatology. 2010;52(3):1124–33.

Chapter 12
Mommy Monitor

Steve Huffman and April R. Daugherty

Isabelle would be lost in this busy world without her smart phone. Work has been intense, trying to coordinate schedules for all the activities of her young son; and now that she is 4 months pregnant she almost forgot about this pregnancy checkup. While thinking it was a routine visit, the time it took for Dr. Smith to come back into the room was a bit concerning. She had things to do, groceries to pick up, a week-end schedule to plan and did not have time to wait. She was not expecting the report that the doctor had when he walked into the room. "You have gestational diabetes." Time seemed to stop; this wasn't in her plan. "Isabelle, I know it's a pain, but you'll need to come in more often, and you'll have to take extra special care of yourself." Dr. Smith went on to instruct her on what to eat, how to take her blood glucose levels, her blood pressure, and what to do if her results became too low or too high.

Isabelle was feeling more confident about the care plan before her, but the cost! As an administrative assistant with limited insurance coverage, she was going to struggle financially. That sinking feeling came back. "How am I going to afford this?"

"Isabelle, would you be interested in home telemonitoring? It would allow us to keep better track of your blood sugar levels, and also inform us of important changes in your blood pressure. We could also look at reducing the number of visits to the office if your test results are consistently not too low or too high. The goal is to keep you and your baby healthy, keep a close eye on your progress, and keep you out of the emergency room until that baby is really ready to come out. This will help your

S. Huffman, MBA(✉) • A.R. Daugherty, B.S. Business, M.S. Technology
Beacon Health System, 615 N. Michigan St.,
South Bend, IN 46601, USA
e-mail: shuffman@memorialsb.org; adaugherty@memorialsb.org

L. Berkowitz, C. McCarthy (eds.),
Innovation with Information Technologies in Healthcare, Health Informatics,
DOI 10.1007/978-1-4471-4327-7_12, © Springer-Verlag London 2013

health and reduce the cost". Isabelle could not help but to cry at those words.
She was so relieved that there would be at least some reprieve to the costs associ-
ated with having a high-risk pregnancy.

Once at home, Isabelle found the setup of the equipment easy. Each day Isabelle
followed the physician's instructions and she was impressed that she didn't have to
enter information; the devices she used did it automatically. When she weighed
herself, the scale uploaded the weight to the telemonitoring system and then right to
the doctor's office. And it was the same for the blood pressure and glucose devices.
"Wow! Now this is cool!" After 5 months of using home telemonitoring, Isabelle
gave birth to a healthy baby boy.

Background

Memorial Health System is a 525 bed, level 2 trauma center located in South Bend, Indiana. It employs over 120 physicians, has a level 2 NICU and a strong Maternal Fetal Medicine practice which works with underprivileged mothers who are identified as having high-risk pregnancies. Memorial is an incredibly innovative corporation and has been featured in the Wall Street Journal for its "Innovation Café", where it brings innovative concepts to the community and its employees are given tools to develop an "Innovation Everywhere" attitude.

The Innovation

Memorial Health created a telehealth system which allows their high-risk obstetrics (OB) clinic to monitor patients with high-risk conditions at home in between office visits. Enrolled patients received an Intel HealthGuide home monitoring device, which was designed to be easy to set up and use. Training was performed by the head nurse at the physician's office and encompassed how to use the device, associated monitoring peripherals and the embedded web camera. The peripheral devices included a glucometer, a blood pressure monitor and a scale.

Once a patient was enrolled, data from the peripheral devices was transferred to a care management web portal, which was viewable by the physician's office staff. In addition, the head nurse would initiate a weekly 10-min teleconference to ensure that the patient was following care guidelines established, such as monitoring their home blood pressure readings and glucose levels. During these weekly teleconferences, the nurses would also allocate time to answer any questions and help patients prepare for their office visits.

Reason for This Innovation

Telemedicine and Medical Home Monitoring have long been discussed as opportunities to leverage technology and reduce cost related to certain medical conditions. Since the medical home concept was initially proposed in 1967 by the American Academy of Pediatrics, there has been a belief that collecting medical record information centrally and enabling accessible and continuous care could positively impact a patient's outcome at a reduced cost. Telemedicine technologies have enabled various medical home projects over the years and have been successfully used in a variety of disease states, ranging from chronic diseases, such as diabetes and congestive heart failure, to short-term conditions, such as acne in dermatology. Additionally, there is increasing market momentum to remotely manage and monitor patients.

In 2008, the Intel Corporation released their "Intel HealthGuide", a hardware and software platform for telemonitoring. Memorial entered into an innovation dialogue with Intel about developing use cases for telemonitoring a subgroup of their patient population. Memorial decided to approach this home monitoring project in a drastically different manner. Instead of focusing on the standard chronic disease states that are typically monitored, they realized that a younger more technologically engaged population with a sub-acute disease state might be a better pilot for this new device. After interviewing a variety of physicians, the choice was to focus on high-risk obstetrics, since the patient population would likely consist of younger women with high interest in their condition and better technology prowess than older patients. In addition, patients were closely aligned with a medical system focused on the time-limited duration of their pregnancy.

Why This Innovation Succeeded

The Innovation Team. Memorial's approach started with the creation of a small team comprised of information systems staff members referred to as the "Innovation Team". Each team member brought an important specialization, including a systems administrator, a programmer analyst, an interface analyst, a clinical systems analyst from the hospital EMR team, and a clinical systems analyst from the outpatient EMR team. This team collectively put in an estimated 400 h prior to the deployment of the pilot program.

The Challenge. The team was challenged to develop a use-case in a 45-day period that was (1) Outside of traditional telemonitoring services and service lines, such as congestive heart failure and diabetes, (2) had a financial return-on-investment, and (3) outcomes that could be measured.

The specific problem chosen was high cost obstetrics care for gestational diabetic mothers who may also have indicators for pre-eclampsia, which is usually diagnosed around the 20th week. For the patient, this is a shocking and unsettling diagnosis, putting her and her fetus at risk. Under the current system, high-risk patients receive a logbook and two devices, a sphygmomanometer and a glucometer. They are asked to monitor their home blood pressure and blood sugar levels on a daily basis, in which the frequency depends based on the patient's clinical requirements.

The Technology. The intervention that was developed was a novel approach to monitoring these high-risk obstetrics patients via the Intel HealthGuide. The goal was to cost-effectively improve the health of the mother and fetus by increasing the dialogue and clinical decision-making between the providers and their patient. Since the patient population in the fetal medicine clinic generally was insured by Medicaid or had no insurance, the financial return-on-investment was based on minimizing complications. In other words, by improving the outcome of the mother and baby, there was the potential to reduce non-reimbursable costs to the Memorial Health System. Thus, the Innovation Team approach was a zero-patient-cost model and the financial benefit targeted was a reduction of visits to the ER prior to birth and a reduction in the number of days in the NICU and in the length-of-stay of the mother post-birth.

Patient Interviews. The Innovation Team conducted interviews with patients who had gestational diabetes in previous pregnancies to gain a better understanding from the patient's viewpoint. They found that when doing the current mode of home monitoring, patients often had a heightened concern that they could not get immediate feedback when questions arose about small increases in blood pressure or decreases in fetal kicks at home. When asked if the use of a tele-home monitoring system would be a viable solution to assist in creating healthier outcomes, the responses from these "Patient Voice' interviews were extremely positive, suggesting that it would lend a source of comfort to mothers while being an excellent educational and monitoring tool as well.

Physician Interviews. During interviews with physicians, the Innovation Team found that this real-time data for high-risk OB patients could provide value in a few ways. For example, if a patient that is being monitored experienced a slight increase in blood pressure over the course of multiple days, a call could be placed to suggest lifestyle changes. And if the blood pressure were higher, a mother might be placed on immediate bed rest in advance of a weekly visit or even told to go directly to the hospital emergency room.

Prototyping. The 45-day innovation period was followed by another 30 days of formalized care plan development, presentations and information-sharing meetings with clinical staff that would be involved in the care of the patient, and development of training material that would be shared with the patients. This was also a time of finalizing costs related to the project as well as developing solid workflows for the nurse, physician, and information systems. During this time, work went into formalizing the expected benefits and how Memorial would track these outcomes.

A small number of Health Guides were purchased along with the associated peripheral devices consisting of glucometers, blood pressure monitors, and weight scales. The funding for the purchase came from the organization's innovation dollars that are annually set aside for innovation ideas worthy of seed funding. The man-hours for implementation were supplied by each department's payroll budgets.

Research. The Innovation Team then engaged a local University to perform an adoption study on the pilot program, and IRB approvals were granted both from the hospital and university. The team also communicated with the physician office regarding how they were planning to handle the research study and how the patient populations would be split between a control group and monitored group. Eligible patients for the pilot were identified during a normal visit. The first five patients who agreed to the study were monitored and the next five were placed in the control group. Both groups received one-on-one interviews, which were performed throughout the pregnancy. They were first informed on the purpose of the study and then given the study survey which explored several attributes including agreeableness, openness to new experiences, and conscientiousness. These questions were to be later used to help understand if and how a mother's personality type might influence the success of the program. The monitored group also received training on the telemonitoring system and the device until after birth. There were no financial incentives for the patient to use the device.

The Pilot Project. The pilot went live in January 2010. The organizational adoption of the pilot was fairly easy as the story behind the potential benefits of the device were great. Various meetings were conducted to inform administration, clinical staff in the office, the emergency room, and the childbirth unit. Training was performed so the childbirth unit could access the patient's home monitored data in the event that the patient came in prior to delivery for emergency care.

Results

This High-Risk Obstetric Telemonitoring project continues today with a total of 24 telehealth kits deployed so far. Although the sample size is still too small to perform significant data analysis, there have been several extremely positive anecdotes which illustrate the power of this innovation. Two of these stories stood out as being particularly useful ones in explaining what this type of home telemonitoring system can do for a high-risk population where two lives can be changed in an instant:

Quickly identifying worsening blood pressure at home. In one situation, an expectant mother was being monitored because her elevated blood pressure meant she was at higher risk for developing pre-eclampsia, a pregnancy related cardio-renal syndrome, which can affect both the mother and child. Soon after receiving the telemonitoring device, her blood pressure rose to dangerously high levels at home. Her physician was alerted to these findings, and he advised her to come to the hospital immediately, and she ended up having to deliver her baby urgently due to her condition. This early warning helped facilitate both the delivery of a healthy baby and the improvement of the mother's health, as her condition resolved once her baby was delivered.

A low glucose emergency. In another case, a patient was considered a "brittle diabetic", meaning her glucose levels could fluctuate quickly. Therefore, she used her telehealth device to regularly submit glucose results for review by the watchful nursing staff. Her blood sugars were dangerously low one particular morning and so her nurse became alarmed and attempted to contact her. Since the patient could not be reached on any of her phone numbers, the increasingly concerned nurse then contacted the mother's partner. Her partner went home to check on her and found her passed out due to her critically low blood sugar. He was able to get her to the hospital and get her stabilized where she remained for several days. Once she returned home, she continued her use of the telemonitoring device right up until she delivered at 40 weeks and she had a healthy full term baby. These two are promising examples that have made Memorial very proud of this project and the potential it has to impact a larger patient population.

Lessons Learned

The lessons learned in this approach with high-risk obstetrics provided a great platform to improve this project as well as expand to other telemonitoring service lines.

Ease of Installation: An important lesson learned during this rollout was the fact that patients could set up the telemonitoring device on their own without Memorial needing to do technical home visits to get it working.

Ensuring Connectivity. Based on a sample of potential patients it was recognized that high speed Internet connectivity in the patient home could be a difficult challenge. The determination was made to include cellular data connectivity on 100 % of the pilot devices to ensure there were no issues with connectivity in patient homes. This allowed Memorial to pre-configure the devices and likely reduced the number of technical questions on connectivity to the Internet.

Rethinking Cost Savings: Memorial learned that the assumption of cost savings is much harder to anticipate because gestational diabetes has long reaching impact to the fetus. In other words, complications to the mother with both gestational diabetes and hypertension could continue for weeks or even months after delivery. Thus an improved financial model would include longer-term outcome data.

Bi-lingual Support: Memorial believes that bi-lingual support of telemonitoring systems is critical. A large population of patients had clinical indications to be included in the study, but due to the device being an English-only device, they were not able to participate in the program. Memorial plans to fully utilize the Spanish version of the device when it is released, which will allow for inclusion of that population going forward.

Device Choices: It was discovered that acceptance of the glucometers could be an obstacle. There were several mothers who utilized a different brand of glucometer prior to being placed in the pilot. Their attachment to their usual devices cannot be underestimated. Once receiving the glucometer that interfaced with the telemonitoring device, several mothers expressed an interest in finding out if they could revert to their previous glucometer and interface it with the telemonitoring device. Unfortunately, the existing FDA approvals for the telemonitoring system only allowed three brands to interface, so all mothers had to adhere to one of those brands

Unfortunately, it appears that when a patient was forced to change their glucometer, it negatively affected their compliance with monitoring their glucose. This was supported by the fact that compliance with the telehealth glucometer was better for mothers who had pregnancy induced diabetes, meaning they had not used a different glucometer on a regular basis beforehand.

A related issue is that Medicaid changes the test strips and glucometers they will support on a yearly basis, and the telehealth device currently being used does not update to accept new glucometers. So even if the health system provides the glucometer for free, there can be cost issue for those patients dependent upon Medicaid to pay for the new type of test strips. Memorial shared the concerns about this issue with the vendor of the telemonitoring device with the hope that they can improve their ability to integrate with multiple glucometers and other devices in the future.

Keeping Project Staff Interested. The Innovation Team viewed this as a fun but difficult project. Along the way countless hurdles were presented that threatened to derail the project. On many occasions, particularly when there was not a lot of critical activity, it would have been easier to set the project aside and focus on other projects or on work supporting the rest of the hospital's information systems. However, when the team heard about the positive patient stories it was easy to keep everyone engaged as they could see the benefit. So even after the project went live, it took regular updates from the physicians' office to keep them interested and engaged in the pilot project.

Compliance Issues: A major hurdle continues to be compliance with patient use of the technology. The team initially made assumptions that compliance with the device would be excellent since they had young and ideally technology savvy mothers, who were already worried about the health of their unborn child and themselves. And while this was true for some patients, the team did find there were still rare patients who were technophobic and did not proceed with the pilot. However, it turned out that the bigger issues was that the additional work of monitoring and working with the telehealth device was just too became burdensome in some situations. As a result of these technical and time issues, 5 of the 24 units deployed were.

To address compliance issues, Memorial decided to provide an award certificate that recognized the mother's dedication to her health, her baby's health, and the betterment of medicine because of her participation in the research. This aided in getting some of the non-compliant mothers to participate more.

Future Plans

Memorial is working on interfacing the results received from the telemonitoring devices into the system's Electronic Medical Record. This will allow more immediate review of results and will complete the patient's chart for review during office visits, adding to the quality of care the patient receives.

Memorial also hopes to further research the factors that affect patient compliance, which would allow a better understanding of which patients might need additional education or incentives based on personality factors or other issues. This data is currently being collected and will be analyzed in more detail once the sample size of the research is sufficient enough to yield accurate results. From a return on investment perspective, as the sample size grows, the plan is to get a more accurate indication of the potential for cost avoidance in the monitored population.

Finally, Memorial will be researching additional disease states, which the program could expand upon. The disease states identified would be those that stand to benefit from the use of the telemedicine technology based on outcomes and/or financial benefits. Based on feedback received while doing interviews with Memorial staff, the diseases currently under consideration for expansion include Chronic Heart Failure and Pediatric Diabetes.

Conclusion

From a clinical perspective, Memorial Health System continues to utilize the telemonitoring device for its high-risk obstetrics population and believes that it will reduce the number of unnecessary emergency room visits prior to birth and reduce the number of NICU days in this targeted population. The survey results from the mothers who have been through the pilot are positive, along with the positive stories like the ones mentioned in the Results section, lead Memorial to believe there will be a beneficial long-term impact on the lives of high-risk obstetric patients and that of their unborn babies.

From an innovation perspective, the approach that Memorial took to get this pilot started, which included creation of a small non-management-led team given a specific challenge and a short time frame to accomplish, is one that will be replicated for future innovation efforts. Memorial looks forward to the continued efforts by members of the hospital's innovative teams to continue to thrust Memorial to the forefront of positive clinical outcomes that are greatly assisted by technology.

Chapter 13
Every Language Now

David D. O'Neill, Susan Anthony, and Margaret Laws

Dr. Rugger, an orthopedist, points to his computer screen, where an X-ray is displayed. "Here we see bone deterioration that is causing your hip pain, Mrs. Martinez. We can treat your discomfort with pain medications and physical therapy. Or, we could do hip replacement surgery. There are pros and cons to both of these, but the decision is going to be up to you."

Juanita Martinez looks quickly back and forth between Dr. Rugger and her daughter Barbara, who is attempting to interpret the doctor's words into Spanish for her mother. Barbara has limited fluency in Spanish. Both women are visibly agitated. They worry that if Mrs. Martinez' mobility is not improved she will no longer be able to manage on her own.

Recognizing the language barrier, Dr. Rugger asks his medical assistant to roll the clinic's portable videoconferencing unit into the room. Moments later he accesses the Health Care Interpreter Network (HCIN) and requests a Spanish interpreter. Almost instantly, an interpreter is visible on the screen. Because the unit is equipped with a camera, the interpreter can make direct eye contact with Dr. Rugger, Mrs. Martínez, and her daughter—almost as if they were in the same room.

The interpreter begins in English. "Hello my name is Ann Galvez, Spanish interpreter number 394. How may I help you?"

Dr. Rugger gives his name, the name of the clinic, and the name of his patient.

"Thank you, Dr. Rugger. Please speak directly to your patient. I will repeat everything you say and everything the patient says back to you. I will ask for a pause or clarification if I need one. The conversation is confidential. I will introduce myself to the patient and tell her the same thing."

"Buen día Sra. Martínez. Mi nombre es Ann y seré su intérprete durante su consulta con el Dr. Rugger para que se puedan comunicar. Repetiré todo lo que usted

D.D. O'Neill, J.D., MPH (✉) • S. Anthony • M. Laws, MPP,
California HealthCare Foundation,
1438 Webster Street, Suite 400, Oakland, CA 94612, USA
e-mail: doneill@chcf.org; santhony@chcf.org; mlaws@chcf.org

L. Berkowitz, C. McCarthy (eds.),
Innovation with Information Technologies in Healthcare, Health Informatics,
DOI 10.1007/978-1-4471-4327-7_13, © Springer-Verlag London 2013

diga en español al inglés, tal como usted lo diga y todo lo que diga el Dr. en inglés al español. Si es necesario, voy a interrumpir. Por favor, háblele directamente al médico como si él hablara español. ¿Le parece bien?"

"Sí, está bien." Mrs Martinez replies.

"Go ahead, Doctor," the interpreter says. "The patient is ready for you."

"Mrs. Martinez, I'm going to describe all of your treatment options in more detail so that you will have the information you will need to consider as you choose how to approach treatment," says Dr. Rugger.

Conversing comfortably in Spanish, Juanita is able to understand what the doctor is telling her and ask the questions that come to her mind. Barbara also asks questions, in English, and the interpreter conveys the doctor's answers to Mrs. Martinez. Another appointment is made, and the patient and her daughter are reassured that video interpretation will be available at that meeting as well. They are given printed materials in Spanish and English to reinforce the information they received verbally.

"I'm confident that we will find a way to manage your hip pain so that you can get back to most or all your activities," concludes Dr. Rugger. As his remark is interpreted into Spanish, he sees a smile appear on his patient's face.

As mother and daughter leave the office, Dr. Rugger thinks back to what it was like before the medical center joined HCIN. Patients routinely experienced long waits for one of the staff interpreters to come to the consulting room. Physician schedules were disrupted and workflow often came to a standstill—even when the language needed was a relatively common one. For seldom-used languages, interpretation relied on voice-only technology, which was often inadequate for dealing with complex or serious medical issues. In all of these cases, the patient experience and quality of care were at risk.

Background

The California HealthCare Foundation (CHCF) works as a catalyst to fulfill the promise of better health care for all Californians. It supports ideas and innovations that improve quality, increase efficiency, and lower the costs of care. CHCF funded much of the initial development of the Health Care Interpreter Network (HCIN) program.

The Innovation

The Health Care Interpreter Network (HCIN) is a collaborative of hospitals and providers that share the services of their trained language interpreters over a video and voice network. Its voice/video technology facilitates very rapid connection (about 12 s) to qualified medical interpreters for 15 spoken languages plus American

Sign Language. The vast majority of the HCIN interpreting is done in the outpatient clinics rung by the county facilities or teaching hospitals.

Two innovations underlie HCIN:

1. Creative use of an existing technology to form a voice/video over IP (V/VoIP) network; and
2. An organizational and governance structure that enables the network to overcome the barriers that frequently stifle innovation in county-operated health systems.

Reason for This Innovation

California is a strikingly diverse state. Almost 40 % of the population (about 12.5 million people) over the age of five speak a language other than English at home and often have limited English proficiency (LEP). Of these, more than 8 million are Spanish speakers, but many other languages—including Armenian, Chinese, Japanese, Korean, Vietnamese, and Tagalog—all have more than 140,000 speakers. Dozens of other languages are also represented in the state [1]. Los Angeles County alone has more than 2.5 million residents with LEP [2]. California is also home to more than 3 million hearing-impaired individuals [3], many of whom use American Sign Language.

Although California's LEP populations generally navigate their work lives and community interactions without undue difficulty, these individuals tend to be at a sharp disadvantage when they interact with the health care system. Not only is the medical terminology likely to be unfamiliar, but the subject matter is both personal and important. To be an effective partner in their care, patients must have a clear understanding of their condition and their treatment choices. This responsibility often overwhelms the ability of adult family members to provide interpretation (there is wide agreement that it is *never* appropriate to place minor children in this role). Hospital or clinic staff interpreters may speak the needed language, but the wait can be long and the interpretation quality uneven.

Aside from inconvenience, the consequences for LEP patients when they cannot communicate adequately with their health providers can be profound in terms of compromised quality and increased cost of care. For example, in a 2005 study of 1,083 adverse events reported by six hospitals, Chandriki Divi reported that, 52.4 % of adverse events experienced by LEP patients were attributable to failure of communication versus only 35.9 % adverse events were related to communication issues for English speaking patients [4].

From the provider perspective, the problems are equally compelling. Hospitals and clinics, particularly those in the public sector—like county-operated facilities— must be able to provide interpreter services for thousands of encounters in dozens of languages around the clock. Beyond issues of quality and efficiency, there are legal requirements that must be met. In 2003, the California legislature passed

Senate Bill 853, which required the Department of Managed Health Care (DMHC) to develop regulations requiring health plans to provide certain translation and interpretation services to LEP enrollees. Between 2004 and 2007, DMHC efforts led to the set of language assistance regulations contained in Section 1300.67.04 of Title 28 of the California Code of Regulations. In addition the Title VI of the Civil Rights Act of 1964 and the California Health & Safety Code §1,259 have language access requirements.

Hospitals and clinics work to meet the needs of LEP patients by attracting bi-lingual providers, hiring staff interpreters, contracting with interpreters, and using commercial voice interpreter services such as Language Line. Each of these approaches is a partial solution, and each has shortcomings [5]. For example, the language proficiency of bi-lingual providers is uneven at best; staff interpreters are often inefficient and may have considerable downtime; contract interpreters must be scheduled and often have significant minimum charges; and voice interpretation alone is not appropriate in many situations.

Why This Innovation Succeeded

The concept behind HCIN is based in part upon initiatives that date back to the late 1990s when the University of California, Davis, established that voice/video can be used at scale for interpreter services. Soon after 2000, San Francisco General Hospital and Alameda County Medical Center established and evaluated a shared interpreter service demonstrating that "videoconferencing technology can enhance access to medical interpretation." [6]

The initiative that became HCIN started in 2004–2005 when a group of county hospitals in Northern California[1] developed the concept of sharing interpreters over a multi-hospital V/VoIP network. The planning for this network was funded by grants from the Department of Commerce Technology Opportunity Program and the California HealthCare Foundation (CHCF).[2] The consultant/facilitator had a clear vision of providing excellent voice/video interpreter services by combining her understanding of the technology with hospital interpreter service experience. The work was supported at a policy level by the CEOs of the public hospitals and agencies involved. These leaders saw the need and had the foresight to encourage and support development of the network. The day-to-day planning was done by directors of interpreter services and others within the participating organizations. Three of the

---

[1]Participating hospitals/health systems included: Alameda County Medical Center, Contra Costa Regional Medical Center, San Francisco General Hospital, San Joaquin General Hospital, San Mateo Medical Center, and Santa Clara Valley Medical Center.

[2]The California HealthCare Foundation (CHCF) works as a catalyst to fulfill the promise of better health care for all Californians. It supports ideas and innovations that improve quality, increase efficiency, and lower the costs of care.

hospitals (Contra Costa Regional Medical Center, San Joaquin Medical Center, and San Mateo Medical Center) established the network and implemented it.

Once the network was functioning, it became clear that it had the potential to serve other hospitals and clinics in California. A series of important questions needed to be addressed:

- Who would own the network?
- How would it be governed?
- Was the underlying technology sound and would it serve in the long run?
- What additional grant funding might be necessary to bring the network to the next level?
- Could the network be financially self-sufficient and sustainable?

These questions were addressed through a series of studies by Deloitte Consulting. Issues of ownership, organizational structure, and governance were resolved by establishing a §501(c)(3) not-for-profit organization and a governance structure/ board in which county hospital leaders could participate.

The client for Deloitte's 2006 "HCIN Scalability Report" [7] was the California Health Care Safety Net Institute (SNI), which is the quality improve- ment partner of the California Association of Public Hospitals. SNI was viewed by many of the CEOs/ agency directors as a logical potential home for the net- work. Based on interviews, Deloitte reported that stakeholders and end-users believed that video-based medical interpretation offered a superior experience for patients and clinicians. Further, Deloitte found that HCIN is a scalable, state-of-the-art technical solution that enhances the productivity of currently employed interpreters and enables providers to share such staff across an IP network that leverages videoconference technology. The strongest case for HCIN was with high-volume users, for whom the financial benefit increased as utilization increased.

Deloitte advised that HCIN would require considerable capital to grow, and that there were multiple business models that could work for HCIN, with each having different implications for governance. The initial economic analysis was done using a number of scenarios regarding member growth, utilization growth, and the extent of programmatic improvement and technological upgrade. The report indicated that HCIN appeared to be profitable at an "accounting level" with seven to eight hospi- tals; however, almost double that number of hospitals would be needed for HCIN to have a positive cash flow.

These findings led to a series of key decisions. A separate §501(c)(3) not-for-profit organization would be formed. The governing board would include public hospital CEOs and agency directors. An executive director who had been a California public hospital CEO was retained.

CHCF funded additional business planning, including modeling of longer-term financial feasibility, and development of an initial marketing plan [8]. This research showed that HCIN would achieve a positive cash flow with approximately 13 hos- pitals and, when including grant funding amortized over 5 years, breakeven at approximately 20 hospitals.

CHCF then funded development of the network through 18 member hospitals, at which point HCIN would be above the baseline of members necessary for financial sustainability. The network grew from three members in 2005 to 18 full members in 2011, and is now sustainable.

Costs to each HCIN member are modest. Each participating member pays an annual membership fee ranging from $40,000 to $60,000 depending upon the size and ownership of the organization. In addition, each member is responsible for providing at least one full-time Spanish language interpreter.

HCIN has provided interpreter services to almost 650,000 people from its inception through the end of 2010. Achieving this growth and sustainability required almost 6 years and approximately $5 million in funding including grants from CHCF, Kaiser Community Benefit, and others.[3]

The results of all of all this work resulted in the following specific aspects of this innovation:

The Technical Innovation

Member hospitals and clinics use an automated V/VoIP call center to leverage their own interpreter resources in order to serve these patients more effectively and economically. American Sign Language is available on HCIN video stations through an outside agency. Languages that are not available and back-up coverage are provided through each member's preferred contracted telephonic language service. HCIN builds on the members' existing interpreter services, optimizes their use, and provides both video and voice modalities. The cost is attractive, particularly to providers who have a staff of employed or contracted interpreters.

The technological innovation entailed placing videoconferencing systems— not originally intended for call center use—onto a call center platform that was not developed for video. It also entailed developing and implementing a call-routing process among unrelated business entities. With these innovations in place, high-quality, portable videoconferencing units are combined with the efficiency of a V/VoIP automated call distributor (ACD) system. This integrated system uses three-tiered points of access. When a request call is made, the ACD system first searches for an interpreter located at the facility that initiated the call. If none is available the system scans the other member hospitals for open interpreters. A successful connection to a hospital-based interpreter takes approximately 12 s. If all local and network hospital-based interpreters are engaged, the system connects with a telephone-contracted interpreter of the facility's choice.

---

[3]Over $3,500,000 of this was provided by CHCF grants. Additional grants or equipment contributions were from the Department of Commerce Technology Opportunity Project and Futijsu.

The Organizational Innovation

The importance of HCIN's organizational and governance structure cannot be overstated. The essential elements include:

- Collaborative of members organized as a § 501 (c)(3) corporation.
- Membership is primarily safety-net hospitals and county health agencies.
- Governing board comprised primarily of the CEOs of the member organizations.
- Requirement that each member have at least one qualified, full-time Spanish interpreter on staff.
- Agreement that each member makes its interpreters available to the network according to a protocol that routs an individual member's calls to its own interpreters first, then makes them available to other members.
- System of compensating for interpreter minutes provided to other members (minutes sold) and of paying for interpreter minutes provided by other members (minutes used).
- Agreement to pay an annual membership fee to help support the management and technological infrastructure of HCIN.

Results

Adoption and Utilization. Patient and provider access to interpreter services has grown both in the number of hospitals/clinics added to the network and in the increasing intensity of use within those organizations. HCIN has expanded from its start-up in 2005 to a robust organization. In 2010, 15 hospital members with 70 HCIN qualified interpreters provided 229,035 interpreting sessions and 1,459,500 min of interpreter services (Fig. 13.1). In early 2011, three additional hospitals joined the network bringing the total to 18. The average number of calls per quarter for hospitals well established on the system is about 3,750; however, the range is from about 1,400 to over 7,000 calls per quarter. Video is used for 45 % of the sessions, of which the majority are used in ambulatory clinics. The remaining 55 % of interpretations are handled by telephone, including situations in which video is not needed or appropriate, such as calls for registration or financial counseling.

Quality and Consistency. One of the most important benefits of HCIN is interpreter quality. All HCIN interpreters are trained and tested in health care and medical interpretation. They must have at least 40 h of formal training in medical interpretation. In addition, most of the interpreters are specially trained for behavioral health interpreting and many are trained for palliative care interpreting.

Efficiency and Cost-Effectiveness. The efficiency of interpreters in member organizations has increased threefold from about eight face-to-face/in-person sessions per day to about 30 sessions using the network. In addition, hospitals that

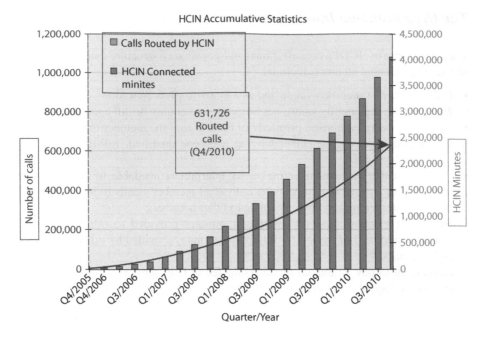

Fig. 13.1 HCIN accumulative statistics

have staff interpreters who are not fully utilized can increase the efficiency of those interpreters by sharing them on the network. Forty percent of participating members are net suppliers of interpreter minutes and 60 % are net users of interpreting services.[4] Furthermore, bi-lingual staff can be used more effectively when there are interpreter services because they are not pulled away from other work to serve as an interpreter.[5]

Return on Investment. Not all members have completed or shared formal return-on-investment analyses. However, one member with significant Spanish interpretation needs shared results of a study. The organization had been paying almost $12,000 per week for an in-person Spanish interpretation consulting service. After hiring two full-time employed Spanish interpreters and paying the annual membership fee, they still saved over $9,000 per week, or $368,000 per year. Additionally, HCIN has enabled hospitals that had no (or few) interpreters to have a basis for hiring interpreters because of the minimum in-house Spanish interpreter requirement. This requirement, along with the availability of HCIN itself, has increased access significantly (Fig. 13.1).

---

[4]HCIN hospitals can also choose to "sell" interpreter minutes to networks outside of HCIN. In the last 8 months of 2010, HCIN member hospitals sold 14,000 min to other network hospitals.

[5]Providers should be tested and qualified to provide care to patients in a language other than English.

Lessons Learned

- **Leadership and Collaboration**. The founders—who were either public hospital CEOs/agency directors or had experience with public hospitals—viewed HCIN as a "public good." This conviction motivated them to persist in developing the venture in spite of the fact that they had no personal economic stake in it. There was exceptional collaboration among the founding member hospital CEOs. Retention of an executive director with county hospital leadership experience facilitated the growth of the membership as well as multiple interfaces with facility staff throughout the decision-making and implementation processes.
- **Need for Quick and Obvious Wins**. Health care providers are often inpatient. They also have long memories about awkward or inadequate interpreter service efforts. Quality and ease of service (single call, rapid connection) and interpretation were essential to give HCIN credibility. Additionally, use of this technology gave hospitals access to new languages and the ability to increase interpreter efficiency. Both were important to winning over hospital executives.
- **Appropriate use of Consultants**. The consultant's financial/business/technical reports gave CEOs and the major funder confidence that the venture was sound. The work plan outlined in the Deloitte reports was followed carefully.
- **Securing Initial Capital**. The "venture capital" provided by CHCF for initial site equipment and initial membership support was an essential building block. The member hospitals could not have supported the development out of their operating budgets.
- **Working with Public Hospitals**. Public-sector decision-making is very slow and complex. One advantage of the collaboration was that public hospital CEOs and agency directors were able to share information and approaches to problem solving.
- **Technology Keeps Getting Cheaper and Smaller**. Throughout HCIN's development, there has been a continuing reduction in size and cost of technology capable of connecting to the network and doing voice/video from quite bulky and complex carts to more compact and portable devices. In fact, reductions in the cost of portable units alone were sufficient to add capacity at many of the participating hospitals and clinics without increasing the overall budget. It is likely that the use of thin, cheap tablets like the iPad will become increasingly utilized. While 4 G phones can be used for American Sign Language interpretation, it is not likely that these smaller screens will be used regularly simply because the images may be too small to be effective. Theft prevention will continue to be an issue.
- **Training**. Training of providers—as well as interpreters—is important; whenever possible providers in member organizations are trained in the appropriate use of interpreters.[6]

---

[6]These provider training programs have received significant funding from Kaiser Permanente Community Benefit Programs.

- **Stable Technology Management**. HCIN's retention of an excellent technology system manager facilitated developing the network. The mutual confidence and commitment underlying this relationship were essential ingredients for success.
- **Conservative Nature of IT Staff**. Installations often took longer than anticipated, in part because IT staff, responsible for protecting firewalls and system integrity, tend to be cautious and conservative when introducing new technology.
- **System Expansion**. As the network evolved, it is become clear that it could be used for more than routine interpreter services. For example, it is also being used for other telehealth services, primarily lactation consultation, psychiatry, and occasionally for endocrinology.

Future Plans

The HCIN plans to continue to expand to hospitals in need throughout California. Additionally, the HCIN technology and strategy is expandable outside of California. In fact, HCIN's technology system manager, Paras and Associates, has developed networks using similar technology in Chicago, Washington DC, New Mexico, Texas, New York, and Pennsylvania [9]. HCIN can link with these networks for additional coverage and access to languages that it does not provide. For example, it uses Mount Sinai Hospital in Chicago and George Washington University Hospital in the District of Columbia for American Sign Language coverage. Likewise, other networks use HCIN for languages that are not readily available in their member organizations, most often Asian languages.

There are plans to continue to expand the concept of shared telehealth services beyond language interpretation, lactation consultancy, and the others mentioned. Trials currently planned include using HCIN to facilitate language access in a post-discharge stroke rehabilitation program, and scheduled behavioral health appointments in addition to on-demand service.

Conclusion

HCIN has been launched and is successful both programmatically and as a business enterprise. It has significant potential to expand its own interpreter services, link with other interpreter networks, and use its technology to couple interpretation with telehealth. HCIN's ultimate success will depend on building on its core network and interpreter services, ongoing innovation as technology and opportunity permit, and the continuing attention of its board and management.

References

1. U.S. Census 2000, table 5. http://www.census.gov/population/www/cen2000/briefs/phc-t37/tables/tab06a.pdf. Accessed on 5 Sept 2012.
2. Speaks LA. Language diversity and English proficiency by Los Angeles county service planning area. Asian Pacific American Legal Center. Mar 2008. http://apalc.org/sites/default/files/LASpeaksLanguageDiversity.pdf. Page 1.
3. Hearing Loss Association of California. The site indicates that hearing loss affects approximately 10 % of the U.S. population. http://hearinglossca.org/information/fact-sheet. Accessed on 22 Apr 2011.
4. Joint Commission. Language proficiency and adverse events in US hospitals: a pilot study. Divi C, Koss R et al. Language proficiency and adverse events in US hospitals. Int J Qual Healthcare 2006;10(2):60–7; Fernandez A, Schillinger D et al. Language barriers, physician-patient language concordance, and glycemic control among insured Latinos with diabetes: the diabetes study of Northern California (DISTANCE). J Gen Intern Med. 2010 Sept 29 [Epub ahead of print].
5. Dower C, Kaiser J. Improving language access in California Hospitals. UCSF Center for Health Professions (2007);6–7. http://thecenter.ucsf.edu/Content/29/2007-09_Improving_Language%20_Access_in_California_Hospitals.pdf. Accessed on 22 Apr 2011.
6. Paras M. Videoconferencing medical interpretation: the results of clinical trials. Oakland: Health Access Foundation; 2002. p. 7.
7. Deloitte Consulting. HCIN scalability report. The report was funded by CHCF. May 2006.
8. Deloitte Consulting. HCIN growth planning report. The report was funded by CHCF. Oct 2008.
9. http://parasandassociates.net/. Accessed on 25 Apr 2011.

Chapter 14
Rise of the ePharmacists

Mark S. Gagnon and Janell Moerer

As the winter months rolled along in Western Kansas the cough and cold season was hitting hard. The Martinez family was no different and had their fair share of runny noses in the house. However, the youngest boy, Mike, did not seem to be recovering as quickly as the rest of the family. Mike continued to run a high fever, feeling extremely tired with a hacky cough and achy muscles. Mike's parents, Barbara and Ray, decided to bring him to the doctor. Dr. Bob ordered a chest X-ray which revealed signs of pneumonia in his lungs, so he decided to admit him into the local hospital to receive IV antibiotics and try to keep his fever down.

At the hospital, Dr. Bob ordered routine antibiotics to treat Mike's pneumonia. However, Dr. Bob did not realize that recent resistant patterns had changed - fortunately, the virtual pharmacist on call was familiar with these patterns and helped suggest a more effective antibiotic regimen. If the routine antibiotics were given, it is likely Mike would have deteriorated and then needed to be transferred to a hospital with an Intensive Care Unit. "It's so nice to be able to keep Mike here. In the past, it was hard for the docs to keep up with all the different drug options and side effects", says Dr. Bob to Barbara and Ray.

"We had to transfer my mother-in-law last year. That was really hard trying to coordinate care, visits and work. What's different now?" says Barbara relieved.

"There were not enough pharmacists to physically staff every hospital in our area 24 hours a day in the past" explained Dr. Bob. "But now we have the 'ePharmacy' program, which lets pharmacists connect with any of our hospitals electronically to help oversee medication ordering and dispensing - even when they are not physically present. It allows our patients to receive better, safer care, and lets them stay in their local hospitals near their families!"

M.S. Gagnon, Pharm.D. (✉) • J. Moerer
Via Christi Health, Inc, 8200 E Thorn, Wichita, KS 67226, USA
e-mail: mark.gagnon@viachristi.org; janellmoerer@centura.org

L. Berkowitz, C. McCarthy (eds.),
Innovation with Information Technologies in Healthcare, Health Informatics,
DOI 10.1007/978-1-4471-4327-7_14, © Springer-Verlag London 2013

Background

Via Christi Health (VCH) is a Catholic nonprofit integrated delivery health system and the largest provider of health care services in Kansas and northern Oklahoma. This includes:

- 12 owned/managed hospitals
- Academic medical center and free standing rehab and behavioral health hospitals
- Via Christi Villages, 17 owned/managed senior communities
- Comprehensive array of ambulatory, post-acute and outpatient centers and services
- Via Christi Physician Services, with more than 300 employed physicians
- Kansas' first Program for All Inclusive Care (PACE)
- 10,000+ employees

Via Christi Health has two key directional strategies: Excellent Performance and Healthcare Transformation. The strategy for transformation is focused on innovations in systems of care and/or care delivery redesign, with objectives to a) improve access, b) improve patient safety and outcome, and c) flatten the cost curve. The VCH Business Development and Innovation Team oversees much of the transformation strategy and provides a comprehensive method of support and development. This team brings new concepts to life through the use of enabling technology, innovation and design techniques in collaboration with core operating leaders.

The Innovation

To address the region's growing hospital pharmacist shortage, VCH developed the ePharmacy program to increase access to highly trained hospital pharmacists in both rural and metropolitan areas across the state for improved patient safety.

An ePharmacist is defined as a hospital trained pharmacist who works from a remote location using secured enabling technology to support bedside clinicians with an effective and timely method of providing medication treatments for patients.

The Via Christi Health ePharmacy system is a telehealth service which enables a pharmacist to provide remote order entry (ROE) services, which is defined as the review and profiling of physician medication orders by a pharmacist from a remote site (e.g. the pharmacist's home), to its ministries and outreach facilities throughout Kansas. Additionally, the ePharmacists can dispense medications using enabling technology. The ePharmacy program also allows pharmacists from a remote location to have a virtual face-to-face visit for a pharmacy consult with the patient, nurses, physicians and other members of the medical staff about a patient's medical condition. Another virtual capability is remote supervision by a hospital pharmacist to an onsite pharmacy technician for drug dispensing oversight and compound mixing oversight. Experienced hospital ePharmacists, with appropriate Kansas state licensure, can reside anywhere in the U.S. and provide the required order review.

Reason for This Innovation

National reports point to a growing nationwide shortage of medical professionals, specifically in the area of pharmacy. In fact, the Pharmacy Manpower Project predicts that by the year 2020, the national supply of pharmacists will fall short of demand by 157,000.[1] At a more local level, a 2007 survey by the Kansas Pharmacy Associate through the Kansas Independent Pharmacy Service Corporation found that six Kansas counties have no pharmacist and thirty-one counties have only one pharmacist. These statistics made Kansas one of nine states experiencing the highest level of pharmacist shortage.

Via Christi began experiencing hospital pharmacist shortages in 2003 and up to five hospital pharmacist shortages were being experienced at any given time. This made it challenging for Via Christi to adhere to the Joint Commission recommendation of a pharmacist prospective review for each medication order before the medication is administered to the patient. Meanwhile, recruitment for highly trained hospital pharmacists became increasingly difficult as competition from large retail pharmacies grew.

In the name of patient safety and staff efficiency, Via Christi needed to develop an innovative model that would close this gap of need in their pharmacy services. To expand access to hospital pharmacists and to provide increased hours of clinical pharmacy support at the bedside to improve patient safety, in 2008 Via Christi developed the ePharmacy program to support hospital order entry services with a new remote "ePharmacist" staffing model.

Why This Innovation Succeeded

The ePharmacy initiative was part of a redesign for VCH pharmacy services led by the pharmacy directors and leaders in coordination with the business development and innovation team. In June 2008, to launch the ePharmacy development, a full-day "decision accelerator" multidisciplinary planning meeting was held with leadership from across the system Outside-thought leaders from pharmacy, telepharmacy, telemedicine and innovation were invited to help identify the strategic direction and design concept for the ePharmacy model.

---

[1](Professionally Determined Need for Pharmacy Services in 2020, David A. Knapp, American Journal of Pharmaceutical Education, Vol. 66, Winter 2002).

The decision accelerator is a concentrated and rapid the development forum for design innovation. This forum set the design for the ePharmacy model and established the milestone roadmap for development, implementation, and ongoing measurement review process. As part of the decision accelerator planning session, a discernment process was held with participants to provide a time for introspection and self reflection regarding the change and disruption this innovative approach would create with staff as well as pharmacy and nursing work flow. Discernment is a term used to describe the activity of determining the value and quality of a certain subject or event. Typically, it is used to describe the activity of going past the mere perception of something, to making detailed judgments about that thing. As a virtue, a discerning individual is considered to possess wisdom, and be of good judgment; especially so with regard to subject matter often overlooked by others. This process helped ensure the major decisions were grounded in reflection, and supported the Via Christi Mission, Vision, Core Values and Catholic identity, while fostering the ability for participants and stakeholders to articulate and communicate the rationale for the direction and decisions — especially where disruption occurs.

Further, the discernment process provided a safe environment for participants to identify the hopes, biases and fears and engaged the team in open dialogue on major concerns such as changes in power and control. Without the discernment process, personal issues often remain unaddressed and can derail or delay the initiative. The group recognized the significant opportunity to improve patient safety and quality and they moved forward in developing a 90 day quick start plan and 1 year roadmap for implementation of the model design.

To recap the decision accelerator planning session, the following represents a high level outline of the steps:

1. Set context and background of the problem or desired future state
2. Present "burning platform"
3. Discernment process: hopes, biases and fears
4. Feature internal and external content experts
5. Frame questions for critical thinking
6. Use small groups for "rapid" design and development sessions
7. Report out/shift and share exercises
8. Create design plan with short term and long term development roadmap with timelines.

The decision accelerator set the design and the development roadmap to begin immediately following this forum. A steering committee of pharmacy leaders and content experts were engaged weekly to review and advise the development team and outline the research study to validate the model impact. The Business Development team supported the pharmacy leaders and steering committee to ensure the value proposition for patients and stakeholders was identified, tested and validated while setting a process for continued model refinement. Rapid prototyping, change management and fail fast techniques are used to move a concept to a viable service.

The timeline outlined below (Fig. 14.1) represents the design, development, and implementation milestones for the ePharmacy remote order entry service.

2008	January January-June June	Problem: Pharmacist shortage escalates Solutions identified technoloty enabled approach Pharmacy decision accelerator resulting in new ePharmacy model &roadmap
	July	Hire ePharmacy Director and develope ePharmacy remote order entry model
	September November	IRB approval for ePharmacy study Engage Kansas Pharmacy Board discussion for remote supervision (telepharmacy) regulations
	December	Hired & trained first ePharmacist (resides in Pennsylvania) Go-live at first Via Christi Hospital
2009	February August September	Expand ePharmacy to other Via Christi Hospital Expand ePharmacy to critical access hospitals ePharmacy study complete; validates value
2010	August September December	Expand ePharmacy for 3rd shift coverage for all Via Christi Hospitals 22 ePharmacists trained ePharmacy published in American Journal of Health System Pharmacists Implement virtual desktop to improve operational efficiency
2011	April December	AHRQ recognizes ePharmacy Pharmacy at critical access hospitals, all Via Christi acute hospitals

Fig. 14.1 Design, development, and implementation milestones for the ePharmacy remote order entry service

In July 2008, a Director of ePharmacy was hired and staff development for the ePharmacy team was initiated. ePharmacy, as a new concept model, has a matrix reporting to both the VP of Business Development and Innovation and to the Executive Pharmacy Director. The matrix reporting ensures accountability and that resources are available for both development and operational adoption while bridging the transformation and performance objectives throughout the health system. This collaborative approach enhances ongoing pilot and prototype testing as well as continued engagement of senior leadership. Creating the matrix reporting structure for ongoing design and development helped the pharmacy team optimize innovation and transformation within the core operations. ePharmacy, as a stable operation, is strongly integrated into, not separate from, hospital pharmacy services, which has accelerated the adoption and diffusion of the service.

The ePharmacy director convened weekly conference calls to establish policies and standard operating procedures. Via Christi Pharmacy leaders also worked with the Kansas State Board of Pharmacy to develop appropriate oversight regulations for remote pharmacy services, e.g. telepharmacy. The first Kansas licensed hospital remote hospital pharmacist (ePharmacist) was hired in Pennsylvania the service was live with the initial prototype within 5 months.

The staffing model is unique in that the "ePharmacist" has to have a Kansas license and 2 years of hospital experience, but the individual can reside anywhere in the U.S. This approach has helped Via Christi leverage experienced, yet geographically distant, hospital pharmacy talent to expand the pharmacy team without the cost and difficulty of bringing pharmacists to a hospital. Remote ePharmacists currently reside in Pennsylvania, California, Minnesota and Colorado. This arrangement can be ideal for a hospital trained pharmacist who wants to "moonlight" after hours from the comfort of their home. Thus, the staffing model leverages scarce hospital pharmacy talent by using both "dual" employees — pharmacists who already work at other locations within Via Christi — and pharmacists who work remotely and hold an active Kansas license.

Results

To evaluate the benefits of the ePharmacy program, a research study was conducted at five of the hospital ministries to validate the value and efficacy of ePharmacy services. The study showed an improvement in patient safety, increased order turnaround, and increased satisfaction among staff. The abstract research protocols for the study were approved by the Via Christi Hospital institutional review board (IRB) and the study was conducted as part of the launch for ePharmacy. Pre ePharmacy and post go live surveys and outcome measures were conducted as part of the study to establish a baseline and to validate value and patient impact. The study was conducted September 2008 through August 2009.

This study found that the program expanded access to hospital pharmacy services, reduced turnaround time for medication orders, freed hospital-based pharmacists for additional quality initiatives, and improved the nurses' satisfaction with pharmacy services. The study was published in the American Journal of Health-System Pharmacy (Sept. 1, 2010) and is recognized on the Innovations Exchange for the Agency for Healthcare Research and Quality (AHRQ). The Innovations Exchange focuses on the improvement in patient education by the hospital pharmacist due to ePharmacy support.

Cost Savings

It was also shown that the ePharmacy program increased the number of documented pharmacy therapeutic interventions with an estimated savings of $1.13 million annually according to ActionOI®. Documented pharmacy interventions indicated that pharmacy has intervened in a potential mistake or adverse action from a written/electronic order. Typically, examples of effective pharmacy intervention are documenting the correction for wrong dose, wrong time or wrong patient. The intervention, then, has a cost or value by preventing a mistake or adverse patient event. Documenting these interventions aides in validating dollar value of order entry services and remote order entry. The ActionOI® tool is a financial and operational comparative database used in the health care industry and by Via Christi to measure cost and impact of clinical services such as pharmacy. ActionOI® uses evidence-based information to assist hospitals in decision-making and prioritization of initiatives. The calculated cost savings from the ePharmacy study were based on metrics established by data collected by ActionOI®.

Increase Efficiency of Onsite Pharmacists and Nurses

Part of the ePharmacy design was to provide support to onsite pharmacists. At the tertiary hospital, two Via Christi hospitals have 24/7 on-site pharmacists. The remote pharmacist was able to help reduce the workload from 5 p.m. to 2 a.m., thus allowing the onsite pharmacists the opportunity to provide more bedside patient education and consultation on Warfarin management on the hospital units.

Meanwhile, two of the Via Christi community hospital pharmacies were only open from 7 a.m. to 7 p.m. This nighttime gap in pharmacy coverage left the nursing staff without access to a pharmacist and required them to write down the medications on a paper medication admission record (MAR) until the pharmacy could enter them the next morning into the electronic medical record (EMR) system. The result was that the nurses could not fully utilize the bedside bar code scanning technology that had been developed to improve patient safety. In other words, since there was not a pharmacist to put the medication on a patient's electronic medication profile, the bar coding system would not provide the medication for the nurse.

The addition of the third-shift ePharmacy service thus allowed the nurses the ability to do bedside medication verification on all shifts and improved the medication order turn around. This also reduced the hospital pharmacists' morning workload, allowing them to spend more time to participate in morning patient care rounds, provide clinical monitoring to help reduce costs, and improve patient safety. While increasing pharmacist coverage during third shift was an additional cost to each facility, the ePharmacy service was provided to the hospitals at half the price it would cost to staff it with pharmacists onsite, due to the shared service model utilized

A New Opportunity Emerges

During the course of ePharmacy development and implementation, monthly and quarterly conference calls were held with the directors of pharmacy. It became apparent during the calls that all of the ministries were working on similar problems and had similar challenges; so, there was opportunity to improve care and operational efficiency among the ministry pharmacy operations. In addition, all of the Via Christi ministries operated on different pharmacy information systems and the medication formularies were not standardized. ePharmacy, however, was the one

2009	October November	Standardization opportunities emerge Pharmacy leaders desire strong collaboration
2010	January February-October November	Pharmacy Decision Accelerator result in new phrmacy services department unit & road map Research best practice and desighn pharmacy service models& ROI Pharmarcy Service Model approved & funded
2011	Janaury February October November	Hire Executive Pharmacy Director Implement Plan & develob reporting Exceeded ROI projections Kansas Pharmacy Board approves hospital remote supervision regulations (telepharmacy)
2012	Janaury February	Pharmacy Services refine ePharmacy and out line telepharmacies (remote dispensing) model 2 telepharmacy pilots go-live through ePharmacy

Fig. 14.2 Development process for Via Christi Pharmacy Services

clinical tool and team that provided a standardized and integrated process with a proven and positive impact on patient care and cost. The standing pharmacy team discussion forums, along with the successful impact of ePharmacy, ultimately led to moving all hospital pharmacy toward stronger integration and standardization.

The model was to integrate Via Christi Health pharmacy services across multiple venues to improve patient safety and quality while increasing access to hospital pharmacists by leveraging the appropriate resources. January 2010, the pharmacy leaders supported by the Business Development team, key leaders throughout the organization, and outside thought leaders gathered, again, for a 2-day decision accelerator planning session to create a phased approach for a new, integrated Pharmacy model within VCH ministries. Since integration would be disruptive to existing operations, the discernment process was helpful in fostering greater trust and openness among stakeholders as it allowed the group time to discuss both negative and positive biases. The team can then focus on the strengths, benefits and value of creating the new, integrated pharmacy service model.

A new steering committee was formed to develop the plan, which received full support of senior leadership and hospital executives and received the funding requested for development and implementation. The pharmacy integration was to increase appropriate standardization to drive down medication costs while improving quality of care and patient safety. Key features were reporting and review patient safety. Year one outcomes resulted in an $800,000 savings and cost avoidance predominately in standardizing drug acquisition. This was achieved by a more focused and centralized process through standard reporting and review by the buyers lead by the Executive Director for Pharmacy. In addition consistent purchasing from the lowest cost, contracting vendor was implemented which is known as optimal purchasing. The timeline below (Fig. 14.2) outlines the development process for Via Christi Pharmacy Services:

Lessons Learned

Lessons learned primarily related to organizational structure and developing new processes and procedures within the organization.

Hiring Policy

The Human Resources department had to develop a new set of hiring practices, standards and policies to enable ePharmacists from across the country to work for Via Christi on a remote basis. Some of the challenges included identifying appropriate facilities in the ePharmacists' area to conduct drug screens, developing new processes and orientation for remote ePharmacist, and applying for workers' compensation in the ePharmacist's state of residence. We learned that the "little" things can create big issues. For example, in some states, workers' compensation rules are monopolistic and include special legislation that requires workers' compensation coverage to be provided exclusively by the state's Designated Workers Compensation program. Via Christi determined that employment of remote staff in these monopolistic states would not be viable. Consequently, as a regional health system, Via Christi's view of a virtual/remote work force has broadened its geographic outreach. In addition, the new "dual" employee pharmacist was developed to provide a specific process for internal full-time hospital pharmacists to also provide services as an ePharmacist. The goal was to retain Via Christi's well trained hospital pharmacists within the service model verses these same pharmacists moonlighting at other locations. Dual pharmacists have a unique hiring and review process to encourage existing pharmacist to stay within the Via Christi family of services.

Regulatory Issues

Collaborating with the Kansas State Board of Pharmacy was one of the most important objectives in developing new and transformational services such as remote order entry and electronic supervision programs. Most states do not have regulations addressing either of these two programs. Via Christi pharmacy leaders and legal counsel assisted the Kansas State board of Pharmacy is developing the remote supervision regulation for the state of Kansas. The Kansas State Board of Pharmacy determined to develop two different sets of regulations for electronic supervision/telepharmacy; one for outpatient and community and the other for hospitals. The rationale for two sets of regulations is due to vast differences in training and market and competitive dynamics between the outpatient and community pharmacy and hospital pharmacy environments. The decision resulted in a more comprehensive regulation that better served the hospital setting.

Securing the System

Finally, the "e" model or remote order entry depended heavily on the use of enabling technology, so a member of the IT team was assigned to assist the Director of ePharmacy in developing the electronic system. The ePharmacy system needed to allow a remote pharmacist access to everything a hospital-based pharmacist would have through a secured connection. The development of such a system had many challenges due to the multiple hospital information systems and lack of standardization among the hospitals both within Via Christi and in outside rural hospitals. A decision was made to "freeze" all the computers so that if a pharmacist downloaded an application that caused another application not to work, he or she could simply shut off their computer and restart it to reset the original system.

The Need for Virtual Desktops

To simplify the remote training and upload of new software, a web-based virtual desktop was installed on all computers to allow the ePharmacists access to all of the applications from any location as long as they had Internet access. The virtual desktop also helped quickly provide updates and new application installations. For example, instead of updating 20 different computers, which could take days and have shipping costs and delays, a single update was applied to the virtual desktop. In an instant, all of the pharmacists had access to the new application with no downtime. The virtual desktop is a key development that has helped sustain the growth of the program and thus save time and frustration for the pharmacist when an update is required.

Using Internet Phones for Communication

Communication was another crucial component of selective service delivery, especially in developing an approach that could connect the on-site hospital team to the right ePharmacist at the right time. Via Christi deployed Internet phones that had a more universal calling process and could be activated with each ePharmacist staffing schedule. Internet created local phone numbers for pharmacists living in different area codes. This gave a more local feel and helped eliminate the fear that a physician might dismiss an out of state call as a wrong number. This capability has been a low cost and reliable method in establishing an effective communication method.

The Importance of eTraining

To train a growing staff of remote ePharmacists, the ePharmacy Director developed a training program that used programs such as WebEx or Go-To-Meeting with

Voice-Over Internet Protocol (VoIP) to communicate to the ePharmacist. The ePharmacy Director is the expert trainer for all information systems and trains remote pharmacists to ensure consistency and quality of service. During training, the ePharmacy Director can view the remote ePharmacist's screen as if they were in the same room with the Director looking over the ePharmacist's shoulder while they train on entering medication orders. The goal of training was to replicate the feel of being face to face. The VoIP allowed both pharmacists to have their hands free and communicate through a headset. This style of training has been critical to the success of the remote order entry service and ensures quality and continuity of the service.

Better Understanding the Value of Pharmacists

Pharmacists often are taken for granted or undervalued as a part of the medical team. And this undervaluing was a major hurdle in promoting the remote order entry program both internally and externally. Many hospitals Via Christi visited across the state have never had a pharmacist onsite. The ePharmacy service provided the value of a low cost option while lifting the bar on patient safety and quality of care.

For example, in an 8-month period a critical access hospital had over 120 medication interventions documented and reported back to the facility by the ePharmacy program. The hospital had the data and the pharmacy support and service to make effective changes to improve the medication treatment process with the staff and for patients. The nursing and staff satisfaction is evident as one critical access hospital nurse told the ePharmacist on the phone, "Wow! You are really taking great care of us. Thank you." It is often difficult to change the culture of a facility and show the value when the service is an added cost that they have never had before. However, when value is demonstrated through increased patient safety then the cost is more than justified.

Future Plans

Via Christi pharmacy will be one of the first teams in the region to provide remote dispensary to community and critical access hospitals. In five to ten years, through enabling technology, VCH plan to bring the hospital pharmacist to the patient's home, car and other areas - all working in concert with their physician and care team. VCH also looks forward to the day when it can help provide weekly health education in all schools to educate the next generation of health and wellness consumers and pharmacy leaders.

Additionally, VCH assisted the Kansas State Board of Pharmacy in developing other remote electronic supervision regulations in Kansas as well. These will allow for the use of two-way audio/visual support for a pharmacist to oversee nurses and/or pharmacy technicians in the timely dispensing of medication and/or compound mixing. As pharmacy shortages grow, the "virtual ePharmacist" will become increasingly necessary for providing safe and effective access to pharmacy services.

Conclusion

In a world where the supply of clinical pharmacists cannot meet the increasing demand for their services, innovative thinking was needed to find a more efficient use of available hospital pharmacists. Via Christi's ePharmacy system has succeeded in allowing remote pharmacists to address some of the clinical needs in a health care organization, thus allowing on-site pharmacists to round with the medical staff and provide more personalized education to patients.

The development of the Via Christi ePharmacy program has provided tremendous opportunities for pharmacy departments across Via Christi Health. On-site pharmacists have been able to round more frequently with the medical team, build stronger relationships with the physicians and care team while gaining the trust in the ePharmacist's ability to provide consultation and medication management.

The shortage of pharmacists may never be eliminated but the development of new innovative technology will continue to provide effective options to fill the gap in the shortage. The use of both the pharmacist and technology will help to improve the care we provide to the patients and communities we serve.

Section III
On the Edge of Edge

The future of healthcare is here, just look around!

What happens when walls come alive? How about when your HIT systems start showing you things you never even imagined in the past? How about instantaneous feedback from your patients? What if losing weight was like an Indiana Jones adventure? Oh, the fabulous places we can go when solving problems with interdisciplinary thinking. And we are not just talking about nurses and doctors on the same team. We are talking about gamers, healthcare gurus, engineers, politicians, savvy business people, and patients mingling minds so that magic can happen.

Although much of HIT innovation takes shape in the EHR and telemedicine worlds, it is starting to blossom in many other surprising areas. Innovators are increasingly taking wild leaps combining technologies, space, and workflow to create superior experiences and better results. This final section of the book is about the future of thinking innovatively with healthcare IT, whether pilfering ideas from other industries or generating radical ideas in this one.

We open with UPMC's SmartRoom: part facility, part technology, part workflow, part patient, part nurse, and all a big bold leap forward. They took the everyday, unnoticed, dumb surface of a wall and coaxed it to life. And through their design process and iterations it picked up more and more intelligence so that the room itself becomes a smart partner to the healthcare team.

From there you will experience pocket-sized EMRs from Partners Healthcare, amazing actionable dashboards from HealthEast Care System and Nebraska Children's Hospital, and the power of the patient's voice made strong from Kaiser Permanente's online "Member Voice Panel". Together they are taking us to the Star Trek world where computers shift from being devices of input to real time guiding assistants which improve the process of care.

We conclude with a trip down the rabbit hole: the Gamification of HealthCare. It is safe to say that none of us know exactly where the rabbit hole will take us, but the exploration of games and game mechanics is getting big. The wellness space is flooded with gadgets, gizmos, and apps that are quantifying just about everything and increasing the motivation and ability of the individual and even of groups to be healthier. Gaming is helping the sick and injured to heal, is increasing chemotherapy compliance for kids with cancer, and is distracting third-degree burn victim during painful dermabrasions. It is indeed a whole new world.

The key concept in this final section is pushing boundaries to get faster and better. Space, technology, workflows and experiences need to be rethought and recreated to wake up from their current dumb, passive states. This is just the beginning of the awakening, and through iteration they will be become smarter, more responsive, more helpful, and more enabling. Explore this section by asking yourself "how might I wake up the things around me?"

Happy Exploring!

Chapter 15
The Smartest Room

Tamra E. Minnier and David T. Sharbaugh

Barbara Martinez woke up early Friday morning determined to get all of her 2nd grade tests graded. She had a lot to do in the upcoming days and needed to stay on task.

After she finished making lunches for her kids, she felt a little tightness in her arm. At school the pain returned and she began to worry. It was just a few months ago that her doctor talked to her about the signs of a heart attack. After a quick phone call to him, she got her husband Ray to drive her to the ER, and her visit there indicated an abnormal EKG. She was admitted to the hospital. "Not again," she mutters. Barb was in this hospital 6 months ago for a 2-day stay following an elective surgical procedure.

After Barb was admitted to her room, she noticed a touch screen monitor on the wall at the foot of her bed. The first caregiver that came in to see Barb was Sue, an admission nurse. When Sue walked into the room, the touch screen automatically showed her name and role. "Wow. I've never seen that before! What is that screen?" asked Barb.

"It's a really cool new technology that our hospital developed. It instantly gives the right information to the right person at the right time. Your TV is hooked in as well. You can now review education materials, medications, and even email! We call it the SmartRoom. OK, now let's start your admission."

Sue looked at the touch screech, "Barb I see here that you are allergic to latex. We'll make sure that no latex is used."

"Amazing", said Barbara relaxing, "this place really does know me."

T.E. Minnier, MSN, RN (✉)
Donald D. Wolff, Jr. Center for Quality, Safety, and Innovation,
University of Pittsburgh Medical Center,
200 Lothrop Street Forbes Tower, Suite 11086, Pittsburgh, PA 15213, USA
e-mail: minnierte@upmc.edu

D.T. Sharbaugh, B.A.
SmartRoom, LLC, 600 Grant Street, 60th Floor USX Tower,
Pittsburgh, PA 15219, USA
e-mail: sharbaugh@smartroomsolutions.com

L. Berkowitz, C. McCarthy (eds.),
Innovation with Information Technologies in Healthcare, Health Informatics,
DOI 10.1007/978-1-4471-4327-7_15, © Springer-Verlag London 2013

Background

UPMC is a $9 billion global health enterprise with more than 50,000 employees headquartered in Pittsburgh, PA. It is transforming health care by integrating more than 20 hospitals, 400 doctors' offices and outpatient sites, a health insurance services division, and international and commercial services. Affiliated with the University of Pittsburgh Schools of the Health Sciences, UPMC is using innovative science, technology, and medicine to create new models of accountable, cost-efficient, and patient-centered care.

UPMC is committed to developing and delivering Life Changing Medicine. Drawing on the power of collaboration and creative thinking, UPMC is taking medicine from where it is to where it needs to be. This commitment has given birth to a new innovation called SmartRoom, which is changing the way care is delivered in hospitals today.

The Innovation

SmartRoom is a computerized system that detects who is in a given hospital room and provides them with the information they need to complete their job efficiently and reliably. The system utilizes a real time locating system (RTLS) and a touch screen user interface designed to make work quick and simple for end users.

The system relies on all staff members wearing tags that can be recognized by sensors in the rooms and in the hallways. Each tag has a unique signal and every staff member has an assigned tag, which they clip to their name badge. When a nurse, doctor, housekeeper or other caregiver walks into the patient's room, the room recognizes the tag and the SmartRoom application is launched on a touch screen monitor. The monitor automatically serves up situation- and role-relevant information as defined by the tag they are wearing. There is no need to find a computer, log on, sort, sift, and fetch; needed information comes to them automatically.

For example, when a dietary hostess enters a room, the SmartRoom screen displays the patient's identifying information, food allergies, dietary orders, and calorie count information. Meanwhile, nurses and nursing assistants would see content and functionality relevant to their jobs, such as allergies, precautions, NPO status, code status, and other key information that they need to keep themselves and their patients safe. Additionally, with the touch of a button on the RTLS tag, the caregiver can change the view on the touch screen and gain immediate access to key clinical information retrieved electronically from the electronic medical record (EMR) system. This includes items such as medications, laboratory results, intake and output balances, and vital signs for the last 48 hours. All of these are presented on the touch screen with easy navigation and drill-down capabilities.

Physicians use the system to check information real-time, such as lab results and vital sign trends. The physician can then use that information to teach the patient about their clinical condition.

In addition to allowing caregivers to see information about their patients, the SmartRoom system can also send information back into the EMR to help ensure fast and consistent documentation. Specifically, the SmartRoom monitor allows caregivers to record data such as vital signs, intake and output, activities of daily living, patient education and other assessments, which are sent to the hospital's EMR system.

The SmartRoom is also used as a tool to help caregivers organize and prioritize their work so they can respond to their most critical tasks first and ensure that all needed tasks for a given patient are accomplished. For example, when a nurse enters a room, the SmartRoom screen shows them the tasks that need to be completed for their specific patient at that moment in time. Additionally, the SmartRoom screen displays information pulled together from the nurse's larger staff assignment to suggest where they should go next based on their staffing assignment and what tasks need to be completed for their other patients.

On a wider scale, the system also powers a SmartBoard at the nurses' station, which replaces the traditional census and assignment board, and it to gets its data from the EMR. Additionally, the SmartBoard knows which nurse is taking care of which patient so that both manual and automatic messages can be sent easily and quickly to the right person at the right time. These features help both the individual nurse and the unit staff ensure that care is provided efficiently.

Finally, in addition to the room-based functions for providers, the SmartRoom includes components for other members of the care team. For the patient and their family, the SmartRoom works with the in-room television, allowing them to view a large variety of pertinent educational and clinical information as well as to access entertainment functions. They can watch education materials, see what tests are being done that day, see when pain medication is due, access emails, play games, and request non-urgent items. Eventually they will be able to order meals and gift shop items and complete surveys. This patient side of the solution is designed to engage the patient and the family in the care process.

Reason for This Innovation

In 2005, a patient who had been to a UPMC hospital many times was admitted again. Because of her clinical condition, it was challenging to get an IV line started, and the specialized IV team was called. The IV team nurse came with her complement of usual equipment: tourniquet, needles, alcohol wipes and other items. As per protocol, she put on a pair of latex gloves and started her process by touching the patient's arm. Unfortunately, she forgot to check the patient's chart for allergies. This patient was allergic to latex and had a severe clinical reaction followed by a severe emotional response to her situation. Not surprisingly, what this patient was most angered about was that she had been to this same hospital many times before but the IV nurse was not aware of her well-documented latex allergy. A review of the hospital's EMR revealed that it did contain the allergies for this patient – but this information was not helpful since it was not presented to the right person at the right time.

At their weekly meetings, the UPMC hospital executive team discusses operational, strategic and tactical issues and reviews all serious events. This event was discussed and the initial response was to blame the nurse for disregarding hospital policy. But, after further discussion, the executive management team discussed how best to ensure that another nurse would not make the same error with another patient. While the nurse broke a policy, the feeling among the management team was that the nurse was not being reckless. Perhaps she was just trying to get through her day – a day that requires caregivers to go out of their way to fetch allergy information before they can do the value-added work of starting IVs. If that was the case, then further steps needed to be taken to ensure that a similar error would not happen again.

In his book, *The High-Velocity Edge*, Dr. Steven Spear recounts a true story in which human error in a complex medication-delivery system led to the unnecessary death of a patient when the nurse mixed two look-alike drugs at the bedside. Spear writes, "You can argue that he should have checked, double checked and even triple checked that he had the right medication, but there is overwhelming evidence that relying on vigilance, monitoring and otherwise being careful is a poor defense against error. People are not wired to be reliably careful" [1]. This perspective on vigilance was shared with the executive team; a system designed around the best efforts and careful attention of the front line is bound to fail over time.

Why This Innovation Succeeded

Executive Support. This project started because of a real error that could have been prevented by appropriate use of the EMR system, but was not. The challenge for hospital leadership was to grapple with the fact that the information systems did exactly what they were designed to do, but the information was too hard to access. A brainstorming session of UPMC quality leaders led to the vision of a system in which the walls could talk and it would be as easy to use as walking into the room. The result was the decision to try and design an innovation based on room-based sensing technologies to provide the caregiver with needed information as they entered the room. The hospital's president has been a strong proponent of simplification in all aspects of systems design, and she gave the approval to start working on an early proof of concept.

The Right People. The Project began when the Senior Director of UPMC's corporate improvement unit received internal grant funding to build a prototype room and was assigned a strong clinical nurse leader and two programming and technical staff as support. Before the staff began designing, they assembled a list of front-line clinicians who they felt could add insight based on their past experiences with the corporate quality group. The team gathered in a room and brainstormed about the project at a very high level over two 2-hour meetings. The design and build team then had enough clarity to begin documenting the requirements for the technical resources.

Improvement Specialists were also essential in fleshing out the vision. They had a range of clinical backgrounds and improvement expertise, and as a part of their job they spend a great deal of time doing first-hand observations of work systems at the point of care. UPMC's Chief Quality Officer assembled and trained this team of Improvement Specialists to help UPMC spread quality and innovation projects across the system. Given their deep experience observing workflow and understanding the front line challenges, their input in those 2-hour design meetings was invaluable.

The Chief Quality Officer assigned a nurse to serve as the clinical design leader. This leader was a bright improvement specialist with a strong advanced clinical background in critical care nursing. She initially spent about half of her time on the initial pilot unit getting feedback, reworking features, and helping to prioritize and define requirements. After three months she became a full-time dedicated leader assigned to the project. She was critical to the success of SmartRoom because her clinical expertise allowed her to talk with front-line caregivers to design a system that would work for them to solve their problems. She would then develop detailed requirements that she would hand off to the two assigned full-time technical resources who worked full time for six months to get an alpha version of the hardware and software deployed on a 24-bed medical-surgical unit at the UPMC Shadyside campus. This unit was selected because of their past experience with the national Transforming Care at the Bedside initiative, meaning they were accustomed to change and disruption.

Within 6 months there were four patient rooms at UPMC Shadyside outfitted with an alpha version of the SmartRoom technology. But over this 6-month design and build phase, there were many forks in the road – sometimes multiple times each day. A key challenge was to keep the scope of the project clearly focused on the initial vision, which required strong leadership.

Making it Easy to Use. From the start, one of the most important outcomes was the degree to which a simplified user interface could be designed to make basic charting tasks quicker for the front line. The system needed to provide a highly usable screen for data entry and send the information back into the hospital's EMR. To design, build and evaluate the SmartRoom Interface, a 10-bed simulation and development lab was used. The space was an old nursing unit with a large nursing station. This simulation lab allowed the team to work out human factors engineering design decisions while simulating and performing time studies to evaluate the SmartRoom without the numerous distractions and confounding factors of a "live" nursing unit.

Another important success factor was the focus on building a system that made it easier for staff to complete their jobs consistently and quickly. This led to several design choices. First, the underlying technology meant that the system was able to

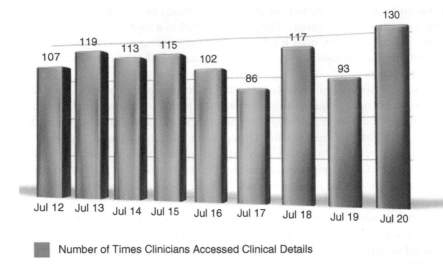

Number of Times Clinicians Accessed Clinical Details

Fig. 15.1 Bedside access to clinical data

interface with the hospital's EMR, apply rules on the patient's data, and deliver relevant instructions on its touch screen for the caregivers at the point of care. But more importantly, the rules were created in such a way to put the burden of remembering, organizing, and prompting on the shoulders on the SmartRoom application – rather than the nurse or other providers. The goal was to reduce the front-line caregiver's worry that something will "fall through the cracks" allowing them to focus time and energy on the more critical aspects of nursing, such as critical thinking, caring, and compassion. The SmartRoom design created a high-reliability organizational environment which unburdens the front-line staff from having to maintain tremendous vigilance for even the most routine tasks, as well as makes any tasks they do quicker and easier to accomplish.

Results

Adoption: Because the SmartRoom creators embraced simplicity in design and focused on decreasing the work burden for staff, adoption has been quick. The use of SmartRoom to document routine tasks has decreased the time spent charting allowing the staff to spend more time at the bedside. The average number of tasks charted in the SmartRoom is about 25 per bed per day. This has remained stable since inception indicating sustainability with the innovation.

The initial screen a user sees contains basic demographic and safety information. By pressing a button on their RTLS tag, a user can get more detailed clinical data (Fig. 15.1). Another measure of adoption was how often a caregiver explored this clinical view function. The graph shows the number of times each day that the

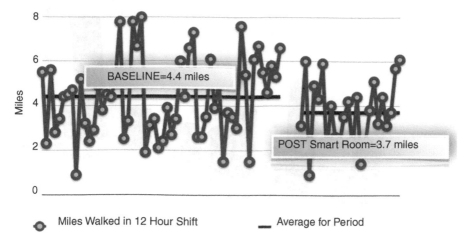

Fig. 15.2 Total miles walked in 12-h shift

button is pushed. On average, for the 129 beds that were live, the caregiver sought out immediate access to deeper clinical data about 105 times a day. Said another way, that is 105 times a day the caregiver isn't leaving the room to look up a lab value, medication list, oxygen order, etc. While this may not seem like a large amount, it's important to remember that the SmartRoom is not the EMR and is not intended to replace the EMR. So when this type of information being used at the bedside, it could signify that something doesn't look right or that a physician would like to double check a lab result or a medication order before making a decision. Having quick access to this type of clinical information at the bedside is thus seen as something that both saves time and improves quality.

A related goal for SmartRoom was to reduce the amount front-line caregivers had to walk so that they could complete their work more efficiently. The vision was that if the work of the nursing team was better organized and coordinated; there would be less foot traffic among the front-line staff. In order to evaluate whether SmartRoom achieved this goal, the nurses and nursing assistants were given pedometers (Fig. 15.2). They wore the pedometer throughout their shift and recorded the value on a data collection sheet at the end of their shift. Most staff on this unit worked a 12-hour shift. For those who did not, the data was normalized to a 12-h shift equivalent. The mean distance walked pre go-live was 4.4 miles in a 12-h shift (55 shifts measured). That dropped to 3.7 miles post go-live (22 shifts measured), a 16 % decrease.

Speed. The following graph shows the time spent charting with and without SmartRoom. The average number of seconds of documentation time is shown on the x-axis. Charting time in SmartRoom was 40–70 % less than traditional inputting with keyboard and mouse. The data was collected using a stopwatch in the SmartRoom simulation lab. The SmartRoom team set up multiple tasks and recorded the time required to complete and document the same tasks with and without the SmartRoom. For example, charting for vital signs decreased from 49 seconds to 11 seconds – a savings of 38 seconds per set (Fig. 15.3). In a 24-bed unit where

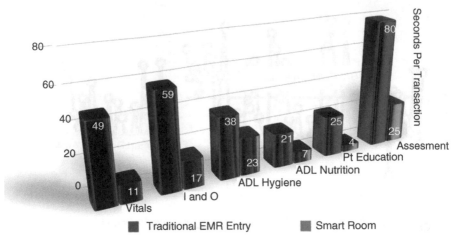

Fig. 15.3 Time saved charting

patients have vital signs checked every 4 hours, this equates to over 90 minutes of time saved each day, just on vital signs alone! More importantly vital signs are now documented at the bedside immediately after they are taken so the data is available to the physicians and other caregivers immediately.

Additionally, it was noticed that some hospital outcome metrics improved after the introduction of the SmartRoom, including a decrease in falls with injury and a decrease in nursing overtime as a percent of direct worked hours. While many factors may affect these clinical and administrative outcomes, one potential contributor may be that the decrease in charting time has an impact on both the nurses' ability to complete other activities and to leave work on time.

Finally, the team is evaluating the impact that SmartRoom has on patients through the Hospital Consumer Assessment of Health Plans Survey (HCAHPS) – a national survey administered by a third party. There are two major questions that assess overall satisfaction with the hospital:

1. On a scale of 1–10 (with 10 being the best) what is your overall rating of this hospital?
2. Would you recommend this hospital to family and friends?

Hospitals use a "top-box" scoring method where they measure and benchmark themselves based on the top score for the question. In the first question, the top-box would be the number of responses that gave a nine or ten. In the second question, the top-box answer is "Definitely Yes". In looking at rooms equipped with SmartRoom, the survey showed the following changes:

1. 8.5 % relative increase in the surveys that scored nine or ten in the "Rate this hospital" question.
2. 12.7 % relative increase in the "Definitely yes" answer for the "Would you recommend" question.

These results were collected by comparing the units in the 12-month period before SmartRoom was installed to the 12-month period after SmartRoom was installed.

Lessons Learned

Lesson #1 – Design simple solutions to solve real problems: While this seems obvious, nothing could be more elusive. Time and time again solutions and interventions designed to address a problem are eventually over designed, overbuilt, overcomplicated, and cumbersome. Somewhere along the line, requirements change and designers begin adding features and functions that give the product many more dimensions than it needs. The final product does too much, is difficult to learn, and often neglects solving the core problem. The SmartRoom was built to achieve its goals with the minimum number of steps. Whenever possible, screen flows were rebuilt to remove extra button pushes in the interest of simplicity. For example, when more than one caregiver is in a patient room, the SmartRoom needs to know which caregiver is using the system so that it can attribute the documentation to the appropriate caregiver. Initially, the programmers built an extra screen that popped up with the names of all the tags detected in the room and the user would select their name from the list. If only one tag was present, the user would still have to select their name. However, over 90 % of the time there is only one tag in the room. Rather than design for the exception, the programmers redesigned the system to know how many people were in the room and only provide the multi-tag prompt if the situation arose. Subtle, but important when 90 % of 100,000 times a month an extra step has been eliminated. Equally important, the SmartRoom leadership set a tone and an expectation that even one extra touch is waste that must be eliminated.

Lesson #2 – Connecting "What" and "How": Healthcare has a lot of technologies and processes that are designed to provide some function or capability. Many of those solutions add work and effort to the front line and their impact is usually much less than expected because the workflow around the innovation has not been well thought out. Systems are designed with the "what" in mind, but if the process is clunky or unreasonable the front line staff reverts to workarounds. This was true in the case of the latex allergy that got the project started. The SmartRoom team tried to remain constantly mindful of the "how". In fact, from piloting it became clear that the workflow design and human factors work are some of the most important aspects to adoption.

For example, many hospitals struggle with hospital acquired pressure ulcers. One of the key interventions is to turn and reposition an at-risk patient every 2 hours. This alleviates the constant pressure on vulnerable skin and helps reduce pressure ulcers – a wound that can be hard to heal and very painful. However, documentation reviews often indicate that amidst the myriad of things that have to get done and documented, turning is one that falls to the bottom of the nurses' list, and sometimes off all together. While the "what" in this instance is clear to front-line caregivers, the "how" is less so, and the work does not happen as a result.

To help ensure that turning would be done reliably, designers strove to design a workflow where the caregiver could be prompted when walking into the room that "it is time to turn the patient" so that the information is given to caregivers when they are ready to take action on it. SmartRoom makes easy for the nurse to document the turning (three button pushes) and once the patient is turned, SmartRoom resets the timer (e.g. for an hour and 45 min) before it prompts the nurse to turn and reposition the patient again. This kind of solution unburdens the care team from having to keep track of a wide range of tasks and allows them to focus their time on more important critical thinking.

Historically nurses have been asked to personally keep track of each task they need to perform for up to six patients, such as who needs to be turned next, who is off for a test, or did their family walk them. This might not be as problematic if it was the only thing they did, but time and again nurses' short-term memories are overburdened with the jobs of remembering, tracking, prioritizing and organizing work. This is a perfect example where, over time, users of EMR systems become focused on documentation rather clinical work. EMRs have worked hard to make documenting easy, perhaps at the expense of building systems that deliver reliable care processes. Hospitals need to do both, ideally at the same time.

Lesson #3. Don't lose sight of the goal. An example of daily work that hospitals struggle with, and that SmartRoom is designed to help with, is hospital acquired infections. This is an elusive problem, but not because there is debate in the literature, in fact it is quite clear that proper hand hygiene will lead to lower hospital acquired infections. As a result, many hospitals have deployed a small army of agents into the field to audit hand hygiene compliance. They go to the nursing floors with clipboards and check boxes based on observation of proper hand hygiene. The Smart Room team realized that with the real-time locating system, the system could track people walking in and out of rooms, and with a tag on the hand sanitizer, the dispenser could signal to the room when it is used. By combining the data and developing behind-the-scenes logic, the system could monitor hand-hygiene utilization. The initial promise of the "what" led quickly to questions about the "how".

1. What if the caregiver just poked his head in to check on the patient but did not touch anything?
2. What if caregiver just walked out of another room and used that hand-hygiene dispenser before entering a room?
3. What if the caregiver washes their hands at the sink in the hallway then walks into a room?
4. What if they use the patient's bathroom sink?
5. What if three people walk into the room and the hand hygiene is only used twice?
6. What if the family (who don't have tags) use the dispenser but caregivers don't, and the system can't tell the difference?

These are all real situations and they are challenges in designing an automated system for capturing hand hygiene compliance. These potential inaccuracies stymied work on hand hygiene until the team refocused attention on the goal – hand-hygiene improvement, not compliance. If the goal was to increase compliance rates from 95.5 % to 99.9 %, then precision would matter. Sadly, hand hygiene compliance is significantly below these figures and the improvements that hospitals need to achieve are significant. So the SmartRoom solution is not focused on compliance, it is focused on improvement.

More specifically, a measurement system is currently under development that will track a numerator and denominator so that the system can calculate a real time hand hygiene rate. Every time someone goes into a room for a minimum specified period of time, their entry and exit count in the denominator as a patient visit. The numerator includes every time that the hand sanitizer is pushed in a room within the window of time that the tag arrives or leaves. In addition, the number of times that the hallway sinks are used, regardless of who uses them, is added to the numerator. This number represents a measure of utilization, but the real intervention is another component of "how". The index will be a rolling index calculated in real time based on the last 25 room visits. The number will be displayed on the SmartBoard in the nursing unit station and on every caregiver touch screen upon room entry. The feedback is immediate, direct, and relevant. It is relevant because using the most recent 25 room visits means that the number actually represents the utilization of the people who are working on the floor at that very moment. The people who are generating the index will see the index all day long. Furthermore, if they use the hand hygiene dispenser or sink, the number will increase. They own it, they control it, and they see it.

Lastly, as part of the "how", the system does not single people out. SmartRoom is intended to be a helpful tool to create safety and simplicity in work by providing alerts and feedback mechanisms that give the care giving team the greatest chance of success every time. SmartRoom is not designed as a system to police staff; that would violate the founding principles of the innovation.

Lesson #4: Allowing for Change. Very little of the original design from the prototype remains in the product 5 years after the first go-live. This is one of the key lessons about early stage innovation. It was challenging, but important, to throw away something that the team had worked passionately on as requirements changed or the front line provided feedback regarding the value of each feature. It is easy to become so attached to parts of an innovation that innovators are unwilling to modify, adjust, or sometimes abandon something that seemed so promising just months earlier. For example, the developers had designed and built a hands-free input mechanism to control the screen. There was a web camera pointing toward the TV. The patient and the caregivers were given a laser pointer which controlled the mouse to allow selections on the screens. While this innovation prevented touching a screen or keyboard, it was not simple to use or to set up and calibrate. At the same time, the Engineering Director had invested so much time and energy developing this solution. It was difficult to accept a change in design that put the web camera and related software on the shelf in the interest of a simpler user interface.

Future Plans

The SmartRoom team has now grown into a separate for-profit company with about 20 developers on staff and growing. UPMC continues to expand the SmartRoom through their UPMC Montefiore campus. When completed, there will be almost 250 beds that are fully SmartRoom operational. UPMC is also building a new 150-bed hospital where the SmartRoom system will be built into all of the medical and surgical rooms.

The SmartRoom continues to add features that are designed to continue to make work easier for the caregivers and safer for patients. This includes work aimed at reducing falls with injury, reducing catheter associated urinary tract infections, reducing hospital length of stay, reducing readmissions and helping with hospital communications and important alerts. The team is also working on an application that will allow video visits with patients from their physician, family, and friends.

Conclusion

The front line of healthcare has seen a tremendous growth in technology over the past decade. Many hospitals have been vigorously implementing EMRs, bar code scanning, CPOE, and bedside technologies including smart pumps and bio-medical device integration. Now even tablets and smart phones are rapidly infiltrating the front line of medicine. The question is whether these technologies have made life easier or more challenging for front-line staff.

The SmartRoom hopes to reverse that trend by creating an environment that allows for immediate access to the right information with the right functionality to the right person at the right time. The result will help drive quality, safety and efficiency projects for years to come.

Reference

1. Spear SJ. The high-velocity edge. New York: McGraw Hill; 2009. p. 54.

Chapter 16
One EMR to Go Please

Steve Flammini and James W. Noga

Buzzzzzzzzzz. Buzzzzzzzzzz.

"Hey John. I'll catch up with you on the court. Just warm up for a few and I'll be right there. I just need to check in," says Dr. Ben Mackie. *Ben has been at Partners Health System for 5 years, caring for patients, and always loving how much easier staying connected gets. Just a year ago, that buzzing noise coming from his iPhone could have meant cancelling his tennis date.*

"Let's see here," Ben murmurs. *Resigned, he slips on his reading glasses. He notices that he received a secure notification regarding one of his patients, Barbara Martinez. Barbara is a new patient, and he had a great appointment with her and her husband Ray yesterday. She seemed pretty stressed, but deeply committed to getting healthier. Based on her first appointment he suspected that she was pre-diabetic, but was keeping his fingers crossed otherwise.* "Come on Barbara… be normal. Be normal," *he thinks as he brings up her recent lab results.* "Excellent. She will be thrilled that there is one less thing to worry about". *He quickly taps the phone icon, and is connected to Barbara.* "Barbara. This is Dr. Mackie; good news! Your labs are normal. I know you were pretty stressed about this, so hopefully this puts your mind to rest." *A few minutes later he is strutting onto the tennis court.*

A surprised John yelps "I didn't even get a chance to warm up this time! You ready for that rematch from last week?"

S. Flammini, B.S., Computer Science (✉)
Partners HealthCare, Inc, 93 Worcester St, Wellesley, MA 02481, USA
e-mail: sflammini@partners.org

J.W. Noga, B.S., MS
Partners HealthCare, Inc, Prudential Tower – Suite 1150 800
Boylston Street, Boston, MA 02119, USA
e-mail: jnoga@partners.org

L. Berkowitz, C. McCarthy (eds.),
Innovation with Information Technologies in Healthcare, Health Informatics,
DOI 10.1007/978-1-4471-4327-7_16, © Springer-Verlag London 2013

Background

Partners HealthCare is a not-for-profit, integrated health care system in Boston, Massachusetts. Founded by Brigham and Women's Hospital and Massachusetts General Hospital – two of the nation's leading academic medical centers – Partners HealthCare includes community and specialty hospitals, a physician network, community health centers, home care and other health related services.

Partners is committed to the community, and dedicated to enhancing patient care, teaching, and research in service to our patients and their families

Partners is the largest private employer in Massachusetts, with more than 60,000 employees, including physicians, nurses, scientists, and caregivers. With a combined research budget of more than $1.5 billion, Massachusetts General Hospital (MGH) and Brigham and Women's Hospital (BWH) are the largest private hospital recipients of National Institutes of Health funding in the nation.

Partners has undertaken the development of a mobile Electronic Health Record (mEHR). This chapter will describe the technical, clinical, and organizational dynamics that have led to the adoption of the mEHR, and that continue to drive its growing popularity.

The Innovation

The confluence of consumer technologies and electronic health records has resulted in levels of mobility for clinicians previously not seen. In the short span of about 90 days, Partners HealthCare delivered a mobile app, enabling providers to use their smart phones to access securely the organization's electronic medical record. The mobile EHR app (mEHR) has heavily leveraged existing enterprise architecture, providing for high levels of security, availability, and agility.

Reason for This Innovation

Partners' founding institutions have a long history of innovation in clinical systems, including groundbreaking work in clinical decision support, medication management, and many other areas of electronic health record development and adoption.

In 1999, the IT group at Partners developed an experimental prototype for a mobile EHR – using early 'Personal Digital Assistant' (PDA) platforms available at the time. The concept was in keeping with the best development practices at the time: Maintain a separation between data, logic, and presentation, so that a mobile version could be provided by leveraging existing clinical data and logic, with an alternative presentation optimized for mobile devices. At the time, the specific mobile platform used was the Palm Pilot, running PalmOS with a fairly primitive

HTML browser. The prototype provided the ability to view visit notes, reports, medications, problems, allergies, and several other clinical data elements. It also provided some limited ability for the entry of this data from the mobile device. While it was an interesting, early demonstration of mobile clinical system capabilities, it quickly became clear that the technologies were not sufficiently mature to provide real value to clinicians. Cellular coverage was spotty at best, battery life was poor, and the capabilities of the device, operating system (OS), and browsers were limited. The prototype provided an informative glimpse into the future of mobile EHRs, but was largely seen as an anachronism – an idea that was ahead of many of the supporting technologies it needed to succeed at scale. It was decided that 1999 was not the time for a mobile EHR at Partners.

The Consumer IT Revolution and Its Impact on the Physician Use of HIT

Fast-forward to 2009, Partners HealthCare, like so many organizations, was in the midst of considering how best to support the explosion of consumer IT capabilities available to its healthcare providers. It had become clear that consumer IT, in the form of smart phones, tablets, social media, collaboration, cloud services, and many others, was changing the game, in terms of user expectations, especially with clinicians. A Manhattan Research Institute study [1] published at the time, showed that:

- The number of physicians using smartphones had surged to 64 %, with iPhones alone more than doubling from 2008 to 2009.
- Physicians were spending more time online, using both computers and smartphones to receive notifications, and access the most up-to-date information at a variety of points throughout the day.
- Mobile technology was allowing doctors to be 'always on' – leading to an expectation of being continuously connected to the clinical systems, regardless of location or end user device.

Given the rapid growth in adoption of consumer IT, especially mobile devices, the IT leadership group decided that it was time to pilot a mobile EHR again. It was becoming clear that major advances in consumer IT had led to a 'critical mass' of diffusion among several complementary technologies – the very thing that was missing back in 1999. Here is a brief summary of how some of these technologies have matured, and when taken together, constitute a good platform for mobile application delivery, including mobile electronic health records:

- Mobile processors: The sophistication of the smartphones has established that they are really no longer phones, but computers.
- Display: For example, the 'Retina display' on the iPhone4 has a 960-by-640-pixel resolution on a 3.5 inch screen – a pixel density of 326 pixels per inch, which

makes for a vivid, natural display compared to previous smart phones, and many computer displays for that matter.

- Operating System: The iOS and Android operating systems for mobile devices are fast, stable, multi-layer, multi-tasking operating systems, with rich SDKs for developers. This has resulted in an explosion of consumer applications with impressive sophistication. This sophistication is also evident in the quality of the web browsers for these platforms, giving users a high-quality web-browsing experience, which is also capable of supporting enterprise-class web applications.

- Power management / battery life: Current mobile battery technology will allow for several hours of continuous use, depending on the various parameters related to power consumption. Smartphones and tablets can go several days in standby mode, and batteries retain 80 % of their original capacity to charge after several hundred full discharge cycles.

- Network technology: Clinicians have come to expect the use of mobile devices on the hospital wireless LAN, and with improvements to WiFi (802.11) protocols, spectrum management practices, and higher systems monitoring and availability, clinicians can expect reasonably good internal WiFi coverage, availability, and speeds up to 54 Mb/s with regular protocols, and up to 300 Mb/s with 802.11n. And separate from WiFi, cellular wireless coverage and performance have improved so most users average speeds in the 1 Mb/s range with 3 G, which may become ten times faster once 4 G is widely available.

- SOA (Service-Oriented Architecture): SOA emphasizes loose technical coupling between services which *provide data and logic*, and the consumer apps that *use the data and logic*. The result is that XML-based software technologies which make up much of the SOA standards really do allow organizations to securely interoperate across technical and organizational boundaries. At Partners, we have invested more than 10 years in developing 'loosely-coupled' SOA-based access to enterprise data and logic, which allows us to heavily leverage our clinical data, and extend it to practically any device and form factor, in a way that provides high levels of security and scalability for a mobile EHR.

- Security / Device Management: Mobile security and device management features have steadily improved, even though these devices were developed for consumer use. The ability to provision devices, integrate them with corporate email/calendaring, manage lost devices, and de-provision is now within reach for organizations.

With these technology advances occurring together, driven heavily by the consumer IT market, the world is now seeing an explosion of mobile applications, ranging in everything from gaming and entertainment, to navigation, to business applications. And with physicians adoption rates now well over 80% for smartphones in 2011 [1], The IT leadership at Partners clearly understood it was time to move, and use this collection of technologies to produce solutions that enable clinicians to access the resources they need to care for patients, around the clock and around the world.

Why This Innovation Succeeded

Agility can be defined as the ability to quickly sense opportunity and respond to it. It is an attribute that is becoming increasingly critical for IT organizations, as business drivers change more quickly, cost pressures increase, and project timetables shrink.

Having made the decision to deliver mobile EHR capabilities, it was important to demonstrate to the organization that we could move quickly on the initiative, and to keep within the spirit of the mobile and consumer technology delivery cycle – specifically, to deliver something useful, fast, and intuitive, and deliver it soon. This would require making sound decisions on the scope of the application, and involving people from the hospitals and the IT organization whom were decisive enough to make good decisions quickly, and whom were influential enough to make those decisions stick. Our goal: to plan, develop, and implement a working mobile EHR, all within 90 days.

Our development team enlisted physician leaders from each of our institutions, and embarked on a planning process that assessed the demand for mobile clinical data and functionality, and the demand for various devices in the physician community. At the same time, we began rapid prototyping sessions with a small, innovative group of developers, folks who were willing to go beyond their 'day job' duties, to push the envelope of what was possible with new technology within a fast timeframe. We also began to work with the broader IT organization to get ready to address issues related to architecture, implementation, and support. Many of the decisions made were unconventional, when compared to how we had traditionally delivered applications, supported devices, and supported users. It was this new orientation, influenced by the values of the Consumer IT market, that really enabled us to move with agility and meet our 90-day goal.

The pilot planning and development began in January 2010, coordinated by the PHS Clinical SOA program. The 'SOA team', already well acquainted with Service-Oriented Architecture, put a strong emphasis on the re-use of existing data, services, and production infrastructure. This high leverage of existing enterprise assets would allow the rapid delivery of a secure, highly available mobile application, while avoiding the necessity to 'reinvent' much of the technology infrastructure. Some examples include existing services for Application Security and Clinical Data Access services:

• Application Security: There are several requirements needed to comply with HIPAA regulations and various organizational policies pertaining to security and privacy. These services are in use within our enterprise clinical application suite, and can be further leveraged by the mobile EHR. *Authentication Services* allow strong user authentication, and are the basis for several other security requirements related to provider identity. *Audit services* provide a facility to record which providers accessed which patient's records, with various indications including timestamp, device id, and overall clinical context. Chart Access control services enforce the access rules to patient records, and help ensure that only

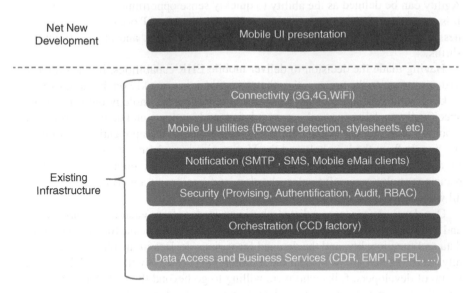

Fig. 16.1 Conceptual approach to the re-use of existing services

those providers with the appropriate relationship to the patient can view the record. This service is already in place for the conventional EMR, and would be extended to the mobile EHR.

- Clinical Data Access Services: Partners has a rich Clinical Data repository (CDR), consisting of the various clinical data on record for its patients from across the entire organization. This data, when produced in the form of results by laboratories, or in the form of reports as a result of clinician documentation, is fed into a central repository, where the patient's global enterprise identity is determined, and the data is permanently associated with that patient, producing a 'longitudinal' record of all clinical data for the patient. The CDR has an extensive, SOA-based collection of clinical data access services. These data access services, implemented as loosely-coupled XML services, can easily be invoked securely by the mobile EHR, allowing it to leverage a vast array of clinical data, taking advantage of many years of development in the access and organization of this data.

The conceptual approach to the re-use of existing services is depicted in Fig. 16.1, which illustrates the relative heavy leverage of existing services and infrastructure, and the relatively small amount of new development required for the mobile presentation (Fig. 16.1).

The planning process involved physicians and IT experts from several of the PHS hospitals. The input received from the planning group helped to define the learning objectives for the pilot, as well as the scope of the data and functionality, the support model, and the enlistment of the pilot participants. It was agreed that the scope would include viewing capability for lab results, reports, problems, medications, allergies, procedures, vital signs, patient demographics, care teams, and several other clinical and administrative data elements. The initial scope would not include data entry, as most of the perceived demand was for mobile viewing of data, not necessarily documentation.

The initial set of mobile devices include the iPhone 3GS, iPhone 4, iPad, and some Blackberry devices. Device selection was based on the security capabilities mentioned earlier, as well as an initial assessment of demand in the physician community. Subsequent assessment of demand among physicians continued to show a strong preference for the Apple iPhone and iPad. This seemed to hold true in the broader healthcare industry, as well. In an April, 2011 article from Healthcare IT News [2], a survey of U.S. physicians by Aptilon Corp. showed that of 341 respondents, 61 % intend to own an iPhone by the end of 2011. This compares with the iPhone's 24.7 % adoption among general U.S. smartphone users. 9 % of physicians plan to use the Android platform, and 9 % plan to use the Blackberry.

For 2011, smartphone adoption will reach 84 % of U.S. physicians, corresponding with Manhattan Research's latest forecast of 82 %. "Healthcare providers have signaled a clear preference for their smartphones," remarks Mark Benthin, Aptilon COO, "Professionals are taking advantage of the latest advancements to connect with information, tools and live resources when, where and how it suits them."

Results

The mobile application was delivered in April 2010, just a little more than 90 days from initial pilot planning. The app was very well-received, and the pilot group grew rapidly from a few dozen initial users, to several hundred by the end of summer. The pilot planning team monitored user feedback, and was pleasantly surprised by the nearly universal enthusiasm expressed by the physician users. A formal user satisfaction survey was performed over the course of the summer, and several benefits have been cited by adopters, and a good initial understanding of the demand for future mobile capabilities has been gained. Some key findings from the survey (150 physicians surveyed, 65 responded):

- Overwhelming device preference for Apple iPhone and iPad among physicians.
- 97 % of respondents view the mEHR as a valuable adjunct to the conventional EHR
- Physicians used the mEHR more frequently when NOT in the Hospital or Clinic

With a successful pilot accomplished, the mobile EHR viewer was released to the general population of clinical users (about 10,000 total) in January, 2011.

As of April 2011, more than 2000 physicians have adopted the mEHR, with their frequency of use ranging from a few patients accesses per month, to many per day. The primary benefit being reported by physicians is the ability to rapidly check clinical data while on the go, whether rounding in the hospital, travelling offsite, or at home. The 'instant on' nature of the mobile device makes it hard to beat for swiftness in accessing the medical record. The following impressions were offered by early physician adopters:

- "The mEHR was a great help to me as a consultant in the hospital by allowing me to check labs and reports during rounds, review the locations of my patients while traveling throughout the hospital, and even look up patient insurance and contact information. Overall, the mEHR improved the efficiency of my daily work schedule and I look forward to its continued development."
- "As a medical resident, the mobile EHR has been extremely useful, pushing the wealth of information on LMR closer to the point of care. I use the mobile EHR on my iPhone to inform clinical decision-making without interrupting rounds, update patients without leaving their room, and check results, notes, and clinic schedules from home. It generates enthusiasm from every clinician I have shown it to, all of whom are seeking ways to access critical information irrespective of time or place."
- "I just set up my iPhone to try out this application. It is GREAT! I am just learning about navigating around it, but already it has been a help. I got paged about a patient during the meeting and was able to log on and check a radiology report. Also, I was in Washington recently at a meeting and was dealing with lab data from one of my patients. I demonstrated it at the meeting – some were saying we weren't at a point where this technology would work yet – and everyone thought it was terrific!!" (Figs. 16.2, 16.3, 16.4, and 16.5).

Lessons Learned

The following lessons have been learned as the mEHR app grows quickly in popularity and is now in its general availability phase:
- Mobile apps should be fast, simple, and intuitive. Many users are already well-acquainted with mobile apps and expect to be able to use a new app with virtually no training. This reflects a set of inherent design principles that is already well-understood by adopters of mobile devices. They will increasingly expect 'enterprise' applications to be as clean, fast, and intuitive. This puts pressure on software vendors to assess the usability of their applications.
- Physicians view smart phones as computers, and will increasingly rely on always being connected to the clinical systems. These expectations will be fulfilled through the use of both traditional IT infrastructure and their own personally owned and managed mobile devices.
- The support of personally owned and managed devices brings different challenges and economies (some favorable) than traditional IT support.

Fig. 16.2 The patient hub
(main menu)

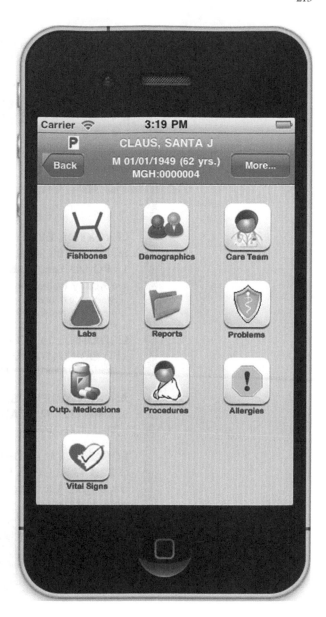

IT organizations must meet the goal of securely extending enterprise resources
to this class of devices, and adjust support models accordingly. IT will not necessarily be responsible for provisioning, break/fix, configuration, etc. They will be
responsible for assuring a sound, high-availability architecture that is flexible
enough to reach a range of non-traditional devices.
- Many physicians prefer mobile apps to be organized by patient lists, such as
  clinic schedules, team lists, or personalized lists. We found it was essential to
  integrate patient lists and care team data to drive the mobile workflow.

Fig. 16.3 Medication list

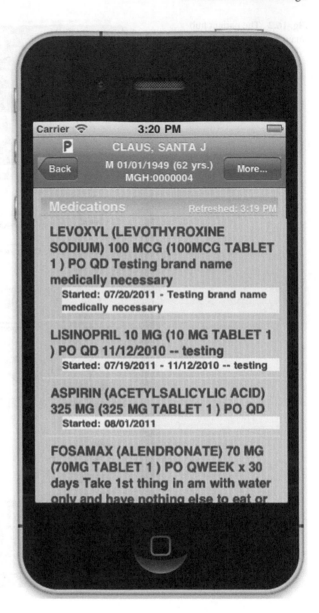

- Mobile apps will increasingly be seen as a valuable adjunct to the traditional EHR, giving clinicians a great degree of freedom to get the information they need, when they need it.
- While mobile apps will not entirely replace traditional EHRs anytime soon, the addition of more capabilities, and the further maturity of the enabling technologies (especially more capable mobile tablets) will drive mobile EHRs beyond simply being a extending technology, to actually causing displacement of the

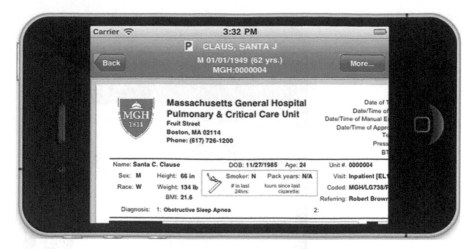

Fig. 16.4 Chemistry panels

traditional enterprise apps and devices. Organizations can move quickly on new technology projects. They should limit the scope of applications, pilot with users who are willing to contribute to innovation, and empower business users (in this case, clinicians) to make decisions and manage the consequences. Rapid cycle times are made possible by understanding which IT assets and processes can be re-used, or extended forward.

- As the IT leadership continued to better understand the impact of consumer IT in the enterprise, one thing was becoming abundantly clear: Users were expecting to gain access to enterprise resources from personally-owned devices. Many of these users (especially clinicians) would take full responsibility for the purchase, use, management, and support of consumer-grade mobile devices. They didn't expect, or even want that from the IT organization. What they did expect was the accessibility of enterprise resources, such as email and calendaring, but more notably – clinical systems functionality. The mEHR planning group recognized this, and agreed that the support model for the mEHR would not extend to the device, or its configuration, or its network connectivity. All of that responsibility would be born by the user. The support model would simply warrant the continuous availability of the application, assuming the user had a device and network connectivity. Given that the production infrastructure supporting the mEHR was the same production infrastructure supporting the conventional EHR application, the team was confident in warranting its continuous availability.
- Given this above arrangement, the team agreed that Mon-Fri, 9a-5p support would be adequate for the pilot. Off hours, the clinicians could forward questions and concerns to an 'mEHR support email account', which would have a 24 h turnaround. These support arrangements are quite different from the usual intensive support agreements usually provided for clinical systems users. Again,

Fig. 16.5 Patient report

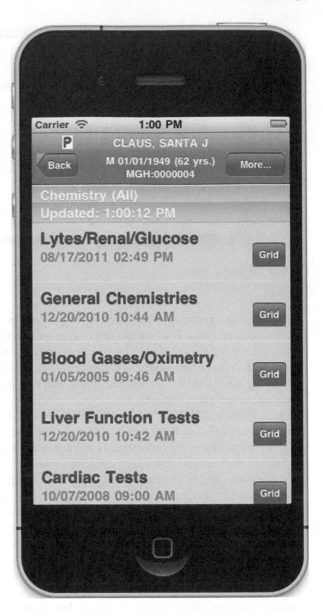

the development orientation, shaped by the consumer IT market, was that the application would be intuitive, easy to use, fast, and available. We thought it was important to reflect this orientation in the support model as well. Moreover, the 'mission' of a mobile application was to supplement the conventional use of the clinical systems while the user was on-the-go. We did not expect the users to depend solely on the mobile functionality, but rather to use it as an adjunct to the traditional EHR.

Future Plans

As we continue to see steady growth of mEHR adoption in the physician community, we see demand for functionality beyond the viewing of patient results and reports. One of the most desired features is the viewing of radiology images. Partners is planning a pilot for Summer, 2011, in which a Radiology imaging viewing component will allow clinicians to access CT, MRI, and PET scans from the mobile device. In fact, in Feb 2011, the FDA approved the iPad for use in Diagnostic Radiology [3] – a validation of the quality of the processor and display.

Clinicians have also clearly expressed their desire to document, not just view, from the mobile platform. Partners is currently assessing opportunities to offer e-Prescribing, clinical notifications, ordering, and structured patient documentation via the mEHR. There is a sentiment among mEHR users that certain transactions and documentation tasks could be handled well with a mobile device.

A shift toward more sophisticated image viewing and physician documentation will require a shift away from simple browser-based rendering on the mobile device (which is the predominant technical approach within the mEHR today). 'Native' apps, using all of the capabilities of the device provided through the software development kit, will be required for operations beyond simple viewing. Of course, with the native device capabilities comes better integration with the device's camera, location services, network connectivity, display, and audio capabilities. This clearly leads to many opportunities to incorporate speech recognition, VOIP, visual recognition, collaboration, and integration with other peripheral devices, including clinical devices.

It is also important to note that the mobile technology innovation driven by the consumer IT market has also begun to benefit healthcare consumers themselves. Partners HealthCare is considering ways to extend its Patient Portal to mobile platforms. The ability to request appointments, refill prescriptions, receive notifications, and view clinical data could all be extended to mobile. In addition, the ability to use the location services on mobile devices could be useful in navigating the hospital setting. Allowing patients to check into clinics, provide insurance information prior to arriving, and accomplish many other useful tasks can be supported with mobile today. Many health care organizations (HCOs) have delivered general consumer apps to the public, that publicize current emergency department wait times, occupancy, and other vital measures of interest to the public. We are only just beginning to witness the impact of consumer IT on the healthcare enterprise, and it is essential for HIT vendors, integrators, and HCOs to understand the potential of these technologies.

Conclusion

The levels of innovation made possible by the economies of the consumer IT revolution are staggering. While the first version of the mEHR has created much excitement in the clinical community at Partners, it is only the very beginning of what is yet to come. Imagine the impact on hospital operations when patients can quickly check in, provide information, and find their way to their clinic with their own personal mobile device. Imagine the positive effect on the meaningful use of EHRs when clinicians can receive notifications wherever they may be, and can act on those events, with much of the functionality of the EHR at their fingertips. In a world where clinicians must face a torrent of new medical knowledge and patient data every day, removing the constraints of time and space by providing instant access, regardless of location, is certainly a strategy Partners HealthCare will continue to develop and refine.

References

1. Healthcare IT News. Physician mobile use grows 45 percent. Healthcare IT News Website. 2011. http://www.healthcareitnews.com/news/physician-mobile-use-grows-45-percent. 7 Apr 2011
2. Manhattan Research Institute. Taking the Pulse® v8.0, healthcare market research. Manhattan Research Institute Website. 2009. http://manhattanresearch.com/Products-and-Services/Physician/Taking-the-Pulse-U-S. Jan 2009
3. US Food and Drug Administration. FDA clears first diagnostic radiology application for mobile devices. US FDA Website.2011. http://www.fda.gov/NewsEvents/Newsroom/PressAnnouncements/ucm242295.htm. 4 Feb 2011

Chapter 17
Real-Time, Right Care

Debra J. Hurd and Brian D. Patty

*"Mom. I'm still not feeling so good. And I'm so tired. I can't keep my eyes open,"
yawed Cindy. That is not like her thought Barbara Martinez, her mom. Cindy was
always so energetic, but it has been a tough few weeks. She went from being a
typical 16-year-old girl to becoming very ill. Barbara and Cindy's father, Ray, had
brought her to the ED the week before with a high fever and flu-like symptoms. She
received IV fluids, antibiotics and was sent home.*

*"Really? Lets take your temperature again," said Barbara, hoping, hoping, hoping
that it would be normal. She knew it wouldn't; Cindy felt hot. The thermometer said 103,
and next thing she knew they were back at the ED and now being admitted to the ICU.
"A ventilator too?!" Barbara couldn't believe what was happening, and was frightened,
but also comforted at the professionalism and caring of Cindy's doctors and nurses.*

*Cindy was placed on several protocols, including those for sedation and ICU,
and because of the ventilator she was also placed on the VAP prevention protocol.
"What's VAP?" asked Barbara, "It doesn't sound good."*

*"Ventilator Associated Pneumonia prevention protocol is used for patients on a
ventilator. It's much easier for patients to get pneumonia when on one, but there are
a few simple things we can do to prevent this," said Cindy's nurse, "Since using the
VAP prevention protocols (VAP Bundle) consistently in our hospitals our VAP infection rate has been zero."*

*"That sounds good to me. Another infection is the last thing any of us needs. But
what is the VAP bundle?"*

D.J. Hurd, RN, MS, NEA, BC (✉)
Nursing Administration, 1575 Beam Avenue,
Maplewood, 55126, MN, USA
e-mail: dhurd@healtheast.org

B.D. Patty, M.D., VP, CMIO
Department of Health Informatics, HealthEast Care System,
1690 University Av W Suite 300,
St. Paul, MN 55104, USA
e-mail: bpatty@healtheast.org

L. Berkowitz, C. McCarthy (eds.),
Innovation with Information Technologies in Healthcare, Health Informatics,
DOI 10.1007/978-1-4471-4327-7_17, © Springer-Verlag London 2013

"Barbara, remember this morning when I started off with Cindy's oral care? Well I knew to do that first because that is a part of the VAP bundle, and the computer helps me decide what to do first to make sure Cindy stays infection free. Its a pretty amazing tool."

"Wow. I didn't realize all the 'behind the scenes' stuff going on." Barbara felt more confident that Cindy was in the right hands. Cindy remained in the hospital for several more weeks, VAP free, and was discharged a healthy, happy teenager. Barbara would be happy to never see a hospital again, but knowing there was one that was so safety conscience, caring and brilliant at what they do, did give her real peace of mind.

Background

HealthEast Care System: HealthEast is a community-focused, non-profit health care organization that provides innovative technology, compassionate care and a full spectrum of family health services. The HealthEast system includes Bethesda Hospital, St. John's Hospital, St. Joseph's Hospital and Woodwinds Health Campus as well as outpatient services, clinics, home care and medical transportation services. HealthEast is the largest, locally-owned health care organization in the Twin Cities' East Metro with 7,300 employees, 1,200 volunteers and 1,500 physicians on staff. HealthEast has won a number of clinical awards including multiple Patient Safety Performance Excellence Awards from the Minnesota Hospital Association and the HealthGrades Patient Safety Excellence Award in 2009. HealthEast was also named one of the "Top 10 Healthcare Systems in the U.S" in the Thomson Reuters *100 Top Hospitals Health Systems Quality/Efficiency Benchmarks Study.*

The Innovation

The VAP Quality Monitor

The Ventilator-Associated Pneumonia (VAP) Quality Monitor is a software tool that monitors clinical transactions as they occur within HealthEast's electronic medical record (EMR) system and uses embedded logic to evaluate the transactions against pre-defined processes of care related to preventing VAP. This tool then presents the status of each process in real time using a red/yellow/green dashboard for each of the VAP bundle elements on each ventilated patient on the unit. The information is constantly available via a wall-mounted monitor, or it can be displayed on demand at any user's desktop.

Caregivers access the VAP results via monitors and PCs throughout their shift, but especially during the multidisciplinary care rounds that occur throughout the day

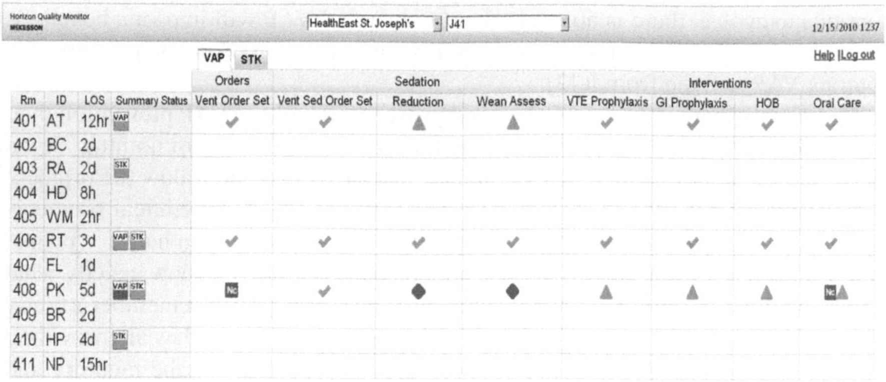
Horizon Quality Monitor
MCKESSON
HealthEast St. Joseph's | J41 | 12/15/2010 1237
Help |Log out
VAP | STK

Rm	ID	LOS	Summary Status	Orders: Vent Order Set	Orders: Vent Sed Order Set	Sedation: Reduction	Sedation: Wean Assess	Interventions: VTE Prophylaxis	Interventions: GI Prophylaxis	Interventions: HOB	Interventions: Oral Care
401	AT	12hr	VAP	✓	✓	▲	▲	✓	✓	✓	✓
402	BC	2d									
403	RA	2d	STK								
404	HD	8h									
405	WM	2hr									
406	RT	3d	VAP STK	✓	✓	✓	✓	✓	✓	✓	✓
407	FL	1d									
408	PK	5d	VAP STK	Nc	✓	◆	◆	▲	▲	▲	Nc ▲
409	BR	2d									
410	HP	4d	STK								
411	NP	15hr									

Fig. 17.1 VAP Quality Monitor screen display

on the ICU. For example, an individual nurse may take a quick glance at the monitor and see that one of his assigned ventilated patients has a "green" status for periodic wean assessment and therefore does not need immediate attention, but another ventilated patient may show a "red" status for daily oral care, meaning the nurse needs to complete that activity. Such immediate feedback helps the nurse prioritize his actions appropriately. Typically the status is green if the task has been completed for the current period, yellow if it has not been completed and red if it has not been completed and there is only 2 hours less until it becomes "non compliant".

Additionally, the charge nurse tracks the VAP monitor and assists the staff nurses who might be falling behind in their charting or their care duties due to other competing priorities. Finally, the system engages physicians by increasing consistent use of the ventilator and sedation order sets and by more active discussions about them at interdisciplinary care rounds (Fig. 17.1).

Reason for This Innovation

As healthcare professionals know all too well, treatment of hospitalized patients involves not only doing the right things to help them get well, but avoiding things which could put their patients at risk of complications. Some patients *must* be ventilated to save their lives, but the process of ventilation itself carries a risk of bacterial pneumonia, specifically identified as VAP.

VAP is an avoidable hospital-acquired condition that exacts a dreadful toll in terms of human lives and healthcare costs. Research has shown that bacterial pneumonia affects between 10 and 20 % of patients who require mechanical ventilation with endotracheal intubation. A patient who contracts VAP will experience an average of 9.6 more ventilator days, 6.1 additional days in the ICU, 11.5 more days in the hospital and incur on average an additional $40,000 in hospital costs [1]. While CMS rules concerning reimbursement for hospital-acquired conditions such as VAP continue to evolve, there is no doubt that treatment of VAP will impact a hospital's bottom line. But saddest of all is the mortality rate – about 70 % of the patients who contract VAP will die from it [2].

Fortunately there is an established and proven protocol for VAP prevention that, when adhered to completely, drives the risk of VAP down to almost nothing. So on the surface, it would seem simple enough to just have everyone follow the protocol and eliminate VAP altogether. However, the reality is that most clinical protocols involve multi-step processes and time-bound tasks that make them hard for people to follow 100 % of the time. Even when physicians and nurses know exactly what should be done to optimize patient outcomes, they struggle to remember exactly which task to do by what time for which of the patients for whom they are providing care. In other words, if adherence to a protocol is dependent on the memory and focus of just one person, the chances for failure are significantly higher than if a whole care team is empowered by technology to know the status of every component of the protocol at any given time.

Due to the multiple care quality and cost-associated reasons discussed, the HealthEast Quality Institute, the body responsible for the strategic oversight of quality outcomes for the organization, identified prevention of VAP as a priority project in 2006. This decision was made due to a higher than expected VAP rate at the hospitals and the alignment with the IHI VAP program. The Quality Institute is made up of a mix of HealthEast Executives, allied independent physician and front-line staff.

Why This Innovation Succeeded

The VAP Bundle Project

For the VAP Bundle Project, HealthEast took its cue from the Institute of Healthcare Improvement (IHI) Ventilator Bundle promoted as part of the IHI "5 Million Lives" campaign. Guidelines for VAP prevention had been published previously by the Center for Disease Control. IHI effectively synthesized their recommendations into a straightforward template designed to facilitate rapid and pragmatic deployment by hospitals.

IHI defined the protocol as follows: "The Ventilator Bundle is a series of interventions related to ventilator care that, when implemented together, will achieve significantly better outcomes than when implemented individually" [3]. According to the published IHI definition, the key components of the Ventilator Bundle are as follows:

- Elevation of the Head of the Bed
- Daily "Sedation Vacations" and Assessment of Readiness to Extubate
- Peptic Ulcer Disease Prophylaxis
- Deep Venous Thrombosis Prophylaxis
- Daily Oral Care with Chlorhexidine

IHI provides many useful tools and suggestions for implementing these components in hospital care, but ultimately each healthcare organization must determine the process specifics, such as frequency of the extubation readiness assessments and recommended medications to be used for peptic ulcer disease prophylaxis, and then drive the changes to clinical practice that are needed for success.

As with adoption of any change, effective measurement of adherence is critical to ongoing improvement. In its initial approach to implementation of the Ventilator Bundle, HealthEast harnessed the capabilities of its EHR to create clinical documentation templates and order sets which mapped to the process components of the bundle. This approach allowed the organization to track adherence through retrospective analysis of electronic elements, such as specific nursing assessments and medication orders.

HealthEast first used the IHI's Ventilator Bundle Checklist to assess adherence with all components of the bundle. As expected, the initial results were not especially good, even after several years of effort with the bundle; overall performance was still lackluster and the organization determined that it was not making adequate progress toward its goals. Analysis conducted through the familiar Plan-Do-Study-Act methodology revealed that despite high levels of enthusiasm and commitment among staff, it was simply too hard for them to remember to complete all the elements of the process all the time. This was felt to be due to the fact that the VAP protocol was one of many that clinical staff were expected to follow in the completion of routine care activities for a variety of different patients, many of whom are on more than one protocol.

For example, consider the experience of a busy nurse who knows she must assess and document head of bed elevation for an assigned ventilated patient every 4 hours. She may be distracted by any number of urgent activities when the end of one of those 4 hours time periods approaches and may even be physically away from the unit for a brief period of time, such as waiting with a patient in the Imaging department. She may not realize the time to achieve the metric has expired until she returns to the unit. A simple alert is not adequate in such a case, as she would not have been able to act on it in time. Missing even one such metric during a shift means that the measure for "compliance with all components of the bundle" has not been achieved. Understanding the cognitive and physical burden experienced by HealthEast clinicians resulted in the genesis of the HIT-fueled VAP Quality Monitor.

The HealthEast Development Process

The development of the VAP Quality Monitor started with brainstorming sessions between HealthEast's Clinical Informatics department, representatives from its Quality Institute, nursing leadership, frontline clinicians, and clinical product development experts from the organization's EHR vendor (McKesson). HealthEast clinical leaders knew having real-time, concurrent information would drive workflow. They were inspired by the work done by a team at Vanderbilt University to create a

Fig. 17.2 VAP Quality
Monitor in use at a nursing
station, HealthEast Care
System

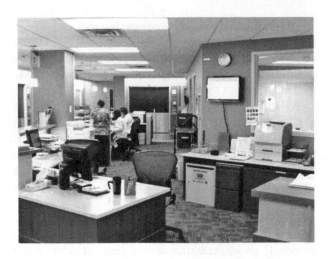

real-time compliance dashboard for VAP reduction in the SICU environment [4, 5]. Through open dialogue and a creative problem solving approach, brainstorming progressed to iterative design sessions. This ultimately lead to a successful pilot of a prototype system within 6 months at one of HealthEast's ICUs. Eventual dissemination to four ICUs in two of the system's three acute care facilities followed.

To refine the tool, HealthEast went through extensive usability testing with end users. This was part of both the iterative design process and feedback from the pilot – which lasted about 3 months. One of the overarching design principles was to avoid any additional work for busy clinicians, so there would be no "new workflow" associated with the VAP Quality Monitor other than looking at the screen. The VAP Quality Monitor does this by constantly analyzing the work that the care team is already doing and then displaying progress relative to that documentation. For example, when the nurse documents the "wean assessment" in the clinical documentation system, the status icon for that component of the bundle automatically updates to green, indicating compliance. There are no additional buttons to click on or boxes to check off (Fig. 17.2).

A second key design objective was to make the user interface as intuitive as possible. Working with the vendor, HealthEast tried out a number of different iconography approaches and display alternatives on users and incorporated their feedback in an iterative fashion to create a clean and straightforward screen. Most new users can learn how to interpret and use the tool in less than an hour, helping affirm its usability.

In terms of everyday clinician workflow, the VAP Quality Monitor makes adherence to the bundle easier by bringing everything front and center. In the past, in order for clinicians to determine whether the VAP bundle elements were met, they needed to look at the physician orders, the medication administration record, the respiratory therapist (RT) assessment and the VAP charting, none of which was accessible in real time. HealthEast would typically not see its failures until the manual chart audits were completed 3 months after the fact. Today anyone on the care team can see the status of all bundle elements in real time.

Resource Requirements

The VAP Quality Monitor project team was made up of individuals from a variety of clinical and information technology backgrounds and leaders at different levels of the organization. The team included an executive sponsor, clinical staff, including unit leaders as well as front-line physicians, nurses and ancillary care providers, and specialists from the informatics and quality department teams. Vendor staff included clinical products managers, IT system architects and software engineers.

Results

The results of the pilot, which was initiated in one ICU in October 2009, were impressive. Prior to the project, the level of compliance with all components of the VAP Bundle ranged between 43 and 74 % across ICUs systemwide. HealthEast saw such a rapid uptick in adherence in that first pilot, 57 % of patients in compliance with the all-or-none bundle the month the pilot started to 100 % of patients in compliance three months into the pilot, that they asked the vendor to deploy the tool in the other ICUs ahead of the planned schedule. They believed it was too important to their patients *not* to implement in all ICUs as quickly as possible. Approximately one year after the pilot, adherence to all components of the bundle across all ICUs was consistently in the 95–100 % range.

However, the outcomes are the real success story. In the year prior to the pilot project, the pilot ICU had 3.07 cases of VAP per 1,000 ventilator. In the year after the onset of the project, there were 0 cases of VAP – none whatsoever. After HealthEast rolled out the tool across all ICUs in its three acute care hospitals, they saw similar success with adherence to all components of the bundle.

A final benefit is that the fantastic results of the VAP Quality Monitor are now used to help educate users and increase adoption. In fact, the training materials for the VAP system start by explaining "why we are doing this", highlighting the improvements in quality outcomes and care documentation.

Lessons Learned

HealthEast has gained many valuable insights through its experiences using the VAP Quality Monitor.

The Importance of Real Life Logic Testing. Prior to the go-live of the VAP Monitor tool, extensive testing was performed based on different scenarios and simulations to assure the logic performed as desired. Once the tool was live, the results of the actual patient data and end user activities did not always match the intent of the logic. For example, hypothermic patients, as denoted by the patient's recorded temperature, were originally excluded from being measured, as defined by how VAP bundle compliance is measured for reporting. However, due to the variation seen in a patient's temperature in the ICU, a patient would go on and off the bundle, causing confusion for the nurses. Ultimately, HealthEast decided to just keep those patients on the bundle at all times to make sure they were always providing the care desired, even though they would be excluded for reporting purposes.

Improving Teamwork. Use of the VAP Quality Monitor has had additional benefits to the way HealthEast provides care. Because it is patient focused and not clinician focused, it improves care team communication and gives the team a systematic approach for assuring that every patient receives appropriate care, every time. Whereas in the past some care team members may not have always completed their respective bundle-associated tasks with awareness of what others were doing, the increased transparency of bundle element status has enhanced collaboration. As one of the ICU Clinical Managers has stated, "The VAP Quality Monitor has fostered teamwork for us. Collaboration between RT and nursing grew. We, *together*, have this person on a vent."

Documentation Standardization. Clinicians quickly began to understand the importance of consistency in the clinical documentation templates and practices, because the logic of the VAP Quality Monitor depends on it. For example, some units had the ability to chart Head of Bed elevation as a type of "yes/no" checkbox whereas others had built the documentation template to require a numerical entry (30°). For the system's logic to work consistently, it must have access to a single "source of truth" in the documentation to analyze. Consistent documentation practices are not typically difficult to standardize at the unit level but may require significant policy review and staff education to standardize across units and facilities.

Documentation Speed and Completeness. Deployment of systems that increase transparency to data may also increase the timeliness and completeness of clinical documentation. For example, one of the staff nurses noted, "The colors [of the icons] are a good visual cue to trigger opportunities to chart in a timely manner." Another ICU nurse explained, "A prompt doesn't mean better patient care—that's from the integrity of the nurse. But sometimes you forget to chart. Then the monitor helps to remind you to chart."

Monitor Placement. In the original pilot unit, the monitor was placed in a rounding room just off of the nurses' station so that it could be referred to during case management rounds. But most of the users wanted it to be more accessible. Nurses would peek around the corner to see their patient's status. Over time the team developed a process by which a charge nurse monitors the board regularly to assist nurses who may be falling behind in completing elements of the bundle. HealthEast has also decided to deploy a HIPAA-compliant desktop version of the display for physicians and case management staff not present on the unit.

Future Plans

While HealthEast has achieved many quality improvements along the "HealthEast Quality Journey" to date, their success with the VAP Quality Monitor has given them confidence that they can attain equally impressive levels of improvement in other areas which they may have struggled with in the past. HealthEast plans to extend these concepts to a number of other care processes, such as preventing catheter associated urinary tract infections and central line infections, as well as care processes for stroke and congestive heart failure. In addition, this type of real-time process visibility allows for novel approaches to patient management, including providing a centralized review of process statuses across a health system or creating an individual caregiver's view of all elements of care processes for which she is responsible. To further streamline workflows, these notifications would ideally be actionable, taking the caregiver to the appropriate next step to advance the care process for their patients.

Conclusion

HealthEast believes the VAP Quality Monitor innovation closes a gap in even the most sophisticated EHR systems. The organization already had the ability to create and deploy advanced decision support tools to help clinicians know exactly what should be done, as well as the tools to measure and analyze performance retrospectively. But caregivers lacked the ability to answer the question, "How are we doing *right now*?" With this innovation, HealthEast has a real-time visual control tool that gives them that knowledge. Every clinician at HealthEast is committed to providing the best possible care to every patient, every time. Now they have another tool to support them in that goal. And patients like Cindy Martinez, as well as their families, can feel confident that they will receive such care.

References

1. Rello J, Ollendorf DA, Oster G, vera-L lonch M, Bellm L, Redman R, Kollef MH. VAP outcomes advisory group. Targeting ventilator-associated pneumonia. Source. 2007;1(3):5.
2. Carr DS. Nonpayment for VAP: management implications. Nurs Manag (CMS Solut Suppl). 2009;40:23–4.Availableonline:http://journals.lww.com/nursingmanagement/Fulltext/2009/06001/Nonpayment_for_VAP__Management_implications.6.aspx.
3. IHI. Implement the ventilator bundle 2009. Institute for Healthcare Improvement website, http://www.ihi.org/IHI/Topics/CriticalCare/IntensiveCare/Changes/Implementthe VentilatorBundle.htm. Accessed on 28 Apr 2011.
4. John Starmer, MD and Dario Giuse, Dr. Ing. A real-time ventilator management dashboard: toward hardwiring compliance with evidence-based guidelines. AMIA. Annu Symp Proc. 2008;702–706. Available online: https://www.ncbi.nlm.nih.gov/pmc/articles/PMC2656080/.
5. William W, Stead MD, (by invitation) Neal R. Patel MD, and John M Starmer MD. Closing the loop in practice to assure the desired performance. Trans American Clin Climatol Assoc. 2008;119:185–195. Available online: http://www.ncbi.nlm.nih.gov/pmc/articles/PMC2394683/.

Chapter 18
Dashboards 2.0

George Reynolds

Barbara helped her son Mike to the ED front desk. He was wheezing pretty badly and his inhaler didn't seem to help. Before she could even yell for help, the woman at the desk called out, "Patty!" and a nurse came around the partition behind the desk. Introducing herself, Patty guided Mike and Barbara to a small room behind the desk. A few quick questions, a quick listen to the lungs, and she had Mike holding an aerosol mask to his face. The woman from the desk wheeled a computer in, asked a few identifying questions and found Mike in the computer system. Patty took over and reviewed the record of Mike's last office visit with Dr. Castle, Mike's pediatrician, read the details of his asthma management plan and confirmed his maintenance and rescue medications. Barbara looked at her watch and smiled. They'd arrived 10 min ago.

As they were led into an exam room, Barbara glanced at the big-screen TV behind the main desk. It was filled with multicolored information about the ED's patients—and it looked like there were a lot of them. As Patty connected Mike up to the monitors, she said, "A doctor will be with you in just a moment." Barbara pressed her lips together grimly; it looked like the ED was having its own rush hour. Fifteen minutes later, Dr. Wyatt entered the exam room and introduced himself briskly. He asked a Barbara a few questions and turned his attention to Mike. Mike was still wheezing loudly, but he was able to complete his sentences, which was a huge relief to Barbara. Dr. Wyatt examined Mike, then picked up the tablet computer that he had brought with him. A few taps on the screen, and the doctor again reviewed Mike's asthma management plan. "I think we're going to be OK, but I'd like to give Mike another breathing treatment and start him on some oral steroids. You're going to be here for a bit," the doctor reported.

The doctor couldn't have been gone more than a minute before a nurse entered, introduced herself as Tara, and gave Mike a little medicine cup with the steroid.

G. Reynolds, M.D., MMM, FAAP, CPHIMS
IT Department, Children's Hospital & Medical Center,
8200 Dodge St, Omaha, NE 68114, USA
e-mail: greynolds@childrensomaha.org

L. Berkowitz, C. McCarthy (eds.),
Innovation with Information Technologies in Healthcare, Health Informatics,
DOI 10.1007/978-1-4471-4327-7_18, © Springer-Verlag London 2013

Mike hated this stuff and made an awful face as he swallowed it. Tara started him on another breathing treatment. With a deep sigh of relief, Barbara gave Mike a hug, "I need to update your dad."

Twenty minutes passed before Tara returned, removed the nebulizer and the oxygen tubes and entered some information into the computer she had wheeled into the room. "Let's watch Mike for a bit off the oxygen before we make any decisions," Tara smiled, "but so far so good." Not long after, Dr. Wyatt returned and listened to Mike's lungs again. "Much better," he declared. "How do you feel now?" Mike gave him a thumbs-up and asked, "Can I go home now?" Dr. Wyatt reviewed his recommendations with Barbara, answered her questions and said goodbye.

A few minutes later, Tara returned with her computer, printed instructions and prescriptions. She reviewed Dr. Wyatt's recommendations again. These people were nothing if not thorough, Barbara thought. Mike was to see Dr. Castle within 48 hours. "When will he get the records from the ED?" Barbara asked. Tara grinned, tapped the enter key on her computer and said, "He just did." Barbara was halfway home before she looked at her watch again and shook her head in surprise—less than 2 hours since they had arrived at the ED's front desk.

Background

Children's Hospital & Medical Center is a 145-bed hospital in Omaha, Nebraska. In partnership with the University of Nebraska School of Medicine, it operates the 126 physician member Children's Specialty Pediatric group. In partnership with Creighton University School of Medicine, it operates the 34-physician Children's Physician group.

Children's Hospital & Medical Center has a rich history based on community involvement and service to children. The original Children's Memorial Hospital was founded in 1948 by Dr. C.W.M. Poynter, dean of the University of Nebraska Medical Center, and Henry Doorly, publisher of the Omaha World-Herald, with a vision that no child in need of medical care would be turned away due to an inability to pay. Today, families from across a five-state region and beyond seek the experience and expertise of Children's Hospital & Medical Center. We provide care to more than 250,000 children each year.

In 2011, Children's Hospital & Medical Center was recognized by healthcare informatics magazine as the healthcare IT Innovator of the Year.

The Innovation

Children's Hospital & Medical Center in Omaha has developed an Analytics program that addresses a variety of clinical, administrative and financial data needs throughout the organization. Over 40 dashboards have been developed that extract

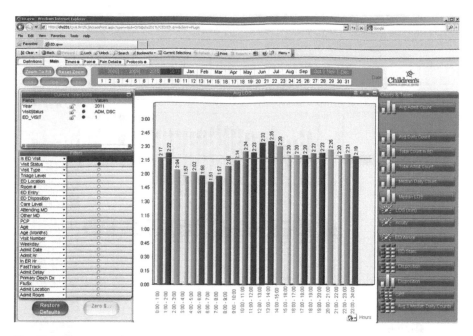

Fig. 18.1 Emergency department dashboard

and analyze data from Children's inpatient and ambulatory electronic medical record (EMR) and associated financial systems. Using off-the-shelf business intelligence technology, these dashboards can be accessed throughout the organization by anyone with a web browser and the appropriate security clearance. Instead of static paper or spreadsheet-based reports, the dashboards allow the user to filter, sort and analyze the data on-the-fly, letting them answer questions they hadn't even thought of when the dashboard was designed. The information technology department (IT) isn't the data gatekeeper anymore—the dashboard users are empowered to come up with creative ways to examine a problem and develop equally creative solutions.

Example: The Emergency Department (ED) Dashboard

The first two things the ED manager reaches for in the morning are a Diet Coke and the ED Dashboard (Fig. 18.1). In a single screen, it gives her an update on the department's activity over the last 24 hours. As with all of the dashboards, it is updated between 2 AM and 4 AM, so the data is never more than a day old. Key metrics such as patient volume and acuity, length of stay, and patients admitted or left-without-being-seen are all presented in a quick summary view. With a single click, she can see the ED census by hour of the day. Another click gives her that

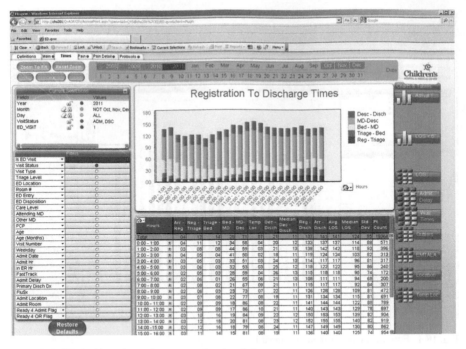

Fig. 18.2 ED dashboard – patient status time breakdown

same view broken down by patient acuity. One more click and she can see the amount of time the average patient spent in each phase of care from arrival to registration to triage to exam room. She can also see the time it took for the doctor to see and treat the patient, make a determination about the patient's disposition and for staff to discharge or admit the patient—all broken down by the hour of the day (Fig. 18.2).

All of this data can be filtered on-the-fly. With a couple of clicks, the view can be limited to only those patients with low acuity scores, since special emphasis has been placed on moving these patients through the system as efficiently as possible. The view could also be changed to look at only those patients who were admitted, or were seen by consultants, or had radiology tests (or a specific kind of radiology test—CT or MRI, for example). The view can be sorted further and filtered by patient diagnosis, time of day, acuity, therapy, age and a number of other parameters. Using these tools, the manager can quickly drill down to identify those patients who are potential outliers and can easily spot potential sources of delay or inefficiency. Another tab in the dashboard focuses on the quality of documentation as it relates to pain scores—another important metric in the ED. Yet another tab focuses on staff performance for specific ED protocols such as the management of infants who may have sepsis or an acute asthma exacerbation.

In the office next to the manager's, the medical director of the ED has his own view of the dashboard data with a specific focus on the performance of the ED doctors, nurse practioners and physician assistants. He can easily drill down to the individual care provider, or look at the patient volume and acuity over the day to be sure the provider staffing and skill mix is optimal. In yet another office, the nurse trauma coordinator has her own dashboard that gives her a very specific view of both the ED and inpatient record designed to monitor all trauma patients. In an entirely different group of offices, another view of the ED patient volume trend is displayed with other census metrics as part of the Chief Financial Officer's dashboard. In this view, charges and revenue are displayed in tandem with patient activity throughout the organization.

However, a snapshot of a day in the life of the ED won't give the ED manager and the department's medical director the information they need to identify trends and measure the success of their efforts over time. Fortunately, the dashboard can answer all of the same questions described above for any period: a week, a month, a quarter, anything up to 3 years. This gives the ED's leaders the ability to spot trends and predict future patient volumes not simply hour-by-hour but to also look at seasonal variations in those patterns. How does the day of the week, the season, or daylight savings time impact patient volume, acuity and flow? All of these questions can be answered using the dashboard. If more detailed analysis is needed, another click exports the table the user has built to an Excel spreadsheet (also known as the Universal Analytics Tool).

Reason for This Innovation

Too often, the data entered into EMR systems remains trapped in those systems or is available to only a few select experts with highly specialized database skills. Unfortunately, the people with those skills are not the same people who are managing departments and caring for patients. As one expert put it, *"Our EMR feels like an ATM that keeps taking money in, but never gives anything back."* In order for EMR implementations to be valuable to the patients, the providers, and society as a whole, executives and providers at Children's became increasingly aware that they must correct this imbalance between the work required to get data into the systems and the value they derived from these systems.

Why This Innovation Succeeded

Obviously, tools like the ED Dashboard were not created on a whim, nor can the Analytics team knock one out in a day. They were developed as a partnership between the data analysts in IT's Data Services division and the end-users, such as the ED manager and her team. This is an iterative process that requires a number of face-to-face meetings as the analysts learn how a specific department or unit works and what the end-users need, while the end-users learn the capabilities and limitations of the dashboard tool and underlying data. But like many innovations, the

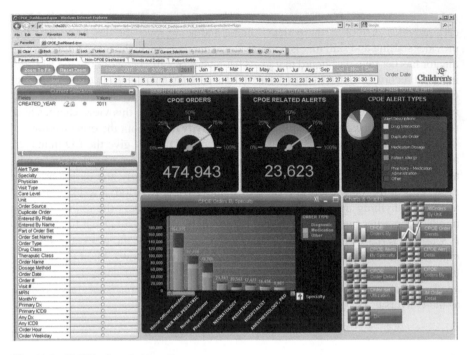

Fig. 18.3 CPOE/orders dashboard

story of the genesis of Children's Analytics program actually began with a simple question, in this case about Computerized Physician Order Entry (CPOE) usage.

In 2007, as CPOE was being rolled-out across the hospital, the Chief Medical Informatics Officer (CMIO) realized he needed a tool to monitor adoption and intervene with providers if adoption was poor to make sure they had the order sets and training they needed. Included in the first iteration of the Orders dashboard was a pie chart showing the number and relative frequency of various types of alerts that were firing in the system, such as whether a drug dose was above the recommended range, if the patient might be allergic to the drug, if the order duplicated another active or recent order, as well as a number of more specialized alerts. Initially, these alert statistics were included in the Orders dashboard so that alerting frequency could be used as a surrogate for the providers' level of skill and training in using CPOE. In other words, providers who got a lot of alerts might be making more mistakes using CPOE and could be targeted for extra help (Fig. 18.3).

However, it was discovered that the alert data could be used for much more than simply identifying providers who were struggling with CPOE. The data could be used to manage the clinical decision support (CDS) associated with CPOE. Instead of focusing on prescribers, the dashboard could be used to focus on the frequency and appropriateness of individual alerts. The Orders dashboard could be used to measure alert frequency, and the CMIO could easily drill down to a specific type of alert (such as duplicate orders) or even to a specific type of alert tied to a specific orderable (such as duplicate orders for albuterol aerosol treatments). This simple tool could identify alerts that might be firing too often, resulting in alert fatigue. In other words, if the system fires a number of alerts that aren't relevant or appropriate, the prescribers quickly learn to ignore *all* the alerts regardless of relevance or appropriateness. So the first goal of the nascent Analytics program was to eliminate as many nuisance alerts as possible.

In order to achieve that goal, a second piece of information was needed. It wasn't enough to simply target the most common alerts. The providers' response to the alerts had to be measured as well. After all, the purpose of an alert is to provide *decision support* to the prescriber. If an alert fires and the prescriber changes the order in some way, then the alert has had an impact on clinical decision-making. If the alert's logic is correct—the prescribed dose actually is too high, for example—then the alert's impact is positive.

Alerts that result in a change in prescriber behavior could be identified in Children's EMR in two ways. First, the Order dashboard could be used to identify all orders that had one or more alerts, were submitted despite the alert, and were subsequently changed or cancelled within 1 hour. The theory here was that a prescriber (often a resident in training) might initially override an alert, then reconsider after looking up the dose or seeking the advice of his supervisor. The second and much more common way to identify effective alerts was to identify all alerts not associated with orders. For example, if a provider attempts to order ampicillin for a patient with a penicillin allergy documented in the EMR, he will get an alert warning him of the allergy *before* he actually submits the order. If the provider then chooses to cancel the order, the order will not ever be recorded in the EMR database—there will be an alert not associated with an order. In order to track these, the Analytics team needed a second dashboard specifically focused on alerts rather than orders. The Alert dashboard tracks all alerts without orders and compares them to alerts with orders (Fig. 18.4).

Combining the number of alerts without orders and the number of orders changed within an hour of an alert, the Analytics team could now identify both the frequency of specific alerts and the effectiveness of those alerts. This was powerful stuff. The dashboards were used (and continue to be used) during Children's Physician Informatics Group (PIG) meetings to refine the CDS program. The CMIO would show the frequency and effectiveness of the most common alerts—duplicate albuterol orders, for example—and the members of the PIG could decide if the alert should be eliminated, modified or left alone. Using this technique, the number of nuisance alerts was greatly reduced.

And while reducing nuisance alerts was incredibly important, the Analytics team and the PIG members came to understand the full potential of their program, that alerts weren't always—or even often—the best way to provide CDS and enhance patient safety. Obviously, this had been well established in the medical informatics literature for years, but the literature was less helpful when it came to the question of what to do about it. Alerts could be made more specific and targeted, but there was no getting around the fact that alerts are disruptive to the prescriber's workflow. The best alert is the alert that doesn't fire because it doesn't have to.

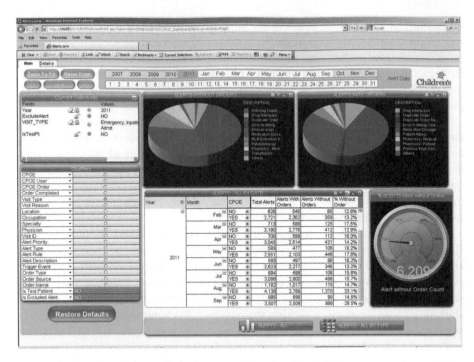

Fig. 18.4 Alerts dashboard showing alerts changing prescribing behavior

The team thus turned its attention from creating more and better alerts to creating order sets and workflows that guided the providers to create better and safer orders. When the team saw that important alerts were being overridden, instead of looking for ways to make the alert more effective, they looked for ways to make the alert unnecessary. PIG members would ask, "How can we make it impossible for anyone to even create an order like that?" If a drug shouldn't ever be given IV (Acetaminophen, for example), make it impossible to ever order it that way. If it can never be ordered IV because the system doesn't offer it as an option, then there is never a need for an alert. In many cases, dosing guidance was automated as part of the order set development—the recommended dose was only a single click away. In other cases, medications were removed from the general order catalog (the so-called "a la carte orders") and limited to an order set. Meanwhile, the system's dashboards are used to monitor the effectiveness of each change that is made.

Results

Decreasing Nuisance Alerts. As the CDS strategy was refined and augmented, the alerting frequency fell steadily from an initial range of 10–12 % of all orders firing an alert to less than 4 % (Fig. 18.5). This represented a combination of

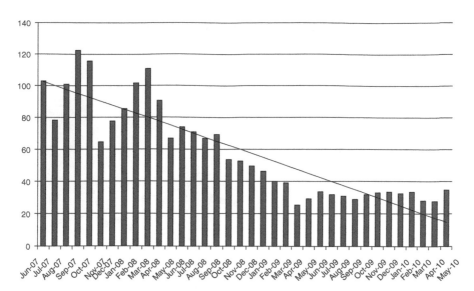

Fig. 18.5 Alert frequency (per 1,000 orders) for CPOE orders

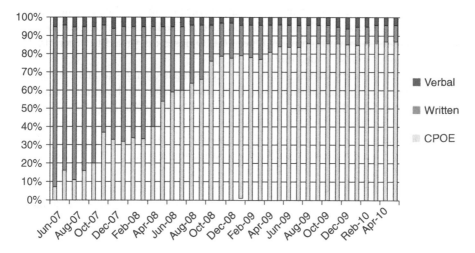

Fig. 18.6 CPOE adoption trend

removing nuisance orders and improving workflows to choose the right order in the first place.

Decreasing Errors. Voluntary inpatient CPOE use rose to over 80 % of all orders placed within 2 years of implementation and almost 90 % by 3 years (Fig. 18.6). Not surprisingly, during the same time, inpatient medication prescribing and transcription errors "reaching the patient" fell by 59 %. Despite the fact that bar-coded medication administration was not in place during this period, dispensing and administration

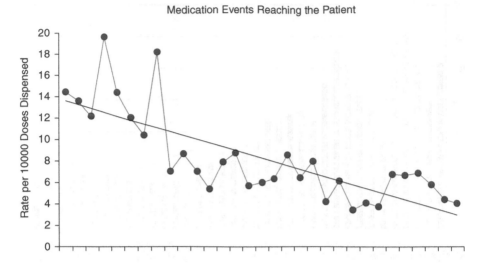

Fig. 18.7 Medication errors reaching the patient per 10,000 doses dispensed

errors also fell—dispensing errors fell by an average of 46 % while administration errors fell by an average of 38 %. As a result, overall medication errors reaching the patient decreased from a high of 19.8 per 10,000 doses dispensed to 4 per 10,000 doses dispensed—an 80 % decline! (Fig. 18.7).

A particularly good example of how Children's made changes to make it hard to do something wrong (i.e. an order which required an alert) is how they created a single order set for the dosing of therapeutic heparin (including low-molecular weight heparins). This order set had CDS imbedded in it in the form of printed guidance on the order set form, automated dose calculation, and a display of relevant lab results. Alerts were not abandoned; there was still a sophisticated set of alerts behind the order set designed to warn the prescriber of potential duplicate or overlapping therapies as well as critical lab results. But the order set was designed to make it very difficult to do the wrong thing—the prescriber has to go out of his way to make an alert fire. As a result, a heparin prescribing error has not reached a patient since the order set was put in place.

Other peripheral benefits attributed at least in part to the analytics program include:

- **ED Length of Stay**. The Children's emergency department's average length of stay decreased over 20 %, taking it from the middle to the shortest of all the Children's hospitals reporting data to the Child healthcare Corporation of America (CHCA), a consortium of 44 such hospitals. Overall, the length of stay in the ED during the first 6 months of 2011 was 146 min (Median: 127 min). For low acuity patients (triage level 4 or 5), the average length of stay was 118 min (Median: 101 min).

- **Patient Satisfaction**. An independent vendor found that the ED patient satisfaction scores are some of the best in the nation, likely in large part due to the shorter lengths of stay and decreased waiting times.
- **Departmental employee engagement**. Children's measures employee engagement annually and tracks performance using three focus questions (e.g. likelihood to refer friends or family members, likelihood to look for/think about another employer). Departmental employee engagement scores for the ED have improved significantly as length of stay (LOS) decreased. One reasonable inference is that a shorter LOS means fewer long waits which can result in fewer dissatisfied families.
- **IT Understanding**. As data analysts got out of IT and into the hospital, they got to see first hand the value of the work they were doing. For example, the analyst who built the ED dashboard met extensively with the ED manager and her staff as they refined and enhanced the dashboard. Instead of simply receiving an e-mail that said, "now, do this," she heard an explanation of the reason the new data or view was needed and the impact it would have on patient flow. And, as changes were made, she could see the data, and hear the ED manager sing her praises, as throughput improved.

Lessons Learned

Correct Data Input is Critical. One lesson that the Analytics team and their clinical and business partners have learned again and again is a seemingly obvious concept: the dashboard cannot report on data that is not stored electronically. A corollary to that lesson: data that is recorded inconsistently or incorrectly will result in faulty analysis. For example, early on in the ED dashboard development, the results displayed in the dashboard did not fit with the manager's understanding of the way patients flowed through the system. She understandably thought that the dashboard builders had made a mistake. However, further investigation revealed that the dashboard was correct; it was the data that was flawed. Short cuts in data entry created patient flow data suggesting patients were stuck in triage. In fact, the time in triage was short, but the change in patient location was not being documented in a timely fashion. Once this problem was corrected, not only was the dashboard data more accurate, the workflow involved in moving the patient from triage to the exam room was improved. The process of building the dashboard actually resulted in more efficient workflows for the ED staff.

End User Engagement. The physicians and other team members who attended the PIG became highly engaged because they had real control of the CPOE and CDS program. They owned the order sets and they controlled the alerts. When a problem alert was identified, changes were usually made within 24 hours—often within an hour or two of the meeting. CPOE with CDS became something that was being done *for* the providers rather than *to* them.

Data-Driven Decisions. Decisions about changes to the CDS system were finally based on data instead of perceptions. If a particular provider complained that an alert about the dose of Vancomicin "always" fired, it only took two or three clicks to display the actual frequency of dose range alerting for that drug on the dashboard displayed on the conference room's large projection screen. A few more clicks and everyone in the conference room could see how effective the alert was. If changes in the logic of the alert were needed, the group could determine the appropriate limits and the could put the changes into place quickly. This data-driven decision model became contagious. Leaders attending the PIG began to see the power of the Orders dashboard, and they started to think of the ways they could use similar dashboards to drive better decisions in the areas they led. In fact, the ED manager was Children's first nursing informaticist before she became the ED manager. The seeds for the ED dashboard were planted in those early PIG meetings.

Future Plans

The analytics program continues to gain momentum and garner leadership support and the list of dashboards in the queue awaiting resources is growing. Here are a few of the mission critical initiatives on which the analytics team is working on for FY 2012:

Hospital Quality Metrics for Meaningful Use Attestation. The ED dashboard described at the outset of this dashboard calculates two of the 15 hospital quality metrics required by the Center for Medicare & Medicaid (CMS) in order to achieve certification of an EMR as the first step in demonstrating meaningful use of an EMR. As a pediatric specialty hospital, many of the other 13 quality metrics are not relevant to our patient population. Nevertheless, Children's must use certified technology in order to qualify for the financial incentive. The analytics team is building a dashboard that will report all 15 metrics, and Children's is working with the Certification Commission for Health Information Technology (CCHIT) to certify the dashboard. This will allow Children's to leverage its core competency in analytics and will save over $250,000 in implementation costs when compared to the solution offered by the core EMR vendor.

Predictive Modeling of Patient Volumes. Accurately matching staffing levels and patient volumes is a challenge for every healthcare organization. Using largely manual data gathering processes, Children's has been quite successful in matching inpatient nursing staffing levels to the inpatient load. However, matching staffing and patient volumes in ambulatory and ancillary departments has proven to be difficult using manual techniques. This dashboard will gather and collate anticipated patient volumes by looking across all scheduling systems including the general pediatric and specialty clinics and out-patient surgery to determine the anticipated patient volumes for the next 1–14 days across the organization. These numbers will be combined with the most recent inpatient, observation and ED patient volumes to create a predictive model that can be used by ancillary departments such as lab and radiology to predict test volume and, by extension, staffing requirements. These results will be compared graphically with departmental staff schedules stored in the organization's time and attendance software allowing managers to see at a glance where there are mismatches between anticipated volume and staffing. This is the first time the analytics program has been used as predictive tool using scheduling data. The project goal is to improve operational efficiency by at least $500,000.

Antibiotic Use & Culture Results. Antibiotic stewardship, that is helping clinicians match the antibiotics their patients receive to the sensitivity profile of the organisms their patients are fighting, is a mission-critical goal for Children's as it continually seeks to improve the care its patients receive. This dashboard will leverage the work already done for the Infection Control department in building their dashboard, and will allow users to quickly view a patient or group of patients who are receiving antibiotics and match those orders to the microbiology results. Patients whose treatment can be changed to less broad-spectrum agents will be highlighted for follow-up by the attending physician or the antibiotic stewardship team. Notices will be sent securely from the dashboard to the attending physician.

Conclusion

Literally thousands of articles have been written about the benefits—both realized and anticipated—of EMRs. The most obvious benefits are the greatly enhanced availability of the medical record across the continuum of care and the enhanced legibility of the record and related orders. And while critically important, these benefits are the low-hanging fruit of EMR initiatives. In order to take EMRs to the next level, CDS programs must be targeted and specific—the clinician must read and find value in the advice being offered. And the designers of these CDS systems must be able to monitor the clinicians' responses and make changes in order to optimize the system.

None of this is possible without data extracted from the EMR systems that is easy to sort, filter, and analyze. This analysis isn't performed just once; it must be an iterative process in which each new answer creates more questions and results in a virtuous cycle of refinements and enhancements.

The key feature of the Analytics Program described in this chapter is that it was created by a very small organization using commercially available tools. It wasn't easy, and it required organizational support, but it represents less than 6 % of the IT Department's operating budget and much less than 1 % of the organization's operating budget. In other words, this is an innovation that can be replicated by healthcare organizations across the country.

The return on investment is hard to calculate. Using "hard dollars", the program has easily paid for itself in enhanced revenue capture and improved operating efficiency. But the "soft dollar" return is probably the more important return. Safer patients, more efficient care, higher patient satisfaction are all inarguably valuable benefits. The Analytics Program didn't create any of these benefits on its own—it merely gave leaders the tools they needed to make improvements.

Chapter 19
The Patient Voice Amplified

Valerie M. Sue and Karen Tsang

For Barbara Martinez, it all began 6 months ago. With the dinner dishes washed, the kids busy with homework, another level of Angry Birds successfully achieved, and the next day's lesson plan for her 2nd grade class completed, Barbara finally had a few minutes to check the family e-mail account. Amid the usual array of e-mails, Barbara noticed a message from the family's health care provider, Kaiser Permanente. She was accustomed to e-mails from Kaiser. Ever since signing up for the organization's Web site two years ago, she had come to expect a few messages from Kaiser every month, more when she needed to schedule appointments for the kids or e-mail their doctors.

But this e-mail from Kaiser was different; its subject line read: "An invitation to join the Kaiser Permanente Member Voice Panel." Even though Barbara wasn't entirely sure what this "panel" was, she decided to open the message. She knew no one else in the family would if she didn't, and it could be something important

The e-mail offered "a unique opportunity to join a community of individuals who will help shape the future of Kaiser Permanente." The opportunity amounted to filling out online surveys and possibly participating in focus groups or interviews. Barbara didn't have time for focus groups, but the idea of providing input to help improve Kaiser intrigued her. The family had been with Kaiser for 14 years and was generally satisfied with the care they received, but Barbara often thought that if Kaiser would listen to her advice, things could improve for all members. And, she rationalized, even if no one acted on her suggestions, they were offering Amazon. com gift certificates for participating in the panel. So she joined.

V.M. Sue, Ph.D. (✉)
National Market Research, Kaiser Permanente,
5820 Owens Drive, Pleasanton, CA 94588, USA
e-mail: valerie.m.sue@kp.org

K. Tsang
National Market Research, Kaiser Permanente,
300 Lakeside Dr. 27th Floor, Oakland, CA, USA
e-mail: karen.tsang@kp.org

L. Berkowitz, C. McCarthy (eds.),
Innovation with Information Technologies in Healthcare, Health Informatics,
DOI 10.1007/978-1-4471-4327-7_19, © Springer-Verlag London 2013

In the six months since joining the KP Member Voice panel, Barbara has told Kaiser what she thinks about the organization's Web site, shared her perceptions of the plan's behavioral health services, provided feedback about a campaign to encourage patients to get flu shots, and let them know that "Mercado de Agricultores" is the best Spanish translation for "Farmers Market." For her input, she's received a total of $15 in Amazon.com gift certificates, for which Barbara is appreciative. But the real reward, it turns out, has been the opportunity to help make Kaiser better. She still doesn't have enough time to exercise or plan healthier meals for the family, but sharing her opinions with Kaiser has given Barbara a sense of empowerment that's motivated her to be even more proactive about her family's health. And as she likes to tell her family and friends, despite being a member of such a large health plan, she feels like her voice is definitely being heard.

Background

Founded in 1945, Kaiser Permanente (KP) is a not-for-profit health-care organization headquartered in Oakland, California. KP serves 8.7 million members in 9 states and the District of Columbia. Nationwide, KP employs approximately 160,000 clinical employees and 14,000 physicians representing all specialties.

The spirit of innovation has defined KP since the founding of the organization and has continued to the present day. Currently, KP physicians and other clinical staff use one of the nation's leading electronic medical records to care for members and KP maintains one of the largest and most used Personal Health Records in the country.

Well ahead of many of its competitors, KP began offering online health services in 1996. "My Health Manager", KP's Personal Health Record, allows members to view parts of their medical record, including laboratory results, immunizations, past office visit information, prescriptions, allergies and health conditions. KP members are also able take care of health care needs via My Health Manager, such as scheduling or canceling appointments, and refilling prescriptions for themselves and other family members. Furthermore, members may e-mail their doctors, ask questions of pharmacists, and act on behalf of another family member. Other features available on KP's member Web site include a host of health and wellness programs, account management services, health and drug encyclopedias, and facility and provider directories.

In addition to ongoing enhancements to the member Web site, KP is continually researching ways to use new technologies to deliver tools that allow KP members to conveniently manage their health, and enable them to become active participants in their health care.

The Innovation

The KP Member Voice panel is an online research panel of more than 25,000 Kaiser Permanente members who contribute their opinions and insights about many aspects of the care and services they receive at Kaiser Permanente. This information helps guide quality improvement and the development of new features and services.

The panel complements existing data sources and provides structured feedback to support business decisions and ultimately improve the health of KP members. The primary goal of the panel project is to achieve a deep and broad understanding of KP members and their experiences with KP. The online panel was identified as a promising venue to collect large volumes of data that could be used across business units for multiple purposes.

Panel members are invited to participate in a variety of studies, such as online surveys, in-person or phone interviews, in-person or online focus groups, and Web site usability tests. Panelists are selected for individual projects based on their demographic and geographic profiles, and, in some cases, answers provided in prior surveys. Participation in individual panel projects is voluntary and panelists sometimes receive incentives (e.g. Amazon.com gift certificates) in appreciation for their time. Incentive amounts range from $5 for short online surveys to approximately $100 for in-person focus groups or in-home interviews.

Panel members were recruited from a random sample of KP members who had registered for the Kaiser Permanente member Web site, www.kp.org. The recruitment campaign began in the fall of 2010 when approximately 200,000 members were invited to join the panel. By the end of the year, more than 21,000 had accepted the invitation. Additional recruitment in early 2011 brought the total number of panelists to more than 25,000. Panelists represent the full-range of KP's membership in terms of gender, age, tenure as a KP member, type of health plan, utilization of KP services, and KP service areas.

As a result of the establishment of the KP Member Voice panel, departments across KP now have access to a pool of research participants who are willing and ready to participate in KP studies. Because extensive profiling data about the panelists have been collected, the KP Member Voice Project Team can identify subgroups for sampling; for example, women of a certain age, married panelists, or members who are managing a chronic condition.

How the Panel Works

To use the KP Member Voice panel, business partners from across KP submit requests to the panel management team. They specify the type of research they are interested in conducting and the participant requirements. If the proposed project is

Flu Campaign Survey Report

A KP Member Voice Project	*June 2011*
Internet Services Group	Web Insights & Analytics

To assist the development of the Kaiser Permanente's 2011 flu campaign, a survey was conducted to test four creative concepts. Members of the KP Member Voice panel were invited to provide feedback about elements of the four concepts and to rank the four concepts relative to each other. Additionally, survey respondents were asked if they received a flu shot in 2010 and if they intended to get one in 2011 after seeing the creative concepts. This report presents the survey results.

More survey participants (37%) ranked the "Remember..." concept over the others as the one they believed to be most persuasive. "Flu myth..." was ranked #1 by 27% of the respondents; 19% thought "You want..." was the most persuasive message; and, 18% said that "Flu cost..." was the most persuasive of the four messages. See below.

Of the three "Remember..." messages tested, 58% of respondents said "Remember the last time you got the flu?" was the most effective of the three; 34% said "Remember the last time your child got the flu?" was most effective. Not surprisingly, only 8% indicated "Remember the last time your wife got the flu?" was most effective. The survey respondents were all women. See pages 2-3 for details.

Got a Flu Shot in 2010
(n=440)

Nearly 3/4 of survey respondents said they got a flu shot in 2010. Of those who got the flu shot, 74% said they did so because they believe it works to prevent the flu. See page 4 for the complete list of reasons for getting (and not getting) a flu shot.

Percent of Respondents Who Ranked the Concept #1

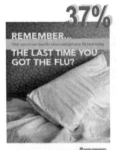
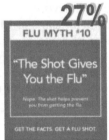
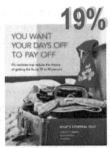
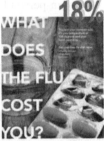

About the Survey

In June 2011, a random sample of 1,000 women on the KP Member Voice panel was invited to participate in an online survey focused on creative concepts for the 2011 flu campaign. The invited panelists represent Northern and Southern California. A total of 440 panelists participated in the survey, 50% are from Northern California. The respondents median age is 56; 75% are married; and 49% have at least a four-year-college degree. Almost half of the survey participants (49%) said they are in very good or excellent health, 38% reported they are in good health, and the remaining 13% described their current health status as fair or poor.

The KP Member Voice panel is an online panel of kp.org registered members who have previously agreed to participate in KP research projects.

KAISER PERMANENTE.

Fig. 19.1 Example of a panel project report. Flu Campaign Survey Report prepared for an internal business partner

suitable for the panel, it is placed on the panel calendar. A member of the panel team works with the business partner to develop and test the study materials, and assists with the launch of the project. There is no cost to individual researchers for using the panel. Panel customers are, however, responsible for providing incentives for study participants. Upon completion of the study, either a complete project report (see Fig. 19.1) or a data file is delivered to the individual researcher.

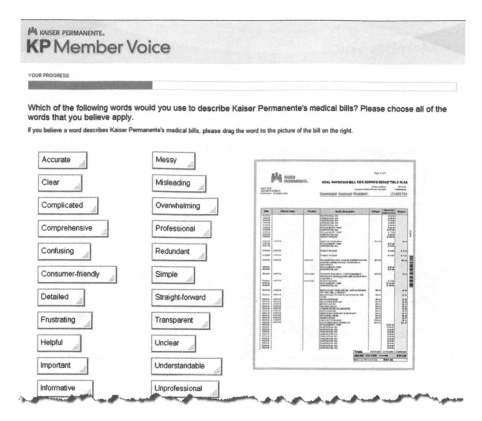

Fig. 19.2 Example of a survey created using panel survey software. Panel survey question

Examples

To date, the KP Member Voice panel has hosted 27 survey projects and provided participants for a dozen research pretests, focus groups, and usability studies. Some examples include:

- An operations leader in Kaiser Permanente's Northwest region wanted to understand why customer service scores had dropped. A survey was developed and launched using the panel survey software (see Fig. 19.2). Within 24 hours of the survey's deployment, more than 400 panelists responded to the survey. The survey revealed substantial incongruence between how members view KP's "customer service" departments and how the departments are actually organized. Shortly after the survey closed, the operations leader was able to recommend that KP focus less on the role of departments and more on content areas. It was also recommended that KP work to educate members about billing issues and improve the hand-off from member services representatives to other employees responsible from bringing resolution to member issues.
- KP's Colorado region needed to conduct a series of tests of a new Facility Locator mobile phone application. A panel survey was created to gauge the ease

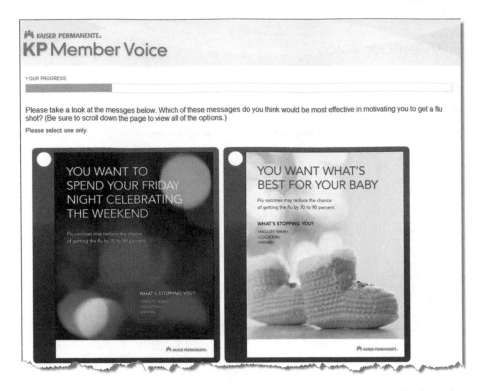

Fig. 19.3 Example of panel survey used to test communication campaign materials. Flu Campaign message testing

with which members were able to download and use the application on their smart phones. The feedback is being used in the development of this and other KP smart phone apps.

- Researchers from KP's Care Management Institute were responsible for evaluating members' perceptions of behavioral health and cancer care at KP. Two surveys were sent to panel members. Responses exceeded the researchers' expectations, causing the team to close the surveys earlier than anticipated. The results from the studies are being used to improve the quality of behavioral health and cancer care KP provides to members. A similar online survey conducted previously using a survey vendor had a budget in excess of $30,000 and required 6 months lead time. Using the panel, the cost of conducting both surveys was reduced to less than $10,000. The elapsed time from the initial request to use the panel to the delivery of the data was 2 months.

- KP's Marketing Communications Department wanted to know if a campaign designed to encourage members to get a flu shot resonated with the target audience. Campaign materials were shown to a sample of panelists who provided feedback about the length, content and tone of the messages (see Fig. 19.3). The feedback was used to direct the redesign and editing of the campaign messages.

These situations all had in common the need for fast and easy access to KP members who were willing to participate in research projects. The KP Member Voice panel filled the needs with minimal effort required on the part of the requester. In each of these situations, the panel provided a convenient and low-cost method by which to recruit research participants and, in many cases, the venue to conduct the research project. If the option of using the KP Member Voice panel had not been available, these researchers most likely would have relied on vendors to contact participants by phone or postal mail. In some cases, the research mentioned above could not have been conducted without access to KP Member Voice panel members.

Reason for This Innovation

With the increasing costs of telephone surveys and dwindling response rates associated with postal mail surveys, it is becoming increasingly difficult for organizations like KP to collect members' feedback. Additionally, a surge in members requesting removal from survey mailing lists because they receive too many surveys from KP was a significant cause for concern. These factors coupled with the continuing desire to incorporate members' voices in the development and execution of new features and services necessitated a novel approach for recruiting research participants.

Widespread Internet use and the rapid adoption of mobile technology (e.g., smart phones) among KP's member population made an online panel an attractive solution for many of the research challenges. The panel offered an avenue for collecting the information needed while respecting members' preferences, including the desire to respond to surveys electronically rather than by postal mail.

Why This Innovation Succeeded

The panel development process began with a series of discussions with key stakeholders representing departments across KP. Although the idea of a pre-recruited research panel was appealing to many of KP's business partners, the effort involved in establishing the panel was substantial and required specialized resources. Out of many discussions, two departments emerged as logical partners: KP's Internet Services Group and the National Market Research Department.

The Internet Services Group is responsible for maintaining Kaiser Permanente's Web site. Department employees are well versed in conducting online surveys and other member-based research focused on KP's online services. National Market Research, KP's department charged with measuring perceptions of the organization's brand in the marketplace, also has extensive survey research expertise as well as experience building an online panel of KP brokers—agents who sell Kaiser Permanente health plans.

Together, four members from the two departments became the panel management team and embarked on a vendor selection process, as it was previously decided that a vendor's product, rather than an application developed in-house, would be

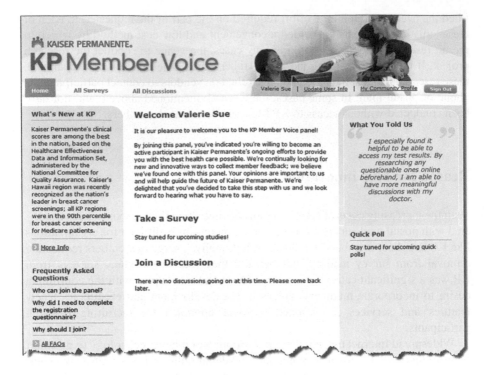

Fig. 19.4 Panelists' website. Landing page of KP Member Voice website

used to build and manage the panel. After several months of vendor interviews, the project team determined that a full-service vendor (one that offered software, survey hosting, and account management services) was the most appropriate for KP's needs.

With the vendors narrowed to three promising options, the project team hosted on-site interviews with the finalists, evaluated their offerings against criteria of needed services, and made a selection. The project team worked with the vendor to develop recruitment materials, a sampling scheme, and a Web site for the panelists (see Fig. 19.4). The vendor also provided guidance regarding panel best practices and discussed such issues as: appropriate incentive amounts, techniques for maintaining panelists' engagement, and content ideas for the panel Web site.

Building the panel required four KP staff members, approximately 12 months, and $100,000 in vendor fees. It is important to note that these staff members were not fully allocated to creating the panel; all had multiple non-panel responsibilities during the panel development period. Additionally, resources from Kaiser Permanente's Information Technology (KPIT) department were needed to evaluate the security of the vendor's software. Associates from Member and Marketing Communications, Brand, and Internet Marketing Services also supported this work by contributing funds, assisting with the vendor selection, and providing advice regarding member outreach.

Results

Adoption

The availability of the panel was communicated to relevant internal audiences via e-mail from departmental executives. A panel Intranet site was also created that allows all KP employees and physicians to learn about the panel, download basic demographic information for each region's recruited panelists, and view a research calendar showing current and upcoming panel projects.

Adoption of the panel as a research resource has been swift. Researchers from a wide variety of KP departments have availed themselves of it. Feedback to the panel team has been overwhelmingly positive and the panel has had numerous repeat customers. During the first year of its availability, KP Member Voice hosted 27 online surveys. The number of panelists responding to individual surveys ranged from 255 to more than 10,000. The typical survey received approximately 400 responses. Additionally, more than 120 participants were recruited for interviews, Web site usability tests, and focus group discussions on a wide variety of topics. For example, seven panelists participated in a KP strategy meeting focused on improving service delivery; six panelists spent a day at the Sydney R. Garfield Health Care Innovation Center testing products and sharing their expectations about the patient room of the future; and, 20 panelists took part in a focus group about how they're using mobile technology to meet their health care needs.

The expectation is that as news of the panel's availability spreads throughout the organization, the volume of requests will increase. This prospect is cause for both celebration and concern. Although the panel management team is delighted by the acceptance and use of the panel, current resources will not be adequate to support the number of anticipated projects. As the panel moves into its second year, the panel team will request additional staff and begin to reevaluate criteria for placing projects in the panel research queue.

Imitation has become another strong measure of success. Two other KP groups are seeking the advice of the KP Member Voice panel team as they develop their own panels - one of KP employees and another of a specialized patient population.

Benefits

- *Speed.* One of the panel's main successes thus far is the speed with which projects have been completed. Using the panel database, samples of participants for research projects may be selected at a moment's notice. Researchers no longer have to endure lengthy recruitment campaigns to identify study participants. Surveys targeted towards specific members (e.g., those who live in the Northwest and have contacted Customer Service) have been completed in a fraction of the time compared to similar non-panel studies. In this Northwest example, 400 completed surveys were desired; the panel provided these results in less than 24 hours. Within 30 hours of the survey deployment, the panel customer was in receipt of the final data file and file of verbatim responses. This type of study would typically take a minimum of 6 weeks from start-to-finish, provided that a vendor contract was already in place.

In another situation, interaction designers from KP's Internet Services Group requested participants from the panel, responding to an unexpected and urgent need to conduct a series of usability tests. Three days after they submitted the request, a list of usability test participants was delivered to the interaction designers. The team was able to begin the usability testing within a week of submitting the initial request. Before the availability of the panel, the user experience team relied on a vendor to recruit participants via telephone outreach, which required 2–3 weeks lead time and cost $135 per participant recruited.

In addition to fast sample selection, panel research projects may be launched as soon as surveys are programmed and tested. And because all members of the panel have previously agreed to participate in surveys and are often eager to do so, responses are returned more quickly than in non-panel online surveys.

One example of quick turnaround was when the KP Web site language experts needed to make a judgment about the Spanish translation of a label, a two-question poll was launched. The poll gathered 279 responses in approximately 12 hours. This allowed the Web site team to make an informed decision about the most appropriate label to use on the Web site. Panelists have responded with similar speed to invitations to participate in telephone interviews and Web site usability testing. With lengthy research timelines no longer a barrier, KP business partners are more likely than before to incorporate member feedback as they plan and execute new programs and services.

- *Cost effectiveness.* The other primary success of the panel has been reduction in research expenditures. The panel significantly reduces KP's reliance on vendors to recruit research participants to conduct surveys and other studies. Study participants recruited by outside vendors cost the organization approximately $135 per person. This expense is eliminated when participants are recruited from the panel database. Since its inception the panel has reduced the cost of participant recruitment by approximately $16,000. Moreover, survey research vendors charge between $10,000 and $15,000 for basic online survey projects. When surveys are conducted using the KP Member Voice panel surveyors are required only to cover the cost of participant incentives, typically between $2,000 and $4,000 for one survey. As more projects are being created and deployed from the panel management software the financial advantage of the panel is becoming evident. The savings in survey vendor and participant recruitment fees during the first year of panel operations more than covered the panel vendor fees.
- *Member Satisfaction and Interaction.* The panel has also given KP the opportunity to prove that it is listening to its members. When panelists are asked to, for example, review marketing materials or redesigned bill statements, they know KP is doing so in response to comments they have previously provided. This 360° feedback process is apparent to panelists and they see how their contributions

are making a difference. In response to a KP Web site evaluation survey one panelist was pleased his suggestion was being followed: *"I can see positive changes, little by little. It looks like you're taking my advice."* On the flu campaign survey another panelist indicated how being part of the panel impacted his health: *"Thanks for asking my opinion. Since joining the KP Member Voice panel I am much more aware of my responsibility in taking care of myself."* Finally, in writing to complain about the wait time at a KP clinic, one panelist said, *"Being part of the KP Member Voice I felt empowered to ask why there was such a long wait at the clinic,"* helping to demonstrate the power and impact of the KP Member Voice panel.

- *Shared resources.* The panel has allowed KP's Internet Services Group and National Market Research Departments to reduce redundancies across the two departments by sharing the panel software, data, and research results. The collaborative environment created by the joint panel work also contributes to improved experiences for all KP members as they are not bombarded with multiple and redundant research requests.

- *Expanded study types.* In addition to standard online surveys, in-person focus groups and interviews, the panel creates new research opportunities. The database holds panelists' responses to all panel projects, making it possible to conduct meta-analyses and longitudinal projects that require tracking responses over time. The panel is also an ideal venue for methodological research, allowing the project team to evaluate the impact of incentives, invitation language, and questionnaire length, for example. Additionally, systematic evaluation of online research methods to complement and/or replace currently used modalities (such as phone interview surveys) is possible.

Lessons Learned

What follows are several lessons the KP Member Voice Project Team has learned during its first year of developing and managing the panel. It is not a comprehensive list, but rather a discussion of some of the highlights that have been especially salient for the project team. These lessons do, however, address many of the common situations faced by panel developers.

Start small and build. In the age of super-sized everything, it is tempting to "think big" when it comes to building a research panel. A reasonable question might be, "Why limit myself to 1,000 panelists when, with a little more effort, I can have 20,000?" If you're sending 10,000 e-mail invitations, it doesn't require too much more work to make that number 100,000. Another attractive feature of the large panel is that you can avoid panelists' burn out because you have many more individuals to whom you can send invitations to participate in research projects. However, regardless of your ultimate goal, it is strongly recommended that first-time panel developers start by creating a small panel, spend some time managing it, and then add members over time.

There are several advantages of this approach. First, errors will be limited to a small proportion of the population. If e-mail invitations to join a panel are sent to 100,000 people, for example, and then a flaw in the panel software is discovered, the same individuals cannot be contacted with a corrected invitation in the future. Discovering errors is disappointing in any event; however, with a smaller sample the impact of the error is minimized. Second, more panelists means increased volume of e-mails (questions, complaints, suggestions) sent to the panel support e-mail inbox. By starting with a smaller number of panelists, panel managers will be able to respond to e-mails in a timely fashion and use the experience to develop standardized responses to common inquiries that can be employed when the panel size is increased. Finally, managing the day-to-day activities of a small panel will provide panel managers with a sense of the range of tasks to be prepared to tackle when the panel grows. With this knowledge, the panel team can be staffed appropriately.

The KP Member Voice panel team employed a tiered approach to gradually build the panel. Phase I was a pilot project where 1,600 members were empanelled. These members were sampled from across KP's eight geographic regions and represented members on several demographic and psychographic characteristics. Empanelling this small proportion of the desired members and conducting a few studies with those panelists allowed the project team time to thoroughly evaluate the internal and external workings of the panel before rolling out the recruitment campaign to a larger sample. Adjustments to panel materials, registration questionnaire, project request process, panel Web site and incentive system were made at the end of phase I. Also, during the post-phase I evaluation, it was determined that the original panel vendor was not a suitable match for KP. The need to select a new vendor delayed the start of phase II by approximately 6 months.

With refreshed materials and a new panel vendor engaged, the team embarked on empanelling 20,000 additional panelists. As with phase I, the team began slowly by launching the recruitment campaign first in KP's Colorado region. When the Colorado region was almost completely empanelled, the team began sending invitations to KP members in Georgia. When Georgia was nearly finished, invitations went to members in Hawaii. And so it went, region by region, until the last group of members from Northern California joined the panel. Although phase II was not without complications, when issues did arise, the experience of the phase I pilot allowed the team to respond swiftly with solutions. At the conclusion of this phase, the team again regrouped to evaluate the successes and problems encountered during this part of the project and to devise solutions that could be addressed in phase III.

The final part of the panel construction (phase III) consisted of recruiting members to fill gaps (e.g., dimensions along which the panel was not representative of the population). During this phase, approximately 5,000 additional members joined the panel. The team also added administrative data to the panel database and implemented a formal process for requesting use of panel resources at this time.

Panel recruitment and refreshment. Panel recruitment and refreshment is an ongoing process. As panelists leave the panel, new members must be invited to join. In addition to the inevitable attrition, panelists are occasionally purged by the panel team. Reasons for purging include: non-response to panel study invitations,

KAISER PERMANENTE.
KP Member Voice

YOUR PROGRESS

Please describe any other activities related to your health care that you would like to perform on a mobile phone.

Please be as specific as possible.

[Previous] [Next]

Fig. 19.5 Example of an open-ended survey question. Open-ended survey question from a panel mobile phone survey

participation in too many panel studies, and no longer being a member of the health plan. The goal of continual panel refreshment is to maintain an active panel that accurately represents the underlying KP population.

An active research panel needs a dedicated staff. Panel management can be completely turned over to a full-service vendor. As mentioned previously, there are many vendors who will develop a client's panel, manage all aspects of it, and produce individual study reports as well as panel health reports. Of course, this usually comes with a hefty price tag. For organizations with no budgetary or legal constraints, nor any desire to be involved in the day-to-day operations of a research panel, this is a sensible path. If, however, there are financial or legal limitations, or perhaps the researchers prefer to be more directly involved with the panel, a panel of approximately 25,000 members will require at least two full-time staff people devoted to its upkeep. This includes: panel communications (periodic newsletters, the panel Web site, and the panel e-mail inbox); vendor management; research consultation with internal business partners; scheduling of panel research projects; programming, or assisting with programming, of panel studies; supervising incentive disbursements; refreshing the panel on a regular basis; and, producing reports describing panel activities and overall health.

This is a guideline. Smaller panels require fewer resources; larger but less active panels, likewise may function well with fewer dedicated staff. It is important to consider not only the size of the panel, but also the number and types of panel communications and research studies planned when determining staffing requirements.

Panelists need variety. To keep panelists engaged, it is best to offer them a variety of research opportunities. Some of the KP Member Voice panelists who were invited to participate in the first online surveys, which contained primarily closed-ended questions, noted that they were hoping for more, and different, opportunities to share their opinions. The project team accommodated the request by including open-ended questions on every subsequent panel survey (see Fig. 19.5). Although not yet implemented with KP Member Voice, other options for free-form feedback include online discussion forums or community blogs.

The project team has not yet conducted a systematic evaluation of panelists' comments, however, they have noted that panelists' comments appear to be longer and more detailed than the comments gathered through non-panel online surveys. Future plans call for an examination of factors such as verbatim content and length and associated demographic and psychographic variables. The lesson here is that when you ask panelists for open-ended feedback, they will provide it. Therefore, researchers need to be prepared to read, analyze, and act on the comments collected from the panel.

Finally, a good fit with the panel vendor is essential for success. Although seemingly obvious, the importance of this factor warrants emphasizing. There are many companies offering a wide range of panel services. At one end of the continuum are those that provide software only, at the other end are full-service vendors that will establish proprietary panels, conduct all panel studies, refresh the panel as participants drop-out, and provide panel reports on a predetermined schedule. Along the continuum are vendors that specialize in particular panel activities, like probability sampling or empanelling hard to reach individuals. One of the keys to a good relationship with a vendor is choosing one that offers the right level of support for your organization. To determine the optimal amount and type of panel services needed, it is helpful to carefully assess the skills and expertise of the in-house panel management team to uncover gaps and potential areas of duplication with what the vendor offers. Asking the following questions during vendor review process may also be useful.

- *How much experience does the vendor have with the survey platform they are offering?* Ideally, the software should be developed by the vendor specifically for panel management. If the vendor uses their own software to conduct surveys and manage their own proprietary panel(s), they will have the requisite familiarity with the tool to assist their customers. It is best to avoid panel vendors that rely on third-party panel software. These vendors will not have the depth of knowledge to answer most questions and "help" or "support" inquiries will take longer to be addressed than when dealing with the software vendor directly.
- *How will incentives be distributed to panelists?* During the sales presentation, almost all vendors will say they have the capacity to "handle" incentive disbursements. This may mean the vendor works through a third-party, perhaps a mailing house or online retailer, to deliver incentives to panelists. Or, it may amount to downloading a list of panelists who are owed incentives and sending that list to the client for further action. It is tempting to accept any general answer offered and move on to more interesting topics. However, in the long run, it will be worth the investment in time to get a step-by-step breakdown of exactly how the vendor proposes incentives be disbursed. In some cases, as when working with sensitive personal health or financial information, for example, sending panelists' names to a third-party will not be an option, and may eliminate the vendor from consideration.
- *Who will be managing the panel account?* When building a large online panel (i.e., a panel with more than 1,000 members), it is important to work with an account manager who has significant experience with large panels. Finding one with experience in your business sector is an added bonus. There are hundreds of details involved in panel development and as many idiosyncrasies associated with

different industries. Working with someone who can point out the potential land mines on the road ahead can greatly reduce the stress associated with building an online research panel. Even the most seasoned panel managers make mistakes; it is wise to ask about the account manager's approach to dealing with problems when they occur. Experienced people will have techniques for rectifying errors and mitigating disasters.

- *Does the vendor maintain their own customer panel?* That is, does the vendor maintain a panel of their own panel customers? A vendor that does this is demonstrating that they are interested in listening to feedback from their customers as they develop new products and services.

Future Plans

Having completed the first three phases of building the KP Member Voice panel, the panel team is poised to embark the first of the post-recruitment phases of the project. As the present panel represents only KP members who are registered to use the KP Web site, the next task is to recruit panelists who are not registered to use the Web site. There are significant challenges associated with empanelling these members. For example, no convenient sampling frame exists; therefore, one must be constructed so that the members can be randomly sampled from the population. Also, additional funding and innovative communication strategies will be necessary to contact these members. The panel team is contemplating a multi-media campaign designed to maximize the likelihood of reaching all sectors of the KP membership. Beyond this, the panel team envisions including non-KP members in the panel. Although non-members would not represent the voice of KP's constituents, this group would serve as a valuable source of comparison against which opinions, attitudes and behaviors of KP members can be evaluated.

While working to construct the next segment of the KP Member Voice panel, the project team will continue to promote the use of the current panel throughout KP, consult with internal business partners regarding specific panel studies and begin to undertake methodological research aimed at maintaining the health of the panel.

Conclusion

Building a large research panel is a challenging, lengthy, resource-intensive process. However, the rewards are substantial. The KP Member Voice Project Team continues to be encouraged by the positive response from business partners across KP. Feedback from panelists has been likewise positive and heartening; many have expressed appreciation for being consulted by KP for their opinions. The KP Member Voice Panel represents the beginning of a paradigm shift in how KP conducts member research. Business leaders across the organization now have access to a convenient, cost-effective method by which to measure members' opinions, attitudes and behaviors. This resource enables them to fulfill their pledge to be active listeners as they strive to continually improve the way KP takes care of its members.

Chapter 20
The Gaming Edge

Alex Tam, Vivian Distler, and Bradley Kreit

Ray Martinez has had a regular game of soccer with his friends for years until a recent ankle injury kept him off the field. His doctor identified some damaged cartilage and Ray went into surgery to get it repaired. Even though it was an outpatient procedure, the doctor said that he wasn't allowed to put weight on the ankle for 3 weeks.

Even after only 3 weeks of staying at home on the couch, Ray had lost significant muscle tone, strength, and balance in his left leg. He started to see a physiotherapist twice a week for hour-long sessions. The physiotherapist told Ray that while he was doing great in the sessions, his real success depended on him doing his own exercises every day at home.

Six weeks after surgery, Ray was able to start walking around without crutches. He couldn't wait to go outside and get back to his regular life. He soon found that he'd rather spend time with friends and family than do the exercise homework. They were becoming a dreaded chore. His therapist could see that his progress had plateaued and Ray confessed that he was having a hard time sticking with the exercises with all the things he was balancing in his life. His therapist suggested that Ray try playing the balance game on the Wii Fit. He made an agreement with Ray that he would reduce the exercise homework if Ray would supplement by playing the Wii Fit.

A little skeptical, Ray tried the Wii Fit, anything to get out of those arduous exercises. Once on the Wii Fit, Ray found that it tapped into that competitive side of him, he even started challenging his daughter Cindy to see who could improve their score more each time. He pushed himself harder and played more often than he thought

A. Tam, BS (✉)
Creative, frog, 660 3rd ST 4th Floor, San Francisco, CA 94107, USA
e-mail: alex.tam@frogdesign.com

V. Distler, JD • B. Kreit, M.A., Anthropology
Health Horizons, Institute for the Future,
124 University Ave, Palo Alto, CA 94301, USA
e-mail: bkreit@iftf.org

L. Berkowitz, C. McCarthy (eds.),
Innovation with Information Technologies in Healthcare, Health Informatics,
DOI 10.1007/978-1-4471-4327-7_20, © Springer-Verlag London 2013

he would. It was fun, and he found himself actually looking forward to playing Wii Fit and then doing the smaller list of exercises. After a few more weeks, the therapist was impressed with his progress and congratulated him on his recovery.

Background

This chapter is different the others… it's OK, innovators get to shake things up now and then! In this chapter, innovators from two pioneering organizations explain how the intersection of gaming and information technologies will increasingly result in truly innovative solutions.

frog: frog works with the world's leading companies, helping them to design, engineer, and bring to market meaningful products and services. With an interdisciplinary team of more than 1,000 designers, strategists, and software engineers, frog delivers connected experiences that span multiple technologies, platforms, and media. frog works across a broad spectrum of industries, including consumer electronics, telecommunications, healthcare, energy, automotive, media, entertainment, education, finance, retail, and fashion. Clients include GE, Intel, Disney, Siemens, Welch Allyn, Amgen, Roche, Humana, and many other Fortune 500 brands.

Institute for the Future: The Institute for the Future (IFTF) is an independent, nonprofit strategic research group with more than 40 years of forecasting experience. We offer clients a deep understanding of global trends and discontinuities that will reshape health and well-being in the coming decade. We work with organizations of all kinds to help them make better, more informed decisions about the future.

What Do Health and Games Have to Do with Each Other?

Ray's experience represents one of the biggest challenges in heath care: how to get patients to adhere to care plans. Physicians meet with a patient, provide a diagnosis, and prescribe a course of treatment. Once a patient leaves the health provider's office, the burden of care falls on them. Patient adherence to taking medication or sticking with a series of tasks—as in Ray's case—can last for weeks, or longer. In many cases, a patient's ability to follow through and stay compliant will determine their health outcome.

By using the Wii Fit, Ray was more engaged in completing his physical therapy regimen. It helped him overcome the burden of doing his exercises, and kept him motivated. The Wii Fit is one of a growing set of digital products and efforts aimed at using games to improve health. Games amplify engagement, and engagement is proving to be a critical element for overcoming a number of health challenges we face.

For most people, health is not something that is top of mind in their day-to-day lives. Health only comes to their attention when something goes wrong and needs to be fixed—or it is a chore that most people know they should do something about but need to find a reason or purpose to pay attention—even though being healthy requires an ongoing investment of time and energy.

Increasing an individual's engagement in their own health is critical to increasing the health and well-being of the population and reducing costs in the long-term. The potential applications of games to health are not limited to rehabilitation. The opportunities are wide ranging, from helping patients adhere to treatment plans to motivating kids and adults in health-building preventive exercise and proper nutrition.

Enter the Power of Games

Games have motivated and engaged people for millennia. They are motivating on a number of different levels because they tap into human needs such as, competition, escape, social interaction, and recognition. They have the ability to capture attention and drive people to push themselves to perform difficult, even frustrating tasks.

Engagement levels with some games even lead to addiction-level behaviors. We've all seen the reports of teenagers that spend countless hours in front of video games and even seniors that spend all of their time at card games and slot machines. Gamers have invested 50 billion hours–6 million years–playing just one game, World of Warcraft. For many people, the instinct is to view this collective effort as a massive waste of time. But what if instead of seeing this time as problematic, we could harness the engaging properties of games to improve health and well-being?

Games have the power to take a treatment that is uncomfortable or frustrating, and motivate a person to see that task as fun and rewarding. The more that patients are engaged with their treatment, the better they will perform and the better the outcomes. As Debra Lieberman, of the Institute for Social, Behavioral, and Economic Research, states "The beauty of a game is that it gives you a goal. People work longer and harder if you give them a goal"

According to game designer Jane McGonigal, one characteristic of gaming is that people willfully choose to perform difficult tasks for no other reason than to complete the task in the game itself. The flow of the game, and those little spikes of endorphins that people get when they overcome mini-challenges, are in themselves a reward for playing. Successful health-related games will be the ones that can harness this benefit of games and direct player energies into positive health benefits.

Compare Efforts for Health with Efforts for Games

A Study in the Journal of the American Medical Association showed that people using pedometers increased their physical activity by 26.9 % over baseline [1]. The study also showed significant decreases in body mass index and blood pressure. An important predictor of increased physical activity was having a step goal such as 10,000 steps/day. Setting and meeting goals is a fundamental game element and begins to illustrate how games can create motivation and results.

It is helpful to compare a health-related situation with a gaming situation to illustrate how games can be effective. Compare the rehab procedure for ankle surgery to the game of Twister. Rehabilitation from surgery requires patients to do a series of exercises on their own several times a week. For these exercises to be effective, there is a level of discipline involved in maintaining a routine. This is difficult, as it is an additional chore and the exercises are physically strenuous. Like a chore, they require extra effort in finding additional time in the day to do these tasks, and they are often frustrating in that you have to stretch beyond your current limits.

Contrast this to the game of Twister™, where players have to contort their bodies into various different positions to win. It captures the full attention of the players and people look forward to the game. Looking closely, you can recognize that the game has incentivized similar challenges to the rehabilitation situation. It is physically strenuous, there's a level of frustration because players need to push themselves to win, and it's extra work—but people will play for hours, even when fatigued. Compare the different attitudes between player and patient (Fig. 20.1a, b).

The physical exertion in the two different situations is the same but the attitudes of the rehab patient are very different to those of the Twister players™. The introduction of play, social competition, and other game elements shifts the mindset from dreaded chore to anticipated fun. Much of this can be attributed to the addition

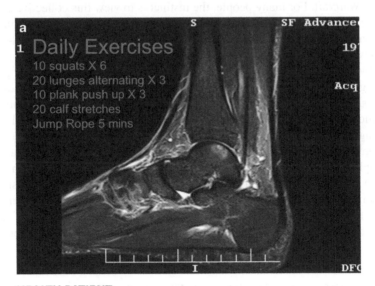

HEALTH PATIENT

Physical Stress: "Unmotivated to do it"
Frustrating: "This is hard"
Extra work: "This is a chore"

Fig. 20.1 (a) MRI of an injured ankle requiring surgery and physical therapy exercises. (b) Twister™ players maintain their interest through difficult tasks (From: http://www.tele–actor. net/tele–twister/

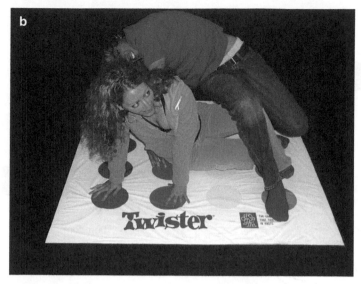

GAME PLAYER

Physical Stress: "Bring on the challenge"
Frustrating: "If I stretch, I can win"
Extra work: "Tired but want to continue!"

Fig. 20.1 (continued)

of those game elements, or game mechanics. It is these game mechanics that make this game interesting and why people continue to play. As Ben Sawyer, cofounder of the Games for Health Conference, puts it "The same mechanics that keep gamers glued to screens of all sizes can be translated to compelling tools for prevention, treatment management and more holistic care."

Why Are Games So Engaging?

Games work because they put players into a zone of complete engagement. American psychologist Mihaly Csikszentmihalyi calls this a "flow experience": a challenging activity that a) requires skills b) provides clear goals and feedback c) requires concentration on the task at hand, d) implies a (partial) loss of self-consciousness and e) a transformation of time.

Maintaining a flow state depends on engaging the player at the right level of challenge balancing between boredom and anxiety. Csikszentmihalyi's graph plots the progression of challenge versus skill in a game (Fig. 20.2). As players increase their skill in the game, they develop mastery over easy tasks and can get bored of the challenges. At this point, successful games dial-up the difficulty to increase the challenge, driving the player to improve their skills even more. This is a fine balance.

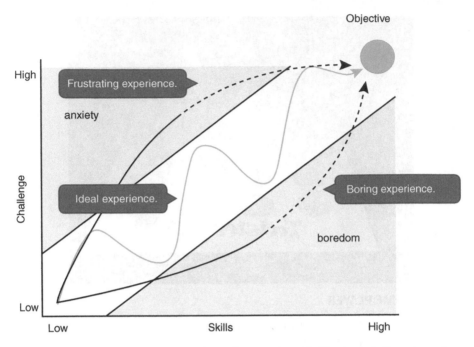

Fig. 20.2 Csikszentmihalyi's flow experience illustrates how ideal levels of challenge keep players engaged

Leave the player unchallenged for too long and they become bored, no longer wishing to continue. Dial up the challenge too quickly, and the player becomes frustrated and no longer feels like they can overcome the challenges.

People in a state of flow are calm, focused, and so completely engaged in an activity that they forget the outside world and lose track of time. The most successful engaging and sticky games do this very well. The key to this is that the game experience is so enjoyable that players feel an overwhelming compulsion to return and continue playing the game.

Getting people to play a game that gets them into a flow state that is also healthy for them, is the holy grail of health games design. By designing the right flow experiences, we can effect behavior change and make it enjoyable at the same time.

Game Foundations

In order to understand how to properly apply game theory in healthcare, it's important to start with the basics of games. In his book, "The Art of Game Design", Jessie Schell describes four fundamental elements of any game. They are mechanics, story, aesthetics, and technology.

- The mechanics are the procedures and rules of the game. They describe the goals of the game and dictate how players can try to succeed or fail at accomplishing those goals. They also describe what happens when players try to take various actions. If you compare games with other forms of entertainment that are more linear, like books and movies, the main differentiators are the mechanics. It is these mechanics that make a game a game.

- The story is the sequence of events that unfolds as the game progresses. This narrative can be linear and pre-scripted or branching and emergent and gives the game a context or backdrop for the activities within the game.
- The aesthetic is how the game looks and feels. It has the most direct relationship to a player's experience as it sets the tone for the game and immerses the player into the world of the game.
- Technology can be high tech or low tech. It can be paper and pencil or animated images from highly rendered graphics engines. It comprises the materials, medium, and interactions that make the game possible.

These four basic elements are tightly related and complement each other in a well-crafted game. Some prerequisites for games already exist in medical and home environments. There are plenty of technology, aesthetics, and narratives that can be used as components to create games. What is necessary is the orchestration of these elements together with mechanics to create engagement.

Game Mechanics

We focus our discussion around game mechanics as they are the building blocks of incentives and motivators and are the major drivers of engagement in games. They are the active ingredients that drive how a game is played and determine the different levels of engagement in the game.

Take Nike Plus as an example. Nike Plus combines pedometer sensor data connected to an iPod and a larger social community to enhance the activity of running. Nike took the activity of running and introduced several layers of game elements to make it much more engaging and compelling to runners of all levels. To date, Nike Plus members have run close to 500 million miles. This success has been built on several key game mechanics (Fig. 20.3).

Team Competition: Players compete as part of teams to collectively run further distances. This creates a sense of shared goals, as team success depends on co-operation. It enriches the social fabric between the players and builds camaraderie.

Countdown: Players are challenged to see who can run further in a fixed amount of time. This introduces a level of intensity that continues to increase until the time runs out.

Surprise/Chance: As players run, and achieve certain milestones, they have a chance to hear congratulatory messages from celebrity sports figures like Lance Armstrong, Paula Radcliff, and Tiger Woods. This mechanic introduces elements of randomness, keeping players wondering what's next and creating anticipation.

Social encouragement: Nike has integrated a player's social community so that they can "Get Cheers" while they run. A runner can expose to their friends in a

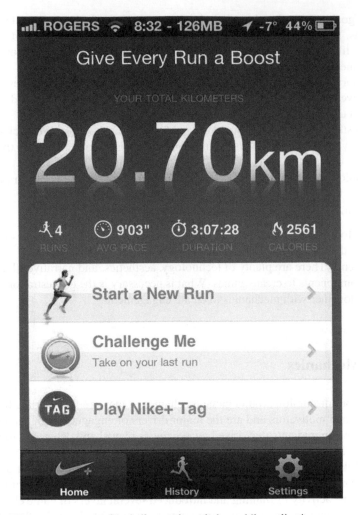

Fig. 20.3 Nike + users engage with challenges through the mobile application

facebook post that they are running, and as their friends like or comment the post, the runner hears cheering over their music as they run.

Nike has taken a simple task of running and applied game elements to make it more fun. The result is an amplification of engagement to the task. Beginner runners are more incentivised to try and stick to running, and advanced runners have additional motivation to push themselves even further.

Consider game mechanics in the context of health and wellness tasks. There is an opportunity to take tasks, where engagement can make a significant difference in treatment and prevention, and amplify and increase the engagement. Tasks like adherence to physical therapy exercises, adherence to medication, meeting nutrition goals, getting regular exercise, all benefit from increased engagement. All of these tasks require effort, however well-designed game mechanics can make completing these tasks feel fun and meaningful rather than feel like a hassle.

The Intersection of Games, Health and Technology

Systems like Nike Plus point toward a future where technology, health, and gaming will converge to form a powerful new kind of initiative and the opportunities that lie at the intersection of all three. In their book Rules of Play: Katie Salen and Eric Zimmerman reviewed the four characteristics of the intersection of games and digital technology. They are immediate and narrow interactivity, information manipulation, automated complex systems, and networked communications. By layering on the lens of health, we can begin to see the landscape for digital health games.

1. Immediate but narrow interactivity: Digital technology allows for immediate and interactive feedback. The response between the player and system is immediate, like playing chess against a computer or pressing buttons to control a character in a video game. However, the interactivity is narrower than real-life as it depends on input devices such as keyboards, mice, and game controllers.	**What this means for health:** There are an increasing number of input and display devices which relate to health. Sensors like the Fitbit pedometer and the networked Withings scale are the new interactive inputs. Even tracking the location of the player can be an input. Feedback comes through any number of digital platforms, in particular the mobile phone that is always present and providing feedback, in context and at points of decision.
2. Information manipulation: Technology can make games richer by accessing, storing, manipulating and rendering vast quantities of data. It alleviates the player from remembering all of the details so that they can focus on the immediate information presented. It also allows for the presentation of rich complex data through high performance graphics engines.	**What this means for health:** Opportunities exist in health to leverage information manipulation to facilitate the interaction between a person and the volumes of data they are gaining about themselves and their communities through emerging practices of self-quantification. This data, presented in a meaningful and digestible format, can help people see patterns of behaviors and understand the health impact of their day-to-day choices over longer time periods.
3. Automated complex systems: Digital games have the advantage that they can automatically process countless game procedures and instructions in real time and without management by the player.	**What this means for health:** Applying this in health, actions by the person can be computed against other goals, their daily schedule, or even actions by their support community to show them the impact and consequence of every decision they make. Complex systems can compute optimal choices along a series of health goals and personal constraints. Real-time feedback on every decision can lead to understanding cause and effect relationships and shape behaviors.
4. Networked communication: Evolving communications technologies, allow players to communicate more than ever before, crossing space and time, mediums and platforms. A person on Facebook can "like" that their friend is running and the runner can hear their friend's cheers over the music in their phone in real time.	**What this means for health:** A person's close relationships are extremely significant in their health. Networked communication dramatically lowers the barriers to connecting people and engaging social groups to play together and support each other. Networks increase the free flow of information, suggestions, encouragement, and helpful nudges between a person and the people that care about them the most, increasing the motivation to engage.

Health Games Today and Tomorrow: Early Signals and Future Directions

Health gaming is still in its infancy—but the opportunities are huge. Already, early gaming efforts have shown promise in applications that range from encouraging behavior change and improving medical outcomes to accelerating brainstorming and R&D.

However, the game industry is a challenging space marked with many products that do not gain critical mass and few blockbuster successes. While there is much literature about designing games, it is a craft that requires expertise and practice, just like health professions. A health game has a better chance for success if it comes from a multidisciplinary team of game designers, health practitioners, technologists and many other disciplines. Fortunately, organizations like the "Games for Health Project", which started in 2004, has been building a community to connect game developers with researchers and medical professionals. They have been supported by grants from the Robert Wood Johnson Foundation's Pioneer Portfolio to bring together people that traditionally did not intersect or even speak the same language.

The rest of this section highlights some of the early successes of health gaming. Think of these as early indicators, or signals, of much broader possibilities to use gaming as a tool to enhance health and well-being. Each example provides a detailed description of the game itself and suggests the kinds of future directions and opportunities that the game represents.

Expresso Fitness: Immersive Gaming Enhances Care and Behavior Change

Cycling is a healthy fitness activity, but there are motivational challenges to getting people to get on a bike in a fitness center. Expresso Fitness has addressed this by combining a spin bike with a video game to increase the engagement in stationary cycling (Fig. 20.4).

In the game, pedaling and steering enables you move around in a virtual game world, with the objective of chasing and catching dragons. The objective is to gather as many dragons as possible within a set time. Keeping the player conscious of time pressure throughout the game maintains a level of intensity and distracts from the effort of pedaling (Fig. 20.5).

The game is set in a fantasy world where the player escapes to an alternate reality and does not consciously focus on the physical exertion of pedaling. The story creates other things for the players to care about and focus on. By using a narrative and introducing game elements, players focus on the game without realizing that they are exerting themselves with more intensity than they would in a normal bicycle ride.

In a study with seniors, published in the American Journal of Preventative Medecine, researchers found that after just 3 months of riding, "Cybercyclists experienced a 23 % reduction in progression to mild cognitive impairment compared to traditional exercisers" [2]. Cybercycling older adults achieved better

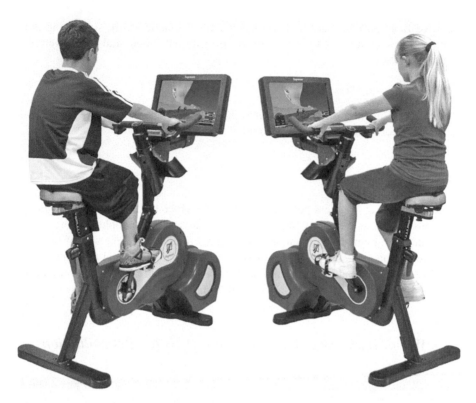

Fig. 20.4 Expresso Fitness users interact with virtual worlds as they exercise

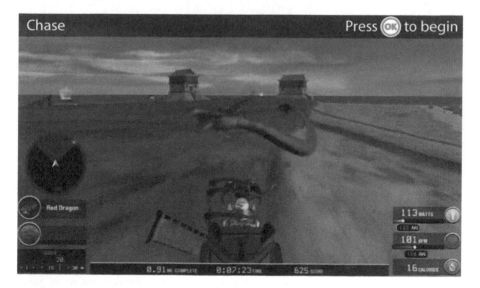

Fig. 20.5 The goal of chasing dragons in the game keeps players focused and motivated

cognitive function than traditional exercisers, for the same effort, suggesting that simultaneous cognitive and physical exercise has greater potential for preventing cognitive decline.

Game Mechanic
Powerup: Touching different elements in the game can multiply the players cycling effort and make them speed up.

Future Directions

Games like Expresso fitness point toward a future where technology-based gaming platforms play an increasingly important role in encouraging people to exercise for health and well-being, rather than as part of rehabilitation or some sort of reactive effort. In the long run, the data from these games have the potential to create a rich digital record of an individual's daily activity levels and fitness efforts, how these vary over time, and their relationship to health outcomes.

SnowWorld: Immersive Games Become Tools for Rehabilitation

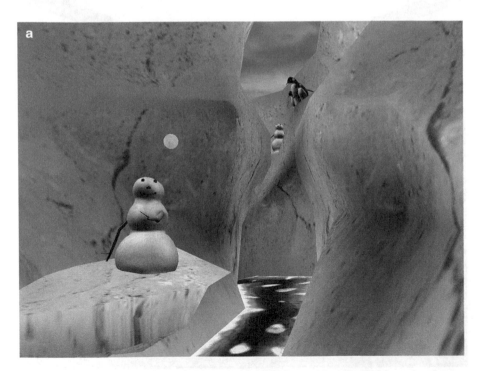

Fig. 20.6 (a) SnowWorld players immerse much of their cognitive attention into virtual game play. (b) Intense visual stimulus and gameplay distracts the pain signals from burn treatment

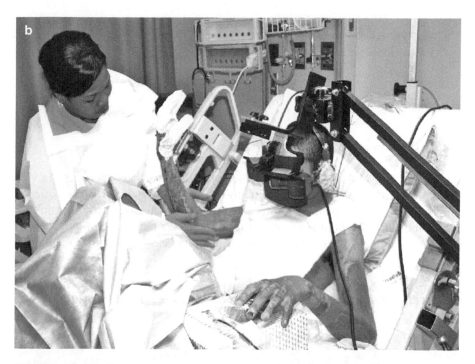

Fig. 20.6 (continued)

Burn victims go through long and painful treatment sessions during recovery. Regular treatments to the wounds can remind patients of traumatic events and anything that is associated with the treatment, such as the treatment room or instruments, becomes a trigger for anxiety in the patient. In some cases, the pain sensations are high enough to overwhelm safe doses of pain medication. To address this issue, researchers at the University of Washington Harborview Burn Centre in Seattle created SnowWorld.

SnowWorld is an immersive game that distracts the brain's attention from pain. Patients wear virtual reality helmets and noise-cancelling headphones to escape to a snow-filled world where they hurl snowballs at penguins and snowmen during treatment.

> "If you hit the penguins, they freeze, and if you hit them a second time, they explode. There's a lot of action in it. You never stop to think about anything else." [3]

This immersive escape into a fantasy game, with many different target objects and objectives for the brain to focus on, reduces the patient's focus on the activated pain receptors. Since the brain can only handle a finite amount of inputs, and is so dominated by visual stimulus, it does not register some of the pain signals. "The idea is that there is so much attention devoted to SnowWorld that there is not enough attention available to process the pain signals anymore."

By treating burns with the help of an engaging virtual game as a distraction, patients need less pain medication and perceive less pain overall. FMRIs have even shown reduced pain-related brain activity during gameplay, and patients are reporting reduced pain and anxiety. "When you compare it to pain stimuli when they were in virtual reality, some regions showed a 50 % reduction in brain activity" [3]

Game Mechanic

Combos: Players have to hit their targets with a series of snowballs before they explode.

Future Directions

Games like Snow World are based on research indicating that experiences in virtual worlds influence our perceptions of physical experience. In particular, patients experience significant benefits for intractable problems like severe burn pain. As these kinds of rehabilitative games get tested and refined, they will lead to new low-cost treatments that can be deployed in-hospital as well as in the home.

Gabarello: Games Aid Physical Recovery and Rehabilitation

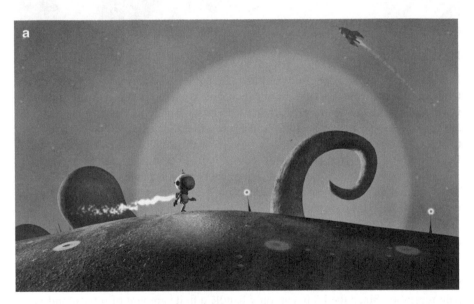

Fig. 20.7 (**a**) Rehabilitation patients use the Lokomat robot to supplement their mobility and use it as a game controller. (**b**) Patients exert more and more of their own strength to move faster through the virtual world

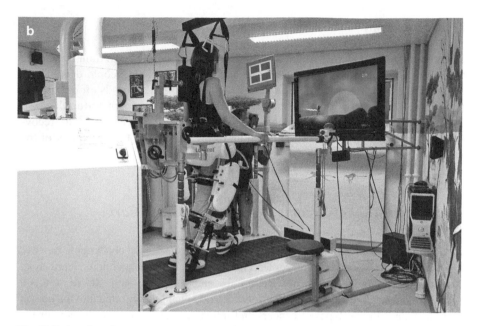

Fig. 20.7 (continued)

Rehabilitation is an involved process which is both mentally and physically challenging. Gabarello engages patients by translating their physical movements and expressing them in the movements of a character in a virtual world. Patients are strapped into a Lokomat robot, which supports and assists their movements as they walk on a treadmill. When the patient takes over more and more of the load from the robot, their character on the screen moves faster. Researchers at the University of Zurich hacked sensors in the robot to record the patient's movements, which serves as biofeedback for how the game works. "We replaced the game controller with a robot" [4] (Fig. 20.7).

"The goal is simple: to walk an astronaut around a planet back to his rocket, along the way freeing it 'from evil little things'" [4]. By having the patient focus on performing actions in the virtual world, their attention is focused on that task rather than on the difficultly of walking. This deflection of attention is more fun and has children actually looking forward to rehabilitation treatment.

Game Mechanic
Discovery: Players explore the world of Gabarello as they walk further in their treatment and jump on to different objects in the game.

Future Directions

In much the same way that simulation games offer opportunities to train clinicians, Gabarello points toward opportunities to use gaming to help people develop, or re-develop, physical skills and capabilities, while taking their minds off of some of the more strenuous work of rehabilitation. Over time, these opportunities will expand to include not only recovering mobility, but also in a variety of injury recovery settings where gaming has the potential to break some of the monotony of the work of rehabilitation.

Re-Mission: Games Become Central to Pediatric Care

Radiation treatment for cancer is an extremely uncomfortable and challenging process, especially for young children and adolescents with cancer. To help children learn about cancer and reframe the treatments, Hope Labs created Re-Mission. Re-Mission is a video game where the players take control of Roxxi, a nanobot injected into the human body to fight different types of cancers and infections. The player must monitor the patient health and report any symptoms back to the in-game doctor. Through playing the levels in the game, children learn about the variety of treatments, how they function, and the importance of being consistent with treatment adherence [5] (Fig. 20.8).

In 2008, Hopelabs conducted an unprecedented randomized trial and proved that by playing Re-Mission, patients demonstrated improved treatment adherence, increased self-efficacy and cancer-related knowledge. Among 200 participants who were prescribed oral antibiotics, MEMS-cap monitoring indicated a 16 % increase in adherence for intervention group [6]. Not only did these randomized trials reveal increased knowledge, but higher levels of chemotherapy were measured in the blood—suggesting that the game had both physiological as well as psychological benefits.

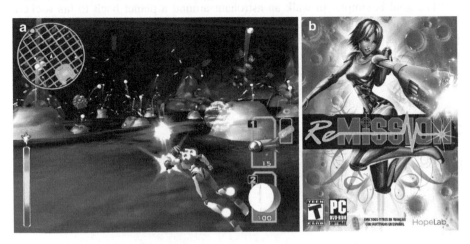

Fig. 20.8 (**a**) Cancer patients travel through pathways in the body to destroy cancer cells, battle infections, and manage side effects of treatment. (**b**) Children gain awareness about cancer by playing the video game

> **Game Mechanic**
> Quests: The character is given specific objectives that are threaded into the narrative of the game.

Future Directions

It's common for parents to complain about the amount of time children devote to video games, but Re-Mission points toward a new model for gaming: one where games, developed thoughtfully and strategically, become an increasingly important tool to encourage young people to engage with their health. Re-Mission is a particularly strong example of the potential for games in pediatric care. Not only does it highlight the potential for games to be used as an educational tool to help children understand a variety of health conditions, but it also highlights opportunities to use games in tandem with other clinical interventions in order to enhance therapeutic effectiveness.

BrainGamers: Gaming Gets Optimized for Mental Fitness

Children with Fetal Alcohol Spectrum Disorder (FASD) are born with damage to certain parts of their brain. As a result, these individuals may have problems with memory, maintaining focus, and behavioral and learning deficiencies. Researchers at NeuroDevNet, in Canada, are exploring a remarkable gaming solution to explore training FASD children to take control of their brain activity levels.

Instead of designing a custom medical treatment game, NeuroDevNet has leveraged existing popular games and added a layer in front of the game. This takes advantage of the extensive development efforts of the game companies, so children play the games they'll be good at. In the study, players wear a headset that monitors brain activity while they are playing the video game. If the player gets too excited, anxious, or unfocused, visual elements like spiders, blurring, or distortion are introduced on a layer in front of the game they are playing (Fig. 20.9). By learning to calm or focus their brain activity, players can make the visual obstructions go away. To the players, the visual obstruction represents just another obstacle in the game to overcome in the course of gameplay, but in reality, they are also training themselves and learning how to consciously control their brain activity.

This research is based on the principle of neuroplasticity, the ability for the brain to change structurally and functionally through training and experience. Over time, the hope is that these children will learn to stay calm and focused in real-life situations that would otherwise present too much stress. This is example of stealth health. The players are directed to focus on one objective, while their actions increase their skills or health at the same time.

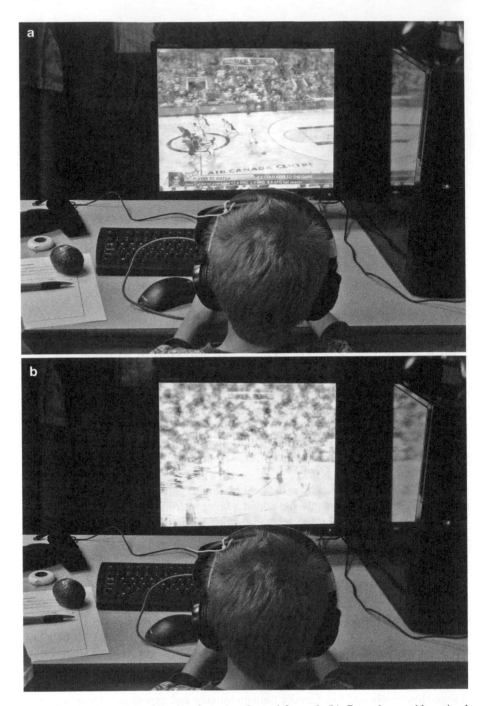

Fig. 20.9 (**a**) Gameplay while the player is calm and focused. (**b**) Gameplay – with a visual obstructions – when the player is too excited, anxious, or unfocused

Game Mechanic
Loss Aversion: The player is incentivized to keep their mind in a state of calm and focus so they don't lose visibility of the screen.

Future Directions

Concepts like BrainGamers point toward a wider variety of initiatives aimed at using game mechanics to enhance mental health and acuity. Known popularly as brain fitness, these sorts of digital based initiatives have a wide variety of potential applications ranging from seniors to educational settings to the workplace. For physicians, these kinds of brain fitness games could be useful in treating conditions ranging from addiction to helping elderly patients ward off some of the cognitive decline of aging.

Dr. Hero®: Simulation Games Hone Practitioner Skills.

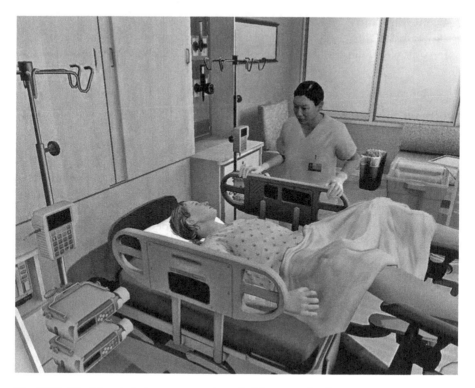

Fig. 20.10 Physicians train in game scenarios to build up procedural memory

Doctors have a wealth of information about procedures, and constantly refresh themselves so that they perform the correct techniques in the appropriate situations. They have a variety of ways to keep up their skills, some easier than others.

Sonia SooHoo, a Kaiser Permanente obstetrician, developed this video game in collaboration with Kaiser Permanente's Innovation Fund for Technology/Innovation & Advanced Technology Group. The video game simulates an obstetrical hemorrhage and takes the physician through the sequence of procedures, based on the protocols established by the California Maternal Quality Care Collaborative.

The player is a labor delivery team member and is presented with multiple medical scenarios. They have access to a care team of nurses and anesthesiologists and a range of techniques and medications at their disposal. By making correct decisions and taking correct actions, they earn points—and the patient survives.

The game is both fun and competitive, and physicians get a chance to practice their response to obstetrical emergencies with the intensity of teenagers playing a video game like Guitar Hero®. Through this intense practice, the skills and decisions become part of "muscle memory" so that in a real emergency situation, the correct procedures and techniques are second nature.

Game Mechanic
Progression: The health of the patient and success of the treatment is granularly displayed through the process of completing smaller specific tasks.

Future Directions

Already, flight simulation technologies are in widespread use in the airline industry as a means to keep pilot skills sharp—and these kinds of simulations have the potential to enhance training initiatives for new as well as veteran practitioners. Over the next decade, as more clinical tools—such as medical imaging technologies—get refined, these sorts of simulations have the potential to not only provide training on generic cases, but could also provide tools for clinical teams to simulate novel or unusually difficult surgeries. These sorts of simulations will not only provide a useful tool for individual doctors, but will provide opportunities for colleagues to train together to refine collaborative approaches to handling emergencies.

Breakthroughs to Cures: Gaming Becomes a Tool for Creative Engagement and Brainstorming

Developed as a collaborative partnership between Institute for the Future, the Robert Wood Johnson Foundation, and the Myelin Repair Foundation, Breakthroughs to Cures was a two-day global initiative aimed at using a massive multiplayer online game to brainstorm new approaches to drug research and development that engaged contributors on five continents.

Based on the concept of using provocative storytelling as a means to get people to rethink their assumptions, the game placed players in an urgent scenario where a deadly disease threatened the lives of tens of millions of people. The game asked participants, in the face of this daunting challenge, to consider how they would reimagine research and innovation processes to ward off the disease. Participants connected virtually during two predetermined 24 hour periods, and over the course of these 2 days, discussed in brief contributions of 140 words or less strategies – and built on each other's ideas at a centralized website that included specific prompts aimed at fostering discussion (Fig. 20.11).

Designed as an open, collaborative environment where models for innovation in medical research can be freely explored—by both experts and non-experts alike—the goal of the game was to generate outlier ideas and strategies that could lead to more effective and efficient strategies for improving medical research models. By connecting hundreds of experts virtually, game participants collectively generated a wide variety of key insights and strategies for accelerating drug development.

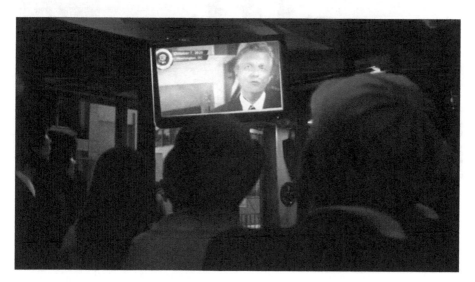

Fig. 20.11   Using a provocative video scenario about an emerging health pandemic, Breakthroughs to Cures engaged hundreds of participants in a virtual game environment to have a global conversation about new approaches to innovating medical research and development

Game Mechanic
Community Collaboration: The entire community of players is rallied to work together to build on each other's ideas towards a shared challenge.

Future Directions

Games like Breakthroughs to Cures highlight an emerging use of crowdsourcing: To tap into the collective, creative conscious to spur collaboration and new ideas. These kinds of crowd sourced initiatives have potential applications as public engagements to spur conversations not just about innovation, but also to gain insight into different meanings of health in different settings. Similarly, hospitals and health systems can explore crowd sourced gaming as a means to quickly and effectively tap into the collective knowledge of their internal teams to drive long-range initiatives.

FoldIt: Gaming Becomes a Platform for Distributed Problem Solving

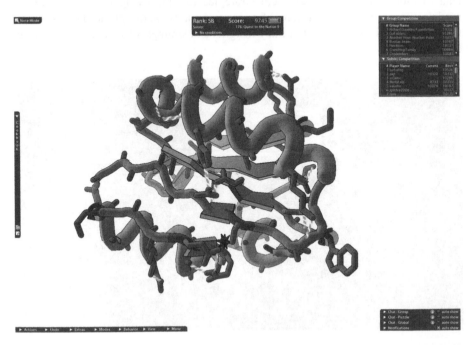

Fig. 20.12 Players work in teams to manipulate protein models to find optimal combinations and achieve higher scores

Protein research is invaluable in identifying molecular targets and structures that can lead to the development of drug treatments. Since proteins are part of so many diseases, they can also be part of the cure. Researchers at the University of Washington have marshaled the efforts of teams of gamers by creating a platform to allow gamers to solve protein-folding puzzles that supercomputers have difficulty solving.

Supercomputers have made great advances, but humans are still better at solving complex problems that require puzzle-solving leaps of insight and 3-D spatial pattern abilities. FoldIt allows players to start off by solving simpler problems, and as they level up, they are introduced to harder and harder problems. As they progress in level, players share strategies with other players to collaboratively solve even more complex problems. This social collaboration of concerted gaming efforts and team competition has had dramatic results, answering some significant questions in scientific research (Fig. 20.12).

For example: on September 18th 2011, gamers and researchers worked together to provide insights about the structure of a protein-sniping enzyme critical for the reproduction of the HIV virus. This decade-old problem was solved in a matter of weeks by teams of gamers, and the discovery will lead to the development of drugs to neutralize this enzyme.

Game Mechanic
Collaborative Competition: Gamers manipulate molecular structures and are scored on various aspects of their solution. When a player achieves a more efficient solution they achieve a higher score. This strategy is then shared with other players so that they can build on the efforts of others.

Future Directions

Projects like FoldIt point toward a future where research and development—even in technical life sciences—emerge not from a single laboratory, but from the distributed work of gamers in a variety of locations. Over the next decade, developing tools and platforms for distributing research and collaboration to nontechnical experts will become a critical tool for enlisting the work of everyday people into critical problem-solving initiatives.

Conclusion

The healthcare system is buckling under numerous strains and costs are continuing to escalate. Meeting these challenges will require creative responses from a variety of stakeholders in health care—including, and perhaps most importantly, patients themselves. Game elements, successfully applied, hold the promise of motivating people to engage more with their health. By adding these elements to desired tasks and behaviors, healthcare practitioners can extend their effectiveness and empower people to stay true to treatment plans and preventative activities.

The application of games in the healthcare space promises to enhance a variety of health interventions, particularly long-term interventions that require patients to play an ongoing role in staying motivated and be capable of making healthy choices. Games shift our mentality when taking part in difficult, undesirable, sometimes even frustrating tasks—transforming them into experiences that we can look forward to and enjoy. At the end of the day, games do something novel: they make health fun. As demands on patients to engage with health continue to escalate, games will provide one of the lowest-cost, yet most effective tools for helping people overcome health challenges and stick with long-term health and wellness goals.

References

1. Bravata DM, Smith-Spangler C, Sundaram V, Gienger AL, Lin N, Lewis R, Stave CD, Olkin I, Sirard JR. Using pedometers to increase physical activity and improve health: a systematic review. JAMA. 2007;298(19):2296–304. doi:10.1001/jama.298.19.2296.
2. http://www.ajpmonline.org/article/S0749-3797(11)00862-2/abstract.
3. Easing pain for burns victims using virtual reality. January 31, 2011. http://www.bbc.co.uk/news/mobile/health-12297569.
4. Wired Magazine October 2010: One small step: Walking with the wearable robot. http://www.wired.co.uk/magazine/archive/2010/10/start/one-small-step.
5. http://en.wikipedia.org/wiki/Re-Mission.
6. http://pediatrics.aappublications.org/content/122/2/e305.full.

Appendices

Appendix A: Meet the Martinez Family

The Martinez family starts with a core of four: Barbara the mom, Ray the dad, Cindy the eldest daughter, and Mike the youngest son. They also have some extended family that you also get a chance to meet. They live in Anywhere, America. They are part Caucasian and part Latino. They are middle-class. They work hard, play as much as they can, but need to be careful with finances as most middle-class families do. They own two cars: a newish SUV and a beat up pickup truck. They live in a three bedroom, two-story home, and owe about $110,000 on their mortgage. Some of their personas are further described in the following paragraphs, and all are detailed in Table A.1.

Barbara Martinez is a second grade teacher, and loves teaching. It's her passion, almost equal to the passion of her family life. She is a supportive wife helping her husband, Ray, stay on top of his plumbing business and diabetes, an energized mother trekking her teenage daughter, Cindy, and her son, Mike, to the myriad of school and after-school activities, and she is also a doting daughter caring for her elderly mother. She is 46 and feels at least that old, but would like to feel 30 again! She has struggled with her weight for a decade, and for the past few years high blood pressure and anxiety have become problems. "I have more lesson planning to do in the evening, but only after fixing dinner for the family in multiple shifts, helping Cindy and Mike with their homework, trying to stay on top of the bills, and hoping to get a minute alone with my husband every few days. I know I should get better exercise, and I wish I could prepare healthier meals for my family, but where's the time for any of that?"

Ray Martinez is a quiet, thoughtful guy. He owns his own plumbing business. For as long as he could remember he wanted to work with his hands, however with his kids needing help with homework he has been exercising his mind more than he cares to. Exercise. He hates that word. It is filled with guilt and failure for him. After helping with homework he loves nothing better than plopping down in front of the

L. Berkowitz, C. McCarthy (eds.),
Innovation with Information Technologies in Healthcare, Health Informatics,
DOI 10.1007/978-1-4471-4327-7, © Springer-Verlag London 2013

Table A.1 Further details for the Martinez family

Name	Family role	Personality	Age	Occupation	Health	Values	Pain points
Barbara	Mom	Frazzled Hard worker Likes to be thorough Uses PC in classroom and for shopping Texts with her daughter and husband	46	Second Grade teacher	40 pounds overweight Stressed Hypertensive	Family Children Proactive about health	Too many things to keep track of
Ray	Dad	No nonsense Kind Loves football and hockey Texts Uses PC for entertainment	47	Plumber	25 pounds overweight Early signs of diabetes	Hard work	Ignores his own health
Juanita	Grandmother (Ray's mother)	Frail Worries Watches a lot of Spanish daytime TV Technology-averse	76	Retired seamstress	Still living independently, but not for much longer	Independence Her grandchildren	Low English proficiency
Cindy	Daughter	Very social Competitive Laptop for school iPhone and mega-texter	14	Ninth Grade student	Lots of activity— Into sports Eats too much junk food	Friends	Wants to be both an adult and a child
Mike	Son	Shy xbox & PC gaming Wants an iPhone but parents won't let him yet	8	Fourth Grade student	Asthma Way too sedentary	Cool new technology	"Everybody's always hassling me to do something"

Name	Relationship	Description	Age	Occupation	Status		Notes
Isabelle	Rays' sister	Single mom, Friendly, Disorganized, Crazy without her iPhone	27	Administrative assistant	Pregnant	Friends, Rest	She's having trouble keeping up with everything now that she's pregnant and a single mom
Stephan	Isabelle's son	Energetic, Zero patience, Plays a few games on his mom's iPhone	3	Getting into trouble	Healthy	Chaos	Time with his mom

television and zoning out. "My doctor tells me I should lose some weight especially since I have diabetes, but what does he know about it—I think my doc could lose some weight himself! And anyway, I feel fine, and my own father lived to the ripe old age of 92, so I figure I'm good for at least another 40 years before my own plumbing gives out."

Cindy Martinez is 14 years old and a star on the Junior Varsity lacrosse team. She is living life loud. She is in the glee and drama clubs. And she loves ninth grade. Mostly because there are so many other kids compared to her middle school. Her iPhone is constantly buzzing and clicking to the point that her dad thought it was broken. She is a mega-texter and doesn't even bother with the PC sitting in her house. Everything she needs is in the palm of her hand.

Mike Martinez is the baby of the family. He is 8 and gets away with everything because he is so darn funny. He idolizes his dad and loves to plop down with him and bait him into a game of Grand Theft Auto. But that is about to change, because his mom bought him the Kinect for his Xbox. "I just got two new games for my Kinect. My mom says Kinect is good because I have to get my butt off the couch to play it. Maybe I can get my dad off the couch too!"

Appendix B: Innovation Glossary

There are hundreds of techniques and methods that can be used to crack the nut of a hard problem, to enhance creativity, and to speed up prototyping. They are as exhaustive as the phone book, however, listed below are some of the ones that our book's authors used to get their ideas moving.

Definitions below are drawn from Wikipedia, KP's Innovation Consultancy, IDEO and the Institute for Healthcare Improvement.

Analogous Observation A research technique used to expand the variety of user inputs into brainstorming thinking. Researchers visit industries that are different from the ones in which their design challenges resides. For example, when working on a healthcare challenge involving high-risk interruptions in the hospital, a team of researchers might visit a flight school to learn from pilots.

Brainstorming A group creativity technique by which a group tries to find a solution for a specific problem by gathering a list of ideas spontaneously contributed by its members. See Business Week Brainstorming for Better Business for an expanded discussion of this technique.[1]

Business Process Redesign The analysis and new design of workflows and processes within an organization.

Cultural Probes Kits A technique whereby a researcher prepares a set of activities for the end-user to complete at home. Examples of activities include collaging, journaling, and photo essays.

Decision Accelerator A method which engages teams, groups and key stakeholders in highly experiential, collaborative processes which accelerate

---

[1]http://www.businessweek.com/innovate/content/jun2009/id2009064_920852.htm

decision-making and alignment around critical issues and opportunities. More details at the Innovation Point website.[2]

Discernment Process An activity of determining the value and quality of a certain subject or event. Typically, it is used to describe the activity of going past the mere perception of something, to making detailed judgments about that thing. As a virtue, a discerning individual is considered to possess wisdom, and be of good judgment; especially so with regard to subject matter often overlooked by others. (Definition from Via Christi Health, Inc.)

Draw Your Experience A technique that asks the end user to draw what comes to mind when thinking about a particular topic, as opposed to talking about the topic. The researcher then interviews the end-user by using the drawing as a vehicle for exploration.

Ethnography A holistic approach that is founded on the idea that humans are best understood in the fullest possible context. It often involves home or work-based interviews and observations.

Expert Cluttering A technique whereby disparate data points are brought together into like-clusters to identify larger themes and root causes in the research. This is usually done with groups to ensure various viewpoints are represented.

Evidence Based Design A field of study that emphasizes the importance of using credible data in order to influence the design process.

Fly-On-The-Wall A technique whereby the research observes an end-user in context (at home, at work, in the car) with minimal interruption.

Handmade Construction A technique whereby ideas are rapidly built out of basic arts and crafts materials.

Human-Centered Design A design philosophy and a process in which the needs, wants, and limitations of end users of a product or service are given extensive attention at each stage of the design process.

Improvisation A technique sometimes called "bodystorming" in which project participants act out new workflows and experiences. This often will help the team work out kinks in a workflow, and help others better understand their overall vision for the ideas.

Iteration The act of repeating and improving an idea, usually with the aim of approaching a desired goal or target or result. Each repetition is called an iteration, and the results of one iteration are used as the starting point for the next.

Lean The removal of "wastages". In simple terms, "wastages" can be explained as the expenditure of resources on other than the end customer product value.

Participatory Design (sometimes called Co-Design) An approach to design attempting to actively involve all stakeholders (e.g. employees, partners, customers, citizens, end users) in the design process in order to help ensure the product designed meets their needs and is usable.

Plan Do Study Act (PDSA) This approach allows for innovators to take prototypes into a live environment for refinement and then piloting. See Institute for HealthCare Improvement's How to Test[3] for more details.

---

[2]http://www.innovation-point.com/lab.htm

[3]http://www.ihi.org/knowledge/Pages/HowtoImprove/ScienceofImprovementTestingChanges.aspx

Pilot A small-scale preliminary study conducted in order to evaluate feasibility, time, cost, adverse events, and/or understand the appropriate size required for a research study.

Positive Deviance An approach to behavioral and social change based on the observation that in any community, there are people whose uncommon but success-ful behaviors or strategies enable them to find better solutions to a problem than their peers, despite facing similar challenges and having no extra resources or knowledge than their peers.

Prototype An early sample or model built to test a concept or process.

Provocation A brainstorming technique whereby the participants are asked to consider outrageous, impossible and sometime nonsensical challenges. For example "Hospital and clinics are outlawed. How will be care be delivered to the community?"

Six Sigma A process improvement methodology that seeks to improve the qual-ity of process outputs by identifying and removing the causes of defects (errors) while minimizing variability in manufacturing and business processes.

Storyboarding A technique by which ideas or a combination of ideas are sketched out comic book style. This is an excellent way to show the ideas overlaid across a visual timeline of experiences.

Storytelling A technique whereby the researcher or others retells key moments and signature events. Storytelling helps to internalize data, build conviction, and surface important connections.

Systems Thinking The process of understanding how things influence one another within a whole. In organizations, systems consist of people, structures, and processes that work together to make an organization healthy or unhealthy.

Voice of the Customer A term used in business and information technology to describe the in-depth process of capturing a customer's expectations, preferences and aversions.

Appendix C: Reading for Inspiration

The following are where the many authors of this book turn to for HIT and innova-tion knowledge and inspiration.

Books

Analytics at Work (Thomas H. Davenport, Jeanne G. Harris and Robert Morison)
   The Art of Game Design (Jesse Schell)
   Art of Innovation (Tom Kelley)
   The Best Practice (Charles Kenney)
   Better (Atul Gawande)

Change by Design (Tim Brown)
The Checklist Manifesto (Atul Gawande)
Competing on Analytics (Thomas H. Davenport and Jeanne G. Harris)
Connected for Health (Louise L. Liang)
The Design of Everyday Things (Donald A. Norman)
Designing Care (Richard M. J. Bohmer)
Gamification by Design (Gabe Zichermann)
Good to Great (Jim Collins)
The Heart of Change (John P. Kotter)
Innovation Driven Health Care (Richard L. Reece)
Innovation in Action: A Practical Guide for Healthcare Teams (D. Scott Endsley)
Innovation Leadership: Creating the Landscape of Healthcare (Tim Porter-O'Grady and Kathy Malloch)
The Innovator's Dilemma (Clayton M. Christensen)
The Innovator's Prescription (Clayton M. Christensen)
IT Governance (Peter Weill and Jeanne Ross)
Made to Stick (Chip Heath and Dan Heath)
Making the Invisible Visible (Donald A. Marchand)
Managing Transitions (William Bridges)
The Myths of Innovation (Scott Berkun)
Practicing Excellence (Stephen C. Beeson)
The Physician-Computer Conundrum (Bria and Rydell)
Redefining HealthCare (Michael E. Porter)
Rules of Play (Katie Salen and Eric Zimmerman)
A Sense of Urgency (John P. Kotter)
Simplicity Shift (Scott Jenson)
Sketching User Experiences (Bill Buxton)
Squirrel Inc (Stephen Denning)
Universal Principles of Design (William Lidwell)

Magazines
Dwell
FastCompany
Good
Harvard Business Review
Health Affairs
Health Informatics
Health Data Management
Journal of the American Medical Informatics Association (JAMIA) Monocle
Presentations Magazine
Survey Magazine
WIRED

Appendix D: Meet the Authors and Their Organizations

Chapter 1

Lyle Berkowitz, M.D., FACP, FHIMSS, is a practicing primary care physician, Founder and Director of the Szollosi Healthcare Innovation Program, Medical Director of IT and Innovation for Northwestern Memorial Physicians Group, and the Associate Chief Medical Officer of Innovation for Northwestern Memorial Hospital in Chicago, IL. He is also a serial HIT entrepreneur and consultant, working with a variety of startups and publicly traded healthcare IT vendors, as well as numerous hospitals, medical groups, pharmaceutical companies and governmental agencies over the past two decades. He serves on the Governance Board of the Innovation Learning Network (ILN), the Advisory Board of the Association of Medical Directors of Information Systems (AMDIS), the Editorial Board of Healthcare Informatics and Clinical Innovation + Technology, and was a member of the Board of Directors for the American Health Information Management Association (AHIMA) Foundation. He wrote the chapter on "Physician Adoption Strategies" for the American College of Physicians' book Electronic Medical Records, and clearly forgot how much work this book writing thing takes! He has been listed as one of HealthLeader's "Twenty People Who Make Healthcare Better"; Healthspottr's "Future Health Top 100", and Modern Healthcare's "Top 25 Clinical Informaticists". Dr. Berkowitz graduated with a Biomedical Engineering degree from the University of Pennsylvania and is an Associate Professor of Clinical Medicine at the Feinberg School of Medicine at Northwestern University. You can find him at www.DrLyle.com.

Chris McCarthy is the Director of the Innovation Learning Network and an Innovation Specialist with Kaiser Permanente's Innovation Consultancy. In this dual role, he innovates at the frontlines of healthcare and he connects innovators across the world to accelerate the spread of design thinking and great ideas; this dual work was featured in the Harvard Business Review (Sept 2010) and in "Pursuing the Triple Aim: Seven Innovators Show the Way to Better Care, Better Health, and Lower Costs" (2012) as well as FastCompany, the New York Times and many more. Some of his innovations include better tools for new moms, safer medication administration for patients, and more robust shift changes for nurses.

Chris was named the 2011 Ellerbe Beckett Lecturer at the University of Minnesota, and is an international speaker on innovation and design. The United Kingdom's National Health Service, the Danish Healthcare System and the Canadian Health System have asked for his insight on innovation and healthcare.

Chris has a master's in business administration from Rensselaer Polytechnic Institute/Copenhagen Business School, and a master's in public health in Health Policy from the University of Massachusetts at Amherst. In his spare time, he obsesses about fitness, movies and home remodels.

You can find him on Twitter: @mccarthychris and his Blog: mccarthychris.com

Chapter 2

Chris McCarthy is the Director of the Innovation Learning Network and an Innovation Specialist with Kaiser Permanente's Innovation Consultancy. In this dual role, he innovates at the frontlines of healthcare and he connects innovators across the world to accelerate the spread of design thinking and great ideas; this dual work was featured in the Harvard Business Review (Sept 2010) and in "Pursuing the Triple Aim: Seven Innovators Show the Way to Better Care, Better Health, and Lower Costs" (2012) as well as FastCompany, the New York Times and many more. Some of his innovations include better tools for new moms, safer medication administration for patients, and more robust shift changes for nurses.

Chris was named the 2011 Ellerbe Beckett Lecturer at the University of Minnesota, and is an international speaker on innovation and design. The United Kingdom's National Health Service, the Danish Healthcare System and the Canadian Health System have asked for his insight on innovation and healthcare.

Chris has a master's in business administration from Rensselaer Polytechnic Institute/Copenhagen Business School, and a master's in public health in Health Policy from the University of Massachusetts at Amherst. In his spare time, he obsesses about fitness, movies and home remodels.

You can find him on Twitter: @mccarthychris and his Blog: mccarthychris.com

Christi Dining Zuber, RN, BSN, M.H.A. Director, Innovation Consultancy, Kaiser Permanente Christi Zuber is a nurse with a passion for design. Zuber has been with Kaiser Permanente since 2001, in roles that have encompassed finance, strategy, facilities design, and her current position, director of Innovation Consultancy which she began to build in 2003. In her innovation and design work, Zuber has partnered with IDEO to learn and internalize a human centered design methodology into Kaiser Permanente. Zuber and her team have spent thousands of hours of time shadowing, conducting ethnographic observations in clinics, hospitals and patient's homes, and field-testing ideas in the front lines of healthcare. Her nursing roots are in home health care. Zuber has a master's degree in Health Administration and a Bachelor of Science in Nursing from the University of Oklahoma.

Chapter 3

Lyle Berkowitz, MD, FACP, FHIMSS, is a practicing primary care physician, Founder and Director of the Szollosi Healthcare Innovation Program, Medical Director of IT and Innovation for Northwestern Memorial Physicians Group, and the Associate Chief Medical Officer of Innovation for Northwestern Memorial Hospital in Chicago, IL. He is also a serial HIT entrepreneur and consultant, working with a variety of startups and publicly traded healthcare IT vendors, as well as numerous hospitals, medical groups, pharmaceutical companies and governmental agencies over the past two decades. He serves on the Governance Board of the Innovation Learning Network (ILN), the Advisory Board of the Association of

Medical Directors of Information Systems (AMDIS), the Editorial Board of Healthcare Informatics and Clinical Innovation + Technology, and was a member of the Board of Directors for the American Health Information Management Association (AHIMA) Foundation. He wrote the chapter on "Physician Adoption Strategies" for the American College of Physicians' book Electronic Medical Records, and clearly forgot how much work this book writing thing takes! He has been listed as one of HealthLeader's "Twenty People Who Make Healthcare Better"; Healthspottr's "Future Health Top 100", and Modern Healthcare's "Top 25 Clinical Informaticists". Dr. Berkowitz graduated with a Biomedical Engineering degree from the University of Pennsylvania and is an Associate Professor of Clinical Medicine at the Feinberg School of Medicine at Northwestern University. You can find him at www.DrLyle.com.

Chapter 4

Peter Basch, M.D., FACP is a general internist practicing in Washington, D.C. and the Medical Director for the Ambulatory EHR eHealth and Health IT Policy for MedStar Health helping to oversee their outpatient EHR, ePrescribing, and Patient Portal systems. He has served as a frequent expert panelist and speaker on issues of EHR adoption and optimization and has been active over the past decade in health IT policy with several organizations, including the American College of Physicians, the Physicians' EHR Coalition, the eHealth Initiative, the Association of Medical Directors of Information Systems, the Center for American Progress, the Brookings Institution, and the Bipartisan Policy Center.

Chapter 5

As a founder of SETMA, James L. Holly, M.D. envisioned a future of health care which would be driven by the power of electronic analysis and documentation. He has been called a visionary for his relentless pursuit of transformation in healthcare and of excellence in healthcare outcomes. Dr. Holly regularly addresses national groups on "electronic patient management" and the "SETMA Model of Care," including the staff of the Office of National Coordinator of HIT, Society for Academic CME, Scottsdale Institute, Updates in Diabetes Care (Joslin Diabetes Center and Harvard Medical School), and many others.

Chapter 6

John W. Trudel, M.D. is a family physician who has been in practice at the Fallon Clinic for 17 years. He is now the chief of a large family practice and internal medicine site. He has always had an interest in computers; with the exception of two entry-level computer programming courses years ago, he has received no formal training other than the Epic Certification Course. He gained his first exposure to an EHR while a resident at the Charleston Naval Hospital in 1991. He found that a difficult and frustrating experience. Dr. Trudel became interested in preventing similar problems and in ensuring that he and his colleagues had procedures in place optimizing efficient, high quality care rather than inhibiting it. He began working with the Fallon Clinic IT department initially as part of the EHR vendor selection committee. During the "pre-go live" period he participated in the "design, build, and validate" sessions, then wrote the adult medicine order sets. Over the past 4 years he has adopted a larger and larger role within the IT department. Currently, as one of two Assistant Medical Directors for Informatics, Dr. Trudel spends his time working on content development, provider support, education, meaningful use, and decision support.

Lloyd D. Fisher, M.D. is a general pediatrician and site chief of one of Fallon Clinic's pediatric practices. While never receiving any formal computer science or informatics training, he has had an interest in information technology (IT) since an early age, teaching himself rudimentary programming languages while still in grade school. During his college years he became one of the web designers for multiple departments at the University of Vermont. Upon entering medical school, Dr. Fisher quickly realized the benefit IT could provide to healthcare and became involved in health IT through the state medical society and a state-wide pilot project to rollout EHRs to small practices. He finished his medical training and joined the Fallon Clinic during the pre "go-live" phase of the Epic EHR. His IT skills were identified and he was charged with developing the documentation templates and order sets for pediatrics. Since then his role has continued to grow as part of the Epic optimization team. In 2009 he became one of the two Assistant Medical Directors for Informatics where he continues to improve efficiency through innovative uses of the EHR. Dr. Fisher is a member of a physician advisory committee to the Massachusetts Regional Extension Center.

Both Drs. Fisher and Trudel maintain a busy and active clinical practice, critical in helping them bridge the gaps and act as translators between the disparate worlds of the provider, the IT analyst, the programmer, and the coding/billing department. Their interests lie in improving the day to day environment of a busy practice, seeing what the real world problems are and finding innovative, sophisticated, yet practical and transparent IT solutions.

Chapter 7

Thomas R. Graf, M.D., is Associate Chief Medical Officer for Population Health and Chairman of the Community Practice Service line for Geisinger Health System. Dr. Graf is responsible for the Value Re-Engineeering of the Care Continuum and other Population health initiatives for Geisinger including the ACO portfolio and Physician Group Practice Transitions Demonstration with CMS. In addition to direct leadership and management of the Community Practice network, he has implemented nearly 40 NCQA Level III accreditation Medical Home sites in the Geisinger ProvenHealth Navigator model. He has extended this to include comprehensive nursing home care with dedicated providers tied to ProvenHealth Navigator clinics. Dr Graf has established innovative care models for optimizing chronic disease with established systems of care enhanced by MyCare modules of care for individual disease parameters lead by mid-levels through the use of the Delta Innovation Incubator program he established. Dr Graf serves as a content expert for the AHRQ's Patient Centered Medical Homes Project, AHRQ's I LIVEPC, international primary care improvement project, AHRQ's Innovation Spread project, and AMGA's Caring for Patients with Multiple Chronic Diseases Collaborative. The Value Re-engineering efforts of Geisinger was recently recognized as the AMGA 2011 Acclaim award winner.

After graduating from University of Michigan Medical School and completing Family Medicine residency training at Henry Ford Health System in Detroit, he served on the faculty of the Henry Ford Family Practice Residency and was Director of the Southwest Georgia Family Practice Residency prior to joining Geisinger.

Chapter 8

David C. Stockwell, M.D., M.B.A. is the Executive Director of Improvement Science as well as the Medical Director of Patient Safety and the Pediatric Intensive Care Unit at Children's National in Washington, D.C.. Dr. Stockwell's research efforts focus on the physician as a leader and manager of the clinical team as well as investigating strategies towards improving patient safety. He is the leader in a multi-hospital collaborative of children's hospitals across the United States investigating automated adverse event detection, identifying novel ways of identifying adverse events via the use of the Electronic Medical Record. Building on an administrative background and interest in quality of care, he has written several peer reviewed articles and textbook chapters on patient safety. He was educated in medicine at the University Of Oklahoma College Of Medicine and trained in pediatrics and critical care at Children's National Medical Center since graduating medical school. He has an M.B.A. from George Washington University.

Brian R. Jacobs, M.D. is Vice President and Chief Medical Information Officer and Executive Director of the Center for Pediatric Informatics at Children's National

Medical Center in Washington, D.C.. In this capacity, he directs the Children's IQ Network® a pediatric health information exchange in the DC metropolitan region. Dr. Jacobs is a Professor of Pediatrics at George Washington University. Prior to joining Children's National Medical Center, Dr. Jacobs was a Professor of Pediatrics at the University of Cincinnati, as well as the Director of Technology and Patient Safety at Cincinnati Children's Hospital Medical Center. While at Cincinnati Children's, he was the principal author of the Healthcare Information and Management Systems (HIMSS) Davies Award. Dr. Jacobs specializes in pediatric critical care medicine and has authored numerous journal articles, book chapters, abstracts, and scientific presentations. He frequently shares his knowledge in the pediatric space as a guest lecturer at conferences, leadership forums, and hospitals. He is a fellow of the American Academy of Pediatrics, HIMSS and the American College of Critical Care Medicine. He also is a member of the Society for Pediatric Research, the Association of Medical Directors of Information Services (AMDIS) and serves on the HIMSS Board of Directors.

Chapter 9

Jonathan S. Wald, M.D., MPH, FACMI, is the Director of Patient-Centered Technologies for an independent non-profit research firm, RTI (Research Triangle Institute), in their Center for the Advancement of Health IT. He spent 10 years (2000–2010) as Associate Director of Clinical Informatics Research and Development at Partners HealthCare, leading the vision and strategy for the enterprise patient portal, Patient Gateway. His experience with physician- and patient-focused clinical systems includes clinical informatics fellowship training at Boston's Beth Israel Hospital (1992–1994), working for a large EHR vendor, Cerner Corporation (1996–2000), serving on national advisory committees for eHealth initiatives with the Markle Foundation and Robert Wood Johnson Foundation, and research at Harvard Medical School. Dr. Wald is a local and national speaker on patient-centered health IT with passion for developing and evaluating innovative health IT applications that enable patients to engage actively in their care.

Chapter 10

Gwendolyn B. O'Keefe, M.D. is the Chief Medical Information Officer and a practicing Internist, and oversees the IT and Informatics teams for the Group Health Delivery System.

Marc Mora, M.D. is a practicing internist and the Medical Director of Consultative Specialties which encompasses all medical and surgical specialty groups in the Delivery System at Group Health.

Tim Scearce, M.D. is Service Line Chief for Neurology as well as Medical Director for Informatics at Group Health Physicians.

Erin DeMarce Leff, M.B.A. is the Vice President of Consultative Specialties.

James Hereford (previously Executive Vice President of the Group Practice Division) is now Chief Operating Officer at Palo Alto Medical Foundation.

Chapter 11

David Aron is a health services researcher and endocrinologist, who along with the help of Renée H. Lawrence and Julie K. Johnson formulated the research project. Katherine S. Thweatt who had managed another IT-related research project joined our group to manage this project. Ajay Sood and Sharon A. Watts are clinicians with major responsibilities in diabetes management. Stacey Hirth is the telemedicine coordinator. They constituted the specialist team (Fig. 11.4). Our perspective is that research must be closely linked to clinical operations. All except Julie K. Johnson are employees of the Veterans Health Administration in the Dept. of Veterans Affairs.

Chapter 12

Steve Huffman currently serves as the Vice President and Chief Information Officer for Memorial Health System located in South Bend, Indiana, a position he has held since 2008. Steve has been in the healthcare technology management field for the last 14 years and currently serves on the Board of Directors for Indiana Healthcare Information Management Systems Society, the Board of Managers for Michiana Health Information Network, the Data Management Council for the Indiana Hospital Association, the Advisory Board for Business Management for Ivy Tech University and is a member of the Advisory Board for Decision Sciences at Indiana University South Bend. Steve completed his undergraduate work at Indiana Wesleyan University with an emphasis in Business Management and completed his MBA at the University of Notre Dame.

April Daugherty has worked in the information technology field for 13 years. The last 7 years she has been serving in the role of a Systems Analyst at Memorial Hospital. April completed her undergraduate work at Bethel College where her concentration was in Business. She completed her graduate education at Purdue University where she obtained a Master's of Science in Technology. April currently works closely with physician practices and their staff to find gaps in what they do that could be complemented by technology. April was on the original Innovation Team that developed the idea to target high-risk obstetrics and pair it with telemedicine in an effort to have an impact on positive outcomes for mother and baby while also furthering the mission of Memorial Hospital. For the work done with this innovative project, the Memorial team was named as a semi-finalist for Healthcare Informatics Magazine's Innovator of the Year award in 2011.

Chapter 13

David D. O'Neill is a senior program officer in the California HealthCare Foundation's Market and Policy Monitor program, which promotes greater transparency and accountability in California's health care system.

Margaret Laws is director of the California Health Care Foundation's Innovations for the Underserved program, which focuses on reducing barriers to efficient, affordable health care for the underserved by encouraging, testing, and promoting lower-cost models of care.

Susan Anthony is an editor in the California HealthCare Foundation's Publishing and Communications Division.

Chapter 14

Mark S. Gagnon, PharmD, received his Doctor of Pharmacy degree and a bachelor's degree in pharmacy from the University of Kansas. Dr. Gagnon is the director of ePharmacy for Via Christi.

Janell Moerer is Vice President of Business Development and Innovation at Via Christi Health. In her role, Janell assesses and develops ongoing growth strategies and opportunities in innovation and care delivery transformation across the health system.

Chapter 15

Tamra E. Minnier has a deep passion for quality improvement, innovation and patient safety. She serves as the Chief Quality Officer for the UPMC system and before that, served as CNO for the UPMC Shadyside campus. She holds several national leadership and committee appointments and has been very active with the Institute for Healthcare Improvement. Tami is well known within the UPMC system as a go-to leader who cuts quickly to the heart of problems and has the tremendous courage needed to tackle the most challenging problems.

David T. Sharbaugh has spent the last 18 years in the quality improvement and innovation field. He has worked in hospitals and health insurance organizations. He spent 3 years with the Pittsburgh Regional Healthcare Initiative, learning about the Toyota Production System and its application to healthcare operations. He served with UPMC as the Senior Director at the Donald D. Wolff, Jr. Center for Quality, Improvement, and Innovation while building the SmartRoom. David is currently the President of SmartRoom, a new organization supported by both UPMC and IBM that exists to see the SmartRoom application expanded beyond UPMC.

Chapter 16

James W. Noga serves as Vice-President and Chief Information Officer of Partners HealthCare assuming the position on April 1, 2011. Mr. Noga comes to this role with a deep and rich history with Partners. He was recruited by Massachusetts General Hospital as Director of Clinical Applications in 1990 and assumed the role CIO of Massachusetts General Hospital and the Massachusetts General Physicians Organization in 1997. Under Mr. Noga's leadership, the MGH has undergone significant technology advances to support all aspects of clinical care and research.

Steve Flammini is the Chief Technology Officer and Director of Application Development for the IT organization at Partners HealthCare. In this role he reports to the CIO and oversees the development of technology strategy and architecture, and is responsible for enterprise application development, delivery, and integration. Mr. Flammini started with Partners in 1989 in the IS group at Brigham and Women's Hospital. He became the Director of Systems Development at BWH in 1992, and the Director of Application development at PHS in 1995. He has been closely involved with many of PHS' groundbreaking initiaitives in advanced clinical systems since 1989. He is a member of the adjunct faculty in the graduate health informatics programs at both Northeastern University and the University of Alabama, Birmingham.

Chapter 17

Brian D. Patty, M.D.: Dr. Patty is a fellow in the American Board of Emergency Medicine and the American Academy of Emergency Medicine. After 4 years as the medical director for Fairview Clinical Information Services (FCIS) in Burnsville, Minnesota, he came to HealthEast Care System in 2005 as the Chief Medical Informatics Officer (CMIO), responsible for championing clinical applications and the use of technology to serve patients, leading computerized provider order entry (CPOE) and electronic health record (EHR) implementations system wide. His long-standing quest to promote evidence-based medicine led to an AMDIS Award in 2005 for his success in a CPOE implementation at a community hospital and ultimately to his role as the CMIO for HealthEast. In 2011 Dr. Patty received another AMDIS award for his role in the quality improvement efforts at HealthEast as described in this chapter.

Debra J. Hurd, RN, MS, NEA-BC: Ms. Hurd is the Patient Care and Nurse Executive of St. John's Hospital in Maplewood, Minnesota, part of the HealthEast Care System. Hurd has held that post since 2002, having served in several leadership roles at HealthEast. She has an extensive background in operational management, quality improvement and organizational growth. Areas of career focus for Hurd include the development and implementation of long-term strategic plans for clinical services and quality improvement. She is a member of the American Organization of Nurse Executives, the Minnesota Organization of Leaders in Nursing and Sigma Theta Tau, Zeta Chapter.

Chapter 18

George Reynolds, M.D., MMM, FAAP, CPHIMS, is the Vice President, Chief Medical Informatics officer and Chief Information Officer of Children's Hospital and Medical Center. He has served as a co-chair of the CCHIT committee on Advanced Clinical Decision Support and has recently served on the NQF Expert Panel on Health IT Utilization. He is an active member and contributor to AMDIS, CHIME and HIMSS. From 1996 to 2008, he served as the Director of Pediatric Critical Care at Children's Hospital and held the same post at the Nebraska Medical Center from 2005 to 2008. He is an Adjunct Associate Professor of the University of Nebraska and Creighton University Schools of Medicine.

He received the AMDIS Award in Applied Medical Informatics in 2007. He has been listed as one of America's Best Doctors every year since 2004. In 2010, he was recognized by Modern Healthcare as one of the 25 top Clinical Informaticists. During his tenure as CMIO and CIO, the Children's and the IT Department have been recognized three times as a Most Wired hospital and twice as one of InformationWeek's top 250 innovators. They received Eclipsys' first Presidents Award. In 2011, Healthcare Informatics awarded Children's first place in their Healthcare IT Innovators Awards.

Dr. Reynolds is board certified in General Pediatrics and Pediatric Critical Care and is a Fellow of the American Academy of Pediatrics. He received his Masters in Medical Management from Carnegie Mellon University, his M.D. from Hahnemann University and his B.A. at the University of California-Davis.

Chapter 19

Valerie M. Sue, Ph.D., is a senior consultant at Kaiser Permanente who specializes in online survey research. She manages a range of survey projects for KP and is one of the lead researchers responsible for the creation and maintenance of KP's nation-wide member research panel. Prior to working at KP, Sue was an Associate Professor of Communication at California State University, East Bay, where she taught communication theory and research methods courses and was director of the Communication Department's graduate program. The second edition of her book, "Conducting Online Surveys," will be published by Sage Publications in fall 2012. Sue has also edited and co-authored a special issue of the journal of the American Evaluation Association focusing on using online surveys in evaluation. Additionally, Sue has authored numerous journal articles and delivered presentations at the conferences of the International Communication Association, American Evaluation Association, the American Public Health Association, and the Healthcare Information and Management Systems Society.

Sue is a graduate of Stanford University where she earned a Ph.D. in Communication.

Karen Tsang is a senior analyst in the National Market Research department at Kaiser Permanente. She works on a wide variety of projects, ranging from brand tracking to Medicare messaging, and is one of the lead researchers responsible for the creation and maintenance of KP's nationwide member research panel. Prior to her time at KP, Tsang worked for a survey research/social marketing firm in San Francisco, CA, where she helped manage projects for many federal and state entities, such as California's Department of Public Health. She has also spent time as part of the research team for a multi-modal treatment study for children with Attention-Deficit Hyperactivity Disorder.

Tsang has a B.A. in Psychology from the University of California, Berkeley

Chapter 20

Alex Tam has been designing products at frog since 2006 and has over a decade of practice bringing products to life that people enjoy using. He leverages design research, concepting, strategy, and interaction design to translate user needs into design solutions. Alex has spent half of his career focused on design for healthcare and continues to drive innovation in this space and speak on topics of rapid ideation and gamification. Through winning a series of hack-a-thons, he's demonstrated how concepting and prototyping with small multi-disciplinary teams can lead to compelling concepts with high impact. Alex hosted Health Games Camp at frog in San Francisco in 2010, bringing together game developers, designers, physicians, and entrepreneurs to explore and develop health games concepts.

Vivian Distler: Upon joining Institute for the Future in 2007, Vivian quickly became the voice of the Health Horizons Program in the blogosphere, writing about trends in the global health economy. As a researcher, Vivian explored the role social media, ubiquitous technology, and how networks can play in personal health management and as valuable new sources of health information. Vivian also led efforts at IFTF in incorporating gaming principles and futures thinking in promoting health and well-being.

Bradley Kreit: Bradley Kreit joined the Institute for the Future in 2009. His research at IFTF builds on his background in anthropology and history by exploring how everyday challenges, decisions and contexts shape long-term futures--both in individual lives and at larger scales. He primarily researches issues involving food, health and biological identity.

Index

L. Berkowitz, C. McCarthy (eds.),
Innovation with Information Technologies in Healthcare, Health Informatics,
DOI 10.1007/978-1-4471-4327-7, © Springer-Verlag London 2013